THE
Psych BOOK

BY:

T MANICKAM, MD

EDITED BY:
DR. P THIRUNAVUKARASU, MBBS, FACS

Author

Dr. Thirunavukarasu Manickam, MD
Founder, Mananalam Clinic, Chennai, India
Contact Email: manamenalamaclinic@gmail.com

Editor

Dr. Pragatheeshwar Thirunavukarasu, MBBS, FACS
Surgical Oncologist and Hepatopancreaticobiliary Surgeon
Medical Director of Surgical Oncology Services
Cape Fear Valley Health System, Fayetteville, NC USA
Contact Email: admin@pragmd.com

Assistant Editors
Aimee Dubin, BS *Campbell University School of Osteopathic Medicine*

Alexis E. Pullizzi, BS *Campbell University School of Osteopathic Medicine*

Artwork Creation
Dr. Jessica Redcay B.S (Education), M Ed, EdD (Doctorate in Education)/
CI (Curriculum in Instructions)
Vice President, Product Owner, RoboKind
Owner of Ludus Learning and Redcay's Resources
Author of STEMoscope Model, VR Acclimation Model, Robokind Phonics,
and IVAKT

Dr. Pragatheeshwar Thirunavukarasu, MBBS, FACS
Adjunct Clinical Assistant Professor of Surgery
Medical Director of Surgical Oncology Services
Cape Fear Valley Health System, Fayetteville, NC USA

Graphic Design and Layout
Jennifer Fisher
Department Chair, Advertising and Graphic Design at
Fayetteville Technical Community College,
Freelance Graphic Designer

Pragatheeshwar Thirunavukarasu, MBBS, FACS
Surgical Oncologist and Hepatopancreaticobiliary Surgeon Medical Director of
Surgical Oncology Services Cape Fear Valley Health System, Fayetteville, NC USA

Acknowledgments for Contributions

Dr. L. Thenmozhi, MD. *Assistant Professor of Psychiatry, Bharat Medical College and Hospital, Chennai*

Dr. V. Venkatesh, Madan Kumar, MD. *Professor of Psychiatry, Institute of Mental Health, Chennai*

Dr. M. Thendral, MD. *Staff Psychiatrist, Al Soor Specialist Clinic, Sharjah, UAE*
Dr V Jayanthini, MD

Dr. Stalin R Subramanian, MD. *Assistant Professor of Medicine, Division of Gastroenterology, Baylor College of Medicine, Houston TX*

Dr. Aimee Dubin, DO. *Medical Student, Campbell College of Osteopathic Medicine, USA*

Dr. Priyanka Ramesh, MBBS.

Mr. R. S. Mani (artwork)

My residents, colleagues and staff at the Department of Psychiatry, SRM Medical College and Hospital.

I thank and dedicate this work to my father, mother, wife, sons, and grandchildren.

Thirunavukarasu Manickam *(Author)*

I dedicate this work to the one woman who has made me the man I am today - my mother, Chithraa.

Pragatheeshwar Thirunavukarasu *(Editor)*

PREFACE

I thought that I could practice Psychiatry effectively after completion of the residency training in Psychiatry. Knowing, learning, and studying Psychiatry was over. After starting practice, the reality was different. I realized that I have to study more and more, know more and more, and learn more in Psychiatry.

It was shocking to me that we, the Mental Health Professionals who are dealing with mental health, normal and abnormality of the mind, do so without knowing what the mind is! We started promoting mental health only by talking about mental illness. This awareness made me feel so low about myself and started discussions with fellow colleagues.

After a couple of years, I realized that most of our colleagues in Medical Practice do not know about mind and mental health either. But they are aware and fairly confident about managing Mental Health problems, which were considered as abnormal behavior.

Very important topics like alcoholism, drug abuse, sexual dysfunction, suicides and attempted suicides/deliberate self harms was not considered as illness and were managed by non-professionals. The complications of the above-mentioned problems are considered as illness, which were managed by medical doctors. All these factors made me introspect why this is happening. The slogan of the World Health Organization was 'Health for all'. Is this Heath for all?

The beauty of Psychiatry is that many of us, including the common man, are unaware that we do not know many things. But we believe that they know many things; it is a paradox.

The common man is able to identify and recognize the altered, deviant, different, and abnormal behavior at the earliest. They seek remedy and help by magico-religious means and non-pharmacological approaches. Because of stigma, they hesitate to approach mental health professionals. Why this denial? Why this apathy? The mistake is not with them. We, the mental health professionals, failed in our duty to educate the common man.

The Government of India launched the National Mental Health Programme to promote Mental Health. In that program, we used to educate physicians, health professionals, paramedics, community workers, and the general public about Mental Health, to create awareness. But most of the lectures delivered to them were on how to identify a mental illness. Not a word about mental health. A local community leader questioned me, 'Why talk about mental illness and not telling us anything about mental health?'.

One of my teachers used to tell me that as one goes up the ladder of knowledge, he has to tell and communicate the knowledge he gained to the benefit of the common man. One has to make a common man understand the difficult issues. My father used to say unless you understand something clearly, you cannot make others understand. This made me understand each word we use in our clinical practice clearly and fully.

I happened to be an expert witness in a case being tried in the District Session Courts. The case was related to Indian Penal Code 302 - murder. In my opinion, I mentioned, "Patient says that he hears voices accusing and threatening him. The patient believes that people are against him and plot to eliminate him". The learned Judge questioned me about how I knew that the patient was hearing those voices. He added that an expert witness should not tell what other people say. He said that an expert witness should be categorically confirmatory on whether the patient heard voices or not. He said that, like other physicians, the psychiatrist must give evidence for the pathology. And then he commented about the mental health of the psychiatrist!

I discussed this situation with the Honorable Justice Venugopal of Madras High Court. We had a couple of hours of interaction over the period of two weeks. He was very impressed with the concepts I put forth to him. He encouraged me to write all of it, in a newspaper continuously, in Tamil. The same was then reproduced in a fortnightly magazine. My writings about the Mind, Mental Health became popular among the common man. But these concepts were not appreciated by my psychiatrist colleagues. Some of my senior colleagues kept antagonizing my concepts, always asking for references for my concepts. These were my concepts, there were no pre-existing references. One of my beloved teachers encouraged me to not stop pursuing these concepts, and that any new things will be quoted as reference only by others in the future.

The majority of my professional time was in the General Hospital set-up, where all specialties are housed. I have to talk and communicate with fellow physicians from other specialties, in a language that they can understand. This effort made me understand psychiatry at a common man level. I had to face media personnel and journalists and educate the public in simple words. I had to find answers and fitting replies to questions from the public. To my surprise, many of my physician colleagues enjoyed those talks and expressed their desire to listen to psychiatry in such a simple manner. This made me write books on psychiatric illnesses in my language, Tamil. Nearly all of them became bestsellers.

At one point, my own students became my colleagues, and we worked together in the same department. They used to sit in my classes and participate in Grand rounds along with the students. They started taking notes verbatim. One of my students recorded most of my lectures. The students then gave all those recordings to me and asked me to write a book on clinical psychiatry.

My son Pragatheeshwar was my student when he was in the same medical school, where I was an Assistant Professor of Psychiatry. He wanted to become a psychiatrist. But I encouraged him to train in surgery. I used to say that surgeons are very good at communication as they are able to convince people to allow them to remove their body parts, often without any questioning. After he became a surgeon, he felt that many of the clinical skills related to interaction with the patients as a surgeon related to how to deal with them psychologically. As he observed me in the department with the patients, he also encouraged me to write a book with my experience.

All these efforts made me to take the decision to go ahead with the book. It took 10 years to complete the book. I completed the chapters and gave them to my son for correction of the language. That was the time of COVID lockdowns, and it made me stay with son for prolonged period of time. We discussed each chapter over several hours, and I clarified to him all the content written. But to my surprise, Prag rewrote the book completely. It took nearly 36 months to complete.

This book is written with the intention that it would be readable by all. It is not only for psychiatrists and mental health professionals. At some time point in everyone's life on this earth, all of us have to deal with mental health. The goal of the book is to identify, recognize, and take steps to interfere with the progression of mental health problems. I did not go with the usual classification system and explain them in that order.

This book will be useful for all Health Professionals, especially Primary Care Physicians. Most of the unknown issues were made known to everybody.

Any work needs suggestions, comments, remarks, etc. Then only the work can be improved further.

T Manickam, MD
Founder, Mananalam Clinic

Editor's Note

The author of this book is Dr. Thirunavukarasu Manickam, my father. I am writing this note to explain my role in creating this book as an obligation to intellectual honesty.

First, a little bit about him: the author was born in 1952 in Madras State, in Southern India, which is now referred to as Tamil Nadu, currently a state in the Union of India. He was born in a Tamil Vellala family, the eighth child of 13 children begotten by Mr. S L Manickam Pillai and his wife, Mrs. Palaniammal. At the age of 16, he was selected based on his educational merit to medical school at Thanjavur Medical College. After graduation, he entered residency training in Psychiatry at the Institute of Mental Health (IMH) in Chennai, likely one of the oldest mental health asylums known in modern history, housing mental health patients since 1795. Notably, residency in psychiatry was introduced four years prior, and he was likely the ninth resident in psychiatry in the state and the youngest to start psychiatry training. He then underwent additional post-doctoral training experience at the Washington University at St. Louis. He worked for the Government of Tamil Nadu, progressing from the position of Assistant Professor of Psychiatry at Madras Medical College in Chennai to Professor of Psychiatry and the Head of the Department of Psychiatry at Stanely Medical College in Chennai. After completing his time with the government, he became the Head of the Department of Psychiatry at SRM Medical College and General Hospital, a private medical university. Throughout his career, he has had a vibrant private practice at his privately owned and operated mental health clinic, *The Mananalam Clinic,* in Chennai. His clinical work extended from the early mornings to afternoons in the university hospitals and from evenings to midnight at his private clinic. He held private practice clinics in other rural towns outside Chennai on 3 out of 4 weekends a month. He would spend one weekend a month with my mother, Mrs. Chithraa Thirunavukarasu, my younger brother, and myself. This was his life for the last 40 years, except when he was vacationing with my mother in places worldwide where psychiatric conferences were held, where he or his trainees were presenting papers, or participating in professional societies.

The author had it both good and bad. The good was the enormous clinical volume, supplied by a flurry of patients at the government university hospitals where free healthcare was delivered and his private clinic, where patients who desired a private setup were seen. He saw it all – the poor, the rich, the wealthy, the ultrawealthy, the educated, the illiterate, the famous, the privileged, the oppressed, the downtrodden, the destitute, and the homeless. He saw the urban folk in Chennai during weekdays and the rural and tribal folk on the weekends. He was surrounded by trainees of all kinds – medical students, nursing students, psychiatry residents, other specialty residents, and post-doctoral fellows. He was exposed to red tape and bureaucracy by being a government employee, politics by being an academic university faculty, and the nuances of finance, business, management, and networking as the owner-operator of his private clinics across the state. In the mornings, he was surrounded by a coterie of trainees in the university hospitals, uttering medical jargon, discussing academic subtleties, and reconciling every patient under the DSM with the luxury of progressing through the published algorithms and guidelines for treatment. In the evenings, he was alone in his private clinic with little to no staff, where prompt clinical diagnosis and predictable clinical improvement were the priorities. In his private practice, no one cared about diagnostic codes or published literature – neither the patient nor the referring doctor. He had to produce durable clinical improvement within a reasonable time to gain credibility.

Furthermore, being one of the earliest graduates in Psychiatry in one of the most populous countries in the world, he was unwittingly sucked into public attention by the media and journalists whenever they needed an expert opinion on mental health-related topics. He was also constantly approached by the judiciary and law enforcement for legal opinions and expert testimonies. The latter exposed him to the general public and positioned him to face their untrained opinions and biases on mental health. The raw material for clinical knowledge is patient volume, and he had no shortage. This allowed him to understand the nature of the entity that drives human activity – the mind. Over several years in the 1980s, by constantly volleying his ideas with the public and academic colleagues, he had summoned a fully formed understanding of the nature of the mind. In subsequent years, he identified clinically applicable criteria for mental health.

The good was the clinical volume and diversity. The bad were many.

First was the time and place of his life. Just a few years before his birth, his homeland transitioned from a colonial presidency under the British Empire to a state under the Union of India. Emerging as a new nation after centuries-old colonial rule, the Indian people were left stricken with poverty, illiteracy, and malnourishment. The meager resources of the government were prioritized to fight malnutrition and infections. The next tier of focus was on prevalent medical and surgical illnesses. The field of psychiatry was very new, and spending time and money on it was prodigal. Mental health was not considered a 'medical' matter. Mental illness was not considered a medical disease. Religious godmen, priests, exorcists, and thugs dealt with mental health patients. Asylums were usually in religious temples and monasteries, where housing conditions were terrible. Psychiatry was viewed as a pseudo-science by the public and as an outcast by the rest of the medical specialists. Being one of the earliest psychiatrists in the country, the author faced this rampant stigma surrounding psychiatry. He had to convince everyone (literally everyone) that the mind was a biological function of the body and could be healthy or diseased like any other organ system. This included most other Indian doctors, who, despite their formal training, subtly yet firmly believed mental health illnesses were not biological. He had to convince people of one of the oldest entrenched societies that it was not evil spirits that made a man hear voices, not a curse that made a person irrevocably sad, but a disease of the brain. And all this, only to convince that the spectacularly disrupted ones – like the paranoid schizophrenic, catatonic, and delirious individuals, were mentally afflicted. Discussing other less dramatic yet highly impactful problems was more controversial. The idea that problems such as alcoholism, drug abuse, violent behavior, marital discord, sexual dysfunction, eating problems, weight abnormalities, delinquency, etc., could have a psychiatric basis was unfathomable. The proposition that children could be mentally affected or that suicide has a psychiatric basis was nothing short of comical and ridiculous to the Indian public.

Furthermore, practicing medicine was (and still is) hazardous in India. An unfavorable outcome, complication, mortality, or even an unsavory comment could lead to a violent mob attack on the doctor or the facility. So, the author had to be extraordinarily diligent in communication skills to avoid conflict.

Another bad thing for him was the geopolitical situation of his homeland

and his people, the Tamil folk. The region encompassed by his home state, Tamil Nadu, being the better disposed and developed relative to the rest of India, was disproportionately hyper-concentrated by anti-superstitious pro-rationalist thinkers, who had ushered in a government whose policies were dramatically outside mainstream Indian cultural thought. They claimed to be 'pro-science', and it was taught to question every existing practice or claim. The Western World, primarily Britain, Europe, and the USA was the source of most scientific research and studies and appeared as the bastion of rationality. The new generation of college-educated Indians and doctors were trained to ask for references and publications to support any claim or assertion. While it was a welcome practice in principle, it manifested immaturely and brutishly. The academic culture eventually came to be that if it had not been written or mentioned in an English publication or textbook by a Western author, it wasn't true! And everything a Western author mentioned in such a textbook was likely true.

So, while his concepts about the definition of the mind and criteria for delineating mental health from mental disorders were received welcomingly by the public, his academic colleagues quickly shot it down. A popular exchange during psychiatry rounds at the end of his lectures would be something like this,

The author: " ... And this is the definition of the mind ... "

His colleague: "Says who?

The author: "I am."

His colleagues: "We don't find any references for this definition in the literature. Do you have any references to support your concept of the mind? Sigmund Freud has explained the components of the mind already."

The author: "What references did Freud provide for his claims?"

His colleague: " ... " (silence)

The crowd of trainees and colleagues would enthusiastically watch this rattling exchange between the professors.

Nevertheless, the antipathy of his colleagues was justified and legitimate. The scientific method requires an unambiguous nomenclature, a declaration of the axioms and hypotheses, and empiric data to support the concept. It needs to be presented among peers and validated prospectively through well-designed studies. The author hadn't done it. So, he had no leg to stand on. He faced multiple practical challenges to publish it, being an emerging psychiatrist and working with bare minimum resources in the governmental university hospital, where research and publishing were rare. But he knew that science takes no excuses. Eventually, he drafted a manuscript and sent it to the *Indian Journal of Psychiatry,* but it was rejected. He tried again and failed. How could he get an audience of psychiatrists in India? He needed a platform. He figured that rising within the ranks of professional societies was the only way to have him heard. Over the next several years, he became more involved in the state and national professional associations.

I was not privy to any of this during my childhood or adolescence. During that time, my father and I barely interacted with each other, and my conversations with him were limited to maybe a few sentences every month. Our home overflowed with books. I grew up reading psychology books to ward away boredom. I started medical school in 1999 at Madras Medical College, where he taught. I sat through his lectures and underwent my psychiatry rotations in his department during this time. I developed an inclination toward psychiatry. As a medical student, I witnessed both endorsement and antagonism to his claims during his lectures. I encountered many people well-managed by the author, leading productive, happy, and successful lives there. I have lost track of the number of people who would randomly walk up to me if they knew I was his son to let me know how grateful they have been to my dad for solving their problems and restoring them to a happy life. He touched many lives and many families. He must be doing something right, I thought. His mental health books for general readership were best-sellers. One of his books, a book on Child Psychiatry, was awarded the State Award by the Government of Tamil Nadu. But his publications sent to peer-review went to the trash. Where is the disconnect? Then, it dawned on me. *The problem was language!*

The author's primary language was Tamil—the medium of instruction throughout his childhood until high school was in Tamil. English became the medium of instruction only in his college years. He had learned English and sailed through his medical education and training in English with the help of a dictionary. His choice of words in English was accurate, but the syntax, grammar, rhetoric, and the mode of presenting an idea were well outside the norm for standard English readership. The ideas that sounded authentic in Tamil came out as silly in his English writings. Translating from English to Tamil is easy, but translating from Tamil to English is no easy task. The English alphabet has 26 letters, and the Tamil alphabet has 247! The English lexicon has roughly 175,000 words, and the Tamil dictionary's headwords range from approximately 300,000 to nearly 1,200,000. Tamil has many sophisticated words to express uniquely different emotions and descriptions with no counterpart in the English lexicon. The other problem was that the culture of scientific research and publications was not prevalent in his medical education time. He was not equipped with the formalities of scientific writing. I discovered this more during my time with him while working on psychiatry topics in medical school. Being instructed in English since kindergarten, I was not as disadvantaged as him in writing English. The author's proficiency level in English writing and unfamiliarity with scientific writing significantly limited academic prolificity. I began to work with him on a few publications, adding significantly to empiric research, data collection, methodology, and analysis. After graduating from medical school, I started residency training in General Surgery in the USA. By this time, I had become more experienced in scientific writing.

In 2010, he became elected President of the *Indian Psychiatric Society*. Yes, the time had come - the opportunity he worked for finally came to fruition nearly 14 years later! He decided to use his time at the slot for the inaugural address by the President-elect to present his ideas on mind and mental health. He contacted me regarding this, and we connected through the Internet and phone. We pulled all the empirical data thus far about the definitions of the mind and consolidated them into a well-articulated model. During this time, we uncovered and fulfilled several unaddressed hollows in the concept. Those days were intense – plenty of developments happened within a short time. Then, he submitted them to the *Indian Journal of Psychiatry*, which was eventually published in 2011, titled '*A utilitarian concept of manas and mental health*'. This paper aimed to define the mind, name its components, and describe its nature. His definition of the mind was meant purely for medical practice. It was meant to consolidate the theory of the mind based on clinical observations, just like the concept of 'circulation' was explained by Dr. William Harvey. We needed another name for the mind to distinguish it as a medical entity from everything else discussed about the mind. We finalized the word 'manas' for this purpose. Another objective of this paper was to identify clinically applicable criteria to delineate mental health vs. mental disorder and to classify those who were not mentally healthy into a few broad groups to strategize management. Following his presentation and subsequent publication, we have witnessed a palpable uptick in using this concept in clinical practice, as reported by them through their personal communications with the author. The citing in academic literature has started but lagging.

During my time as a surgical resident and as a surgeon, I have encouraged him to work on a simple survival guide for trainees containing all the nuances he had learned from decades of busy clinical practice. The author had been compiling something of this sort for years, and the objective was to make it a narrative guide for trainees at all stages. Along the way, he had designated some of his trainees and colleagues to contribute to these chapters. However, he felt it wasn't what he expected.

At this point, he sought my partnership in creating this book. I drew inspiration from the book *'Top Knife'*, written by the famous trauma surgeon Dr. Kenneth Mattox. The book is a must-read for general surgeons. It is written in narrative style, and reading it sounds like a mentor surgeon leaning over his mentee's shoulder during an operation, whispering high-yield points of wisdom into the ears. I felt that the author's work could be similar to it. The author gave me his rough drafts of chapters, some in English and some in Tamil. I reviewed it with him, added relevant content for an academic English readership, removed redundancies, reorganized the flow of the content, consolidated dispersed high-yield points into topic-specific lists and tables, and fixed the language. As a sample of his English drafts for articles, I have reproduced his writing for the Preface, fixing only unacceptable grammatical mistakes. Nevertheless, after my editorial work, the author has reviewed all the chapters thoroughly and has approved the final version published here. The chapters are now totally different from the initial drafts. Nevertheless, the contributors to the initial drafts are recognized here as additional contributors. I intend to publish his original drafts later as a separate booklet.

All said and done, I have not been formally trained in psychiatry. I have been humble through this process and have been further humbled by this experience at the vastness of impact of psychiatry in our lives. Over the last few years, working on this book has consumed more time than my time in writing on surgical topics. Yet, it has been a rewarding and enriching experience.

So, my role in this book is that the author provided the eggs, and I made them into an omelet for your palatability. I hope you enjoy reading this book.

Dr Pragatheeshwar Thirunavukarasu, MBBS, FACS
Surgical Oncologist and Hepatopancreaticobiliary Surgeon
Medical Director of Surgical Oncology Services
Cape Fear Valley Health System, Fayetteville, NC USA

How to use this book?

This book is meant to be a primer on mental health. So, the author focused on the definitions, fundamentals, pathophysiology, and clinical examination of major psychiatric topics only. Details on management were outside the scope of this book.

Over the years, subsequent authors who cited the author's initial publication noted that the word 'manas' has also been used in non-medical and philosophical contexts. We also noticed that they had been misled by the word 'manas', as though the author's concept of the mind reflected some Asian, Eastern, or Indian philosophy. On the contrary, we drew nothing from any cultural or religious ideas. It was a purely biological definition that could be consistent with the scientific method prevalent in modern medicine and generalizable across different societies. So, we have discarded that label in favor of a new word of the author's choice, 'Ulan', which we feel has yet to be corrupted and can be a safe alternative for the mind in academic medical usage. 'Ulan' means 'the inside' or 'that which is inside'. Wherever the *Ulan* concept is used to discuss the pathophysiology of a disorder, this symbol is used.

The author had come up with multiple tips and tricks up his sleeve for prompt clinical diagnosis necessary in everyday busy practice. He has identified areas of frequent blunders leading to misdiagnosis and strategic errors. These points would be most beneficial to private psychiatrists worldwide who need to prioritize the ends of good clinical outcomes over the means of statistically ritual diagnosis that can only be afforded by the salaried university physician. As an editor, I have consolidated these concepts from written drafts and discussions as the 'Mananalam Clinic Experience' (MCE) to distinguish it from the rest of the published literature so that future psychiatrists may test these clinical concepts and techniques in their research. These high-yield concepts, developed at the Mananalam clinic by the author, are highlighted with the logo

Foreword by Dr. M. Riba

About 25 years ago, I was asked to give a presentation in Athens, Greece, about collaborative care – where a psychiatrist provides medication while another mental health clinician, such as a social worker or psychologist, provides psychotherapy. My colleagues and I were doing some research in this area, and it was a growing type of care in the United States. After the presentation, a psychiatrist from Ghana came up to me and shared that there were no social workers in Ghana, that the total number of psychiatrists in the entire country was about 6, no child psychiatrists, and that what I was talking about was probably interesting in high-income countries, but had little relevance in low-income countries, such as Ghana.

I came away from that interchange with a deep appreciation for my Ghanian colleague who was respectful, thoughtful, clear, and courageous in letting me know that if I wanted to speak and do research on such a mental health topic, I should consider cross-cultural and demographic issues, as well as differential privileges and resources. I took his recommendations very seriously and became quite active in the World Psychiatric Association. With the support of colleagues at the University of Michigan and Kumasi Teaching Hospital in Ghana, we have tried to build an ongoing academic relationship, learning from each other. My Ghanaian colleague shaped much of the trajectory of my work in psychiatry, with a strong emphasis on Global Mental Health.

In reading The Psych Book by Dr. T. Manickam, MD, edited by his son, Dr. P. Thirunavukarasu, MBBS FACS, I again appreciate the importance of learning from colleagues who have much clinician experience and wisdom, and who trained and worked in different cultures, with limited resources. The introductions/preface provided by Dr. Manickam and the loving tribute and history given by Dr. Thirunavukarasu speak to the contributions of historical context and ways to understand how we all come to where we are and the attending circumstances. Just as we take histories of patients and their families, this author and editor help us contextualize this very rich book, filled with personal anecdotes and ways to understand "the why." In this day of books with hundreds of references (that are probably not primary sources), replete with metanalyses, and out of date almost from the time of publication, this book is so personalized that many of its clinical pearls can live on and on. It is also quite enjoyable and readable.

The Psych Book is a short, but skillful book. Certainly, having it on your bookshelf ensures that you appreciate the need for all of us, across cultures, religions, ethnicities, countries and boundaries, to work together in the interest of our patients and their families, regarding mental health. The Psych Book is a reminder of the wisdom and experience so many of our colleagues are willing to share with us, across oceans.

With sincere thanks and appreciation to Dr. Manickam and Dr. Thirunavukarasu, their patients and their students.

Michelle B. Riba, M.D., M.S.
Professor of Psychiatry
University of Michigan
Past President, American Psychiatric Association

Foreword by Dr. M. Posner

What Psychiatry Needs

This remarkable book emphasizes the critical need for relating mental illness to the normal function of the mind. The first four chapters place understanding the mind at the center of psychiatry. The progress that has been made in understanding the function of the human mind in relation to the structure of the brain is critical if psychiatry is to succeed in the treatment of mental disorders.

In Chapter 5, the book turns to the practical issue of the clinical examination of adults and in Chapter 6, to the examination of child patients. Chapters 7 through 20 deal with the diagnosis and treatment of disorders usually seen as central to psychiatry. The centrality of the mind makes psychiatry a much more integrated and appealing profession. Indeed, the book ends with an appeal to the young, quoted below:

"There has never been a better time to be a psychiatrist in human history. And it is only slated to get better. Psychiatry is on its way up. I have been thoroughly fulfilled and personally enriched by being a psychiatrist. I encourage everyone to take a close and serious look at psychiatry before passing it up for another choice of profession."

My training is as a psychologist, but I worked for several years in the Department of Neurology and Neurosurgery, where my research involved the early days of cognitive brain imaging. Later, I spent several years in a Psychiatry Deptartment at the Weill-Cornell School of Medicine. I was recruited there to start an institute devoted to the development of the brain and mind in infancy and early childhood. In both places, I worked with young neurologists and psychiatrists being trained to carry out clinical and research functions in their field. Like Prof. Manickam, I felt these researchers needed to understand recent developments in the science of the mind in relation to the brain to treat their patients and to move forward with the research on whatever disorder they were to study.

Prof. T. Manickam provides a useful definition of the mind in terms of its function. In behavioral psychology, it was thought that the mind must be active and produce behavior to be observed. According to this view, psychology must be a science limited to behavior. Cognitive psychologists emphasized methods to make mental processes observable. This effort was enhanced by the development of brain imaging. The view that the mind at rest could not be observed was questioned by imaging studies (Raichle 2009). Brain networks active during mental tasks remained correlated at rest allowing us to view some aspects of the mind even when it is not engaged in any task. I agree with Prof. Manickam when he says in Chapter 1,

"There is strong evidence in the field of biology for the brain being the predominant seat of faculties attributable to the mind, but it might be premature to conclude that anatomical and chemical characters of the brain alone can explain all that is encompassed by what we term as mind"

Cognitive neuroscience tries to integrate the functional and structural aspects of the normal mind that can then illuminate our ability to understand its disorders.

Of the many psychiatric disorders covered in this book, I have chosen only three for comment. These three are linked to attention, and with colleagues, I have conducted original research and am thus somewhat able to evaluate the chapters and comment on what in the future might be possible. These three chosen areas are anxiety, substance abuse, and personality disorders.

Chapter 10 deals with anxiety which is among the most prevalent of psychiatric disorders. The chapter lists the following categories of anxiety: Phobias, Panic disorder with or without Agoraphobia, Generalized Anxiety Disorder (GAD), Obsessive Compulsive Disorder (OCD), Acute Stress Disorder, and Post Traumatic Stress Disorder (PTSD). Anxiety is a normal emotion but can become excessive and, in extreme versions, can severely impact one's life.

There is a long history of identification of anxiety as closely tied to attention since obsessive attention to negative affect can be a cause of abnormal anxiety. The role of attentional control networks goes beyond diagnosis to suggest possible treatments. The pathway between the mid-prefrontal cortex (adjacent to the ventral anterior cingulate) and the amygdala has identified key structures in the executive network with high trait anxiety

(Kim & Whelan, 2009). Thus, several forms of anxiety may be closely tied to the ventral anterior cingulate's control of limbic activity (Bush, Luu & Posner, 2000). In one study of social anxiety, there is a significant difference between the orienting network in patients and controls (Heeren, Maurage & Philippot, 2015). Therapies for anxiety involve training people to avoid attending to negative affect and using the executive attention network to reframe the context in a way that reduces the tendency to produce anxiety (Ghassemzadeh, Rothbart, & Posner, 2019). In the next section, we describe some evidence that enhancement of control by the anterior cingulate through meditation may be useful in improving control of substance abuse. Improvements in executive attention through meditation might also allow enhanced control of anxiety.

In his very helpful chapter 13 on substance abuse, Prof. T. Manickam argues:

"The stigma associated with substance abuse is that they would be considered 'weak in willpower' unable to exercise moral restraint, unreliable, immoral ..."

This idea fits well with a deficit in the ability to regulate behavior (Baler & Volkow 2006). The attentional brain network involved in such regulation includes the anterior cingulate gyrus (Petersen & Posner, 2012) and this network has been shown to be improved in connectivity in humans through meditation (Tang et al, 2010) and in mice by low-frequency stimulation (Piscopo et al, 2018) Moreover, in the case of tobacco (Tang et al 2013) and opioid addiction (Hudak et al 2021) meditation has been shown to lead to a reduction in the addiction. A possible mechanism proposed is low-frequency stimulation found in mice to foster connectivity by increasing the myelin sheath (Piscopo et al., 2018). In the case of tobacco addiction, the reduced smoking did not depend upon the desires of the addicted person, but only on the improvement in network conduction. With opioid addiction those persons with a larger amount of theta 4-8 Hz) oscillations showed a greater reduction in opioid usage (Hudak et al, 2021). While this research needs more replication it suggests a way of reducing addictions by changing the brain network involved that could be a general tool for reducing substance abuse and other disorders involving self-regulation.

Personality disorders are an especially complex form of disability, as Chapter 17 points out.

In the case of Borderline personality disorder Chapter 17 outlines the potential harm:

"Repeated deliberate self-harm and premature death from suicide are consequences of BPD. Reportedly, there is an overall 8-10% risk of suicide associated with borderline PD, and hence suicidal gestures must be taken seriously."

An underlying cause of the disorder might be the same brain network as was found for some forms of addiction (Posner et al, 2002) when those diagnosed with Borderline Personality Disorder (BPD) were compared with people with high affect and low effortful control but no evidence of BPD. Those with the disorder showed significantly longer times to resolve conflict. This suggested that BPD involved poor self-regulation. If this is true, it might help those with BPD to undergo meditation training to strengthen their regulatory abilities.

Increased emphasis on mental health problems has created a scarcity of people trained to provide care (Weiner, 2022). This book could lead to greater interest on the part of young people in the field. This may be just the right moment for this book to interest the general public as well as newly trained physicians in the field of psychiatry and help those already practicing psychiatry to profit from the author's wise approach to the field.

Michael I. Posner
University of Oregon

References

- Baler,R.D. & Volkow, N.D. (2006) Drug addiction: the neurobiology of disrupted self control Trends in Molecular Medincine 12/12, 559-565.
- Bush, G., Luu, P. & Posner, M.I. (2000). Cognitive and emotional influences in the anterior cingulate cortex. ***Trends in Cognitive Science*** , 4/6:215-222.
- Ghassemzadeh, H. Rothbart, M.K. & Posner, M.I.(2019)

Anxiety and brain networks of attentional control. Cognitive and Behavioral Neurology 32/1, 54-62.

- Heeren A, Maurage P, Philippot P. (2015) Revisiting attentional processing of non-emotional cues in social anxiety: a specific impairment for the orienting network of attention. Psychiatry Research 228:136–142.
- Hudak, J., Hanley, A.W., Marchand, W.R. et al. Endogenous theta stimulation during meditation predicts reduced opioid dosing following treatment with Mindfulness-Oriented Recovery Enhancement. *Neuropsychopharmacol.* 46, 836–843 (2021).
- Kim MJ, Whalen PJ. 2009. The structural integrity of an amygdala prefrontal pathway. J Neurosci. 29:11614–11618.
- Petersen, S.E. & Posner, M.I. (2012) The attention system of the human brain: 20 years after. Annual Review of Neuroscience 35, 71-89.
- Posner, M.I., Rothbart, M.K., Vizueta, N., Levy,K., Thomas, K.M. & Clarkin, J. (2002).
- Attentional mechanisms of borderline personality disorder. Proceedings of the National Academy of Sciences USA, 99 (25):16366-16370.
- Piscopo, D., Weible, A., Rothbart, M.K., Posner, M.I. & Niell,C.M. (2018) Changes in white matter in mice resulting from low frequency brain stimulation Proceedings of the National Academy of Sciences USA 115/27 6639-6646.
- Raichle, M,E. (2009) A paradigm shift in functional brain imaging. Journal of Neuroscience 29/41 12729-12734.
- Tang, Y., Lu, Q., Geng, X., Stein, E.A., Yang, Y., & Posner, M.I. (2010) Short term mental training induces white-matter changes in the anterior cingulate PNAS 107/35 15649-15652.
- Tang, Y-Y, Tang, R., & Posner, M.I. (2013) Brief meditation training induces smoking reduction. Proceedings of the US National Academy 110/34 13971-13975.
- Weiner, S (2022) A growing psychiatric shortage and increased demand for mental health services AAMC News Aug. 9, 2022.

Foreword by Dr. V. Irai Anbu

Dr. T. Manickam is a renowned psychiatrist practicing for a long time, and his services are highly applauded by the people of Tamil Nadu. He has had a rich academic experience by virtue of his faculty positions in various medical institutions. He has consolidated his knowledge and wisdom gained over the years and has authored an elaborate guide dealing with various facets of mental health.

I was entrusted with the pleasant task of writing a foreword for this mammoth book and I am sure my comprehension would be like a seashell holding ocean water as much as it could.

I had the joy of going through this book prior to publication, perusing each word meticulously with the fervor of a student preparing for a competitive examination. The book has been carefully drafted, its sentences pregnant with meaning and significance. Despite his mastery of Western psychology and psychiatry, the author has corroborated from literature and proverbs native to his fatherland.

The book begins with the basic yet challenging proposition of deciphering the mind using the mind. The difficulties are epitomized with astounding logic and irrefutable reasoning. In the initial few pages, conceptualizations of Sigmund Freud and his delineation of the Id, Ego, and Superego have been dealt with concisely. He concludes that suppression of the libidinal energy or the disobedience of the Super Ego in any form does not disappear silently into the night. It will come back to take its pound of flesh at some point. He also explains about the subconscious mind and its nature. The Humanist School advocated by Abraham Maslow has also been briefed. The statement 'there is no health without mental health' is a powerful statement deserving universal comprehension.

The chapter 'What is Mind?' is quite interesting with the introduction of the word 'Manas' propounded by the author at the Indian Psychiatric Society convention. His original article on this matter has been included to make the readers understand the rationale behind the choice of the name 'Manas', which the author later disregarded in favor of the name 'Ulan'. The mood, thought and intellect always exist in any Manas/Ulan.

The author cautions against labeling individuals as 'normal' or 'abnormal'. We can distinguish them as 'mentally healthy', 'mentally not healthy' and 'mentally unhealthy' individuals. He defines mental health as the fulfillment of three characteristics -(a) Awareness about one's own self, (b) Ability to relate well with fellow human beings and (c) All of one's deeds and activities are useful to one's own self as well as others, at least not detrimental to self as well as others.

The author clearly states that the patient may use words such as 'psycho', 'hysterical' or 'narcissistic' to describe others or oneself based on what they read on the Internet and that the psychiatrist must avoid endorsing such descriptions unless medically accurate. The 'Big 9' fundamentals of psychiatric clinical interview would be highly useful to the tyros commencing psychiatric clinical practice. Various delusions, obsessions, phobias, illusions, and hallucinations have been beautifully explained in this book.

The differentiation between child psychiatry and adult psychiatry is quite interesting. As the author warns, many parents presume that their children will outgrow their abnormal behavior with time. Ultimately, they end up with a complex problem involving multiple complications.

Depression is a term often misused by people without understanding that pervasiveness is the crucial factor for considering it as a medical condition. Depressive disorders, symptoms, and related issues have been enlisted with examples. The chapter on bipolar disorder, coupled with experience gained from Mananalam Clinic, will be immensely useful for both psychologists and budding psychiatrists. Mood contagion is an important caution given by the author for examining patients with bipolar disorders.

The chapter on Psychosis begins with the essential difference between the psychiatric patients and the psychotic patients. He also mentions that while schizophrenia often responds well to treatment, there are situations where patients may never return to complete normalcy. I enjoyed his statement, 'the patient not answering a question is also an answer'. It reminded me of the famous quote 'Not making a choice is also a choice' from Jean-Paul Satre's 'Being and Nothingness'.

The six different clinical categories of anxiety have been elaborately described in an intelligible manner with examples. The author cautions that anxiety could be an early symptom of dementia. He makes it a point to educate the readers with the etymology of various terms used in psychiatric medicine. Obsessive Compulsory Disorder has been unambiguously differentiated from schizophrenia. He also mentions that people with obsessive traits are incredible assets in governmental leadership positions and law enforcement.

The book is not devoid of humor. The author mentions his physician colleague who had the habit of repeatedly asking for the details of dog bites to make sure rabies was not missed in the differential diagnosis. His patients used to complain that dog bites were more tolerable than the doctor's.

While narrating the features of Post-Traumatic Stress Disorder, he gives a novel reason for the adage 'Child is the father of man,' echoed by William Wordsworth in his 'My heart leaps up'. The Concentration Camp Syndrome and its relevance will enlighten the readers on the impact of life's unprecedented disasters on mental well-being.

The author has already written a book in Tamil for general readers on the topic of addiction and substance abuse, and its evils. In this book, he categorically states that no substance other than a wholesome diet and clean drinking water is needed for healthy living. Various stages of drug addiction, such as the contact phase, euphoria, user phase, problem user phase, tolerance phase, and dependence phase, have been outlined in simple terms. This chapter should reach not only psychiatrists but also the people responsible for pedagogy. The next chapter on Alcohol Use and Addiction is equally a mind-opener.

Many young men and women are now addicted to Gaming and Internet-related use. The author contrasts gaming with gambling while asserting that the basic concepts of Substance Abuse Disorder and Addiction are applicable to Gaming Disorders as the biochemical pathways involved in reward and punishment that get hijacked are similar.

The chapter on somatoform disorders specifically states that manifestations related to the disorders in the mind would not improve with physiological treatments. Personality and Personality Disorders have been explained through the five major personality trait dimensions. One could easily understand the symptoms of personality disorders and their implications.

The chapter on suicidal behavior is extremely important in the current day as suicide rates are increasing worldwide along with changes in lifestyle. Similarly, the chapter on violent behavior is also crucial for the psychiatrists who deal with such patients. Longevity has increased due to the advancements in medical care, and we come across numerous instances related to the bizarre behavior of octogenarians and nonagenarians.
The author has traced possible reasons, including dementia, for sexual misbehavior in older adults, which may explain why some older age adults get charged with POCSO (Protection of Children from Sexual Offences) Act-related offenses.

The last chapter is a capsule of wisdom gained due to the continuous practice and diligent studies done by Dr. T. Manickam. They shall be noble commandments for beginners.

The Psych book is a highly informative and educative piece of academic literature and would certainly stand testimony to the brilliance of the author. It would become his masterpiece on deciphering the mind and its ramifications.

V Irai Anbu, M.A., M.Sc., M.B.A, PhD
Former Chief Secretary to The Government of Tamil Nadu, India

Foreword by Dr. Lakshmi Narasimhan Ranganathan

With great pleasure, I introduce you to 'The Psych Book', a unique and insightful work authored by the esteemed psychiatrist Dr. Thirunavukarasu Manickam and edited by Dr. Pragatheeshwar Thirunavukarasu. With its distinct approach and comprehensive content, this book is a valuable addition to psychiatry.

The book opens with a captivating exploration of the mind, using the age-old proverb, 'pasithaalum puli pullai thingaathu,' to challenge the behavioristic school of thought. The second chapter (the million-dollar question), the third chapter (the billion-dollar question), and the fourth chapter (the trillion-dollar question) are all gems that warrant zillion readings!

The concepts of 'Manas' and 'Ulan' are exciting, clearly explained, and evidence of the author's wisdom. I encourage every reader to read thoroughly the author's original work, 'A Utilitarian Concept of Manas and Mental Health', which was published in 2011 and reproduced in this book.

The 'nine gems of clinical psychiatry' discussed in Chapter 5 are fantabulous. The discussion on the importance of 'dependable love' in children's mental development and the tips for dealing with the 'silent child' and the 'angry child' found in Chapter 6 would be beneficial to the practicing psychiatrist. The MCE tables on Depression are wonderful accompaniments to Chapter 7. The Common clinical narratives encountered in Bipolar disorder and the description of the common temperament types are excellent discussions in Chapter 8. The importance of using the word 'Ulan' and the challenges experienced in managing psychosis are well-elucidated in Chapter 9. The highlights of Chapter 10 are the author's unique medical and behavioral perspective on anxiety. I enjoyed the discussion on the various 'flavors' of OCD in Chapter 11 and nearly chuckled at the humorous reference to one of his colleague's obsession while eliciting dog-bite histories. I found the author's nuances in understanding post-traumatic stress disorder and its overlap with anxiety disorder in Chapter 12 to be an elegant display of the wisdom available in this book. Chapters 13 through 15 discuss the most relevant aspects of addictive behavior in clinical practice. Chapter 16 makes the reader realize how somatoform disorders could contribute to building a psychiatric practice in the community and could be a very gratifying experience for the psychiatrist to treat these patients. Chapter 17 is a beautiful rendition of the fundamental principles of personality and personality disorders.

I considered Chapter 18, which discusses suicide, to be an absolute gem and a must-read for all medical professionals. The differentiation of violent behavior into maleficent vs. non-maleficent is novel and remarkable. Chapter 20 briefly discusses critical aspects of geriatric psychiatry, which is essential in today's increasingly older population.

The points of wisdom from the author found in Chapter 21 is a concentrate of the author's wisdom derived from nearly three decades of busy clinical practice in psychiatry. Reading this chapter was akin to drinking the Amruth (the immortal elixir of life). The book culminated in Chapter 22, a short note on the joy of psychiatry, which again was a pleasure to read.

In short, as a practicing neurologist, I find this book extraordinarily useful because of its clarity and brevity. It carries the wisdom of Prof. T Manickam and Dr. P Thirunavukarasu, the author's many years of experience, and provides invaluable tips for the practicing neurologist.

I strongly recommend that every neurologist read this excellent book.

I wish 'The Psych Book' a great success.

Professor Lakshmi Narasimhan Ranganathan, MD, DM, PhD, FAAN, FRCP, FEBN, FIAN
Head of the Department of Neurology
SRIHER, Chennai.

Contents

Chapter 1
The Mind:What We Know So Far...   *1*

Chapter 2
The Million-Dollar Question – What Is The Mind?   *37*

Chapter 3
The Billion-Dollar Question - What Is 'Normal'?   *73*

Chapter 4
The Trillion-Dollar Question - What is Mental health?   *85*

Chapter 5
The Toolbox - Psychiatric Clinical Examination   *119*

Chapter 6
The Child Patient   *153*

Chapter 7
Depression   *185*

Chapter 8
Bipolar Disorder   *211*

Chapter 9
Psychosis   *231*

Chapter 10
Anxiety Disorder   *255*

Chapter 11
Obsessive-CompulsiveDisorder   *271*

Chapter 12
Post-Traumatic StressDisorder   *299*

Chapter 13
Addiction and Substance Abuse   *315*

Chapter 14
Alcohol Use and Addiction   *335*

Chapter 15
Gaming and Internet-Related Disorders   *347*

Chapter 16
Somatoform Disorders   *361*

Chapter 17
Personality and Personality Disorders   *381*

Chapter 18
Suicidal Behavior   *405*

Chapter 19
Violent Behavior   *433*

Chapter 20
Geriatric Psychiatry   *447*

Chapter 21
Points of Wisdom for thePracticing Psychiatrist   *455*

Chapter 22
The Joy Of Psychiatry   *463*

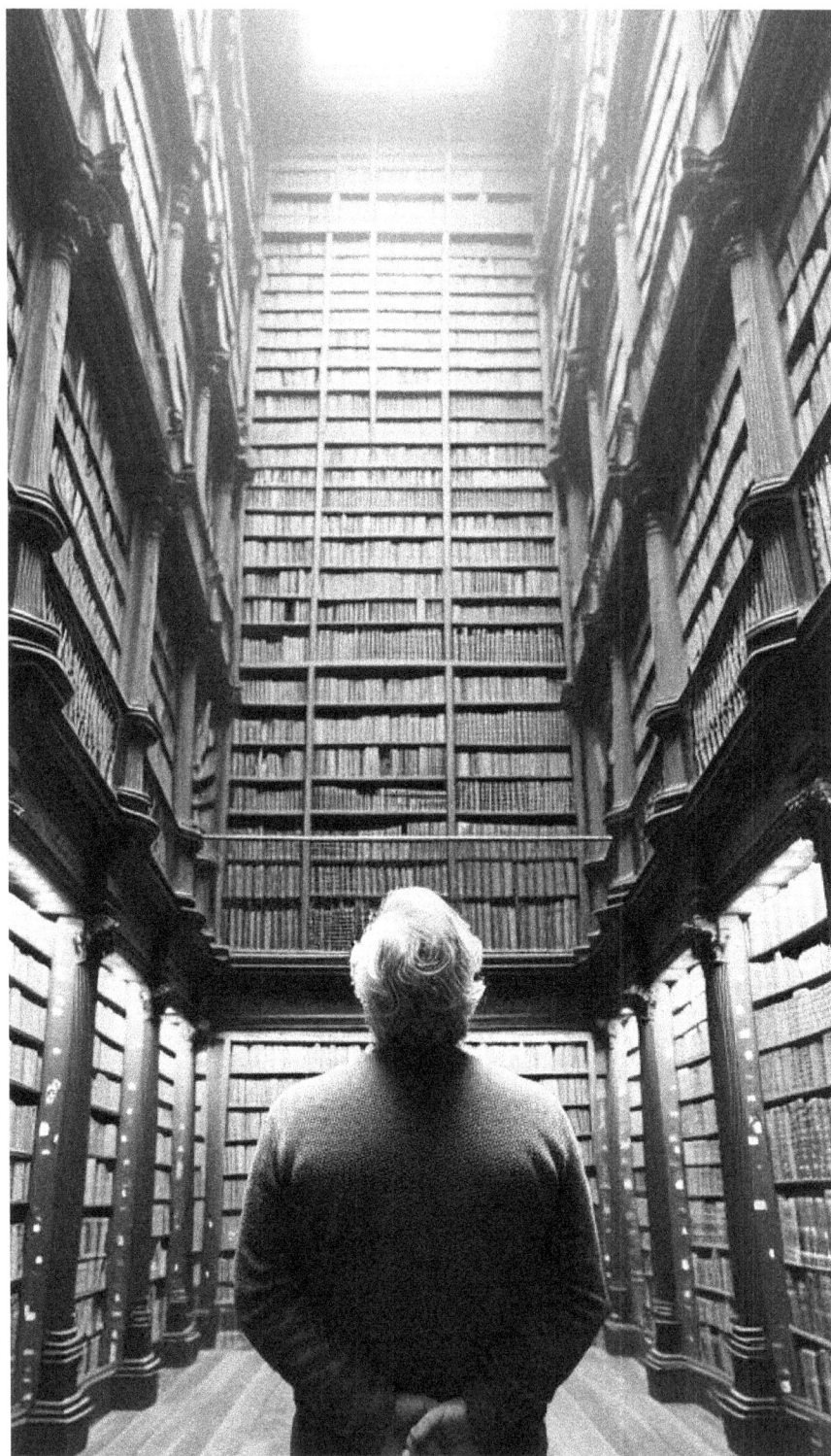

CHAPTER 1

The Mind:
What We Know So Far...

The scope of this chapter is to make the reader understand the 'mind' from a medical standpoint. It may be impossible to understand the mind in the context of all that has been said and written about it, but as doctors, we don't need to reconcile all of it. We only need to understand the mind from the medical standpoint, and we must do it without ambiguity, as academic discussion would be futile if we do not come to terms with the definition of the mind.

Plenty has been said about the mind in scriptures, literature, poetry, popular media, and art. Philosophers, artists, religious icons, prophets, politicians, priests, kings, lawmakers, judiciary, etc. have all had much to say about the reason directly or indirectly. In the current age of widespread use of public platforms for interaction, such as social media, everyone has something to say about the mind – not just their two cents, but their grand theories. However, the overwhelming majority of the content said and written about the mind has contributed little to the understanding what the mind is or how it operates. Instead, it simply glorifies the influence of the human mind over worldly matters and various aspects of life. For example, religious thinkers and scriptures use 'faith' (a mental ability) and 'prayer' (a mental activity) to advance their mission. Politicians and lawmakers use the emotions (a mental ability) of the people to reach their agenda. Philosophers primarily depend on various mental skills to explain life's multiple phenomena. Artists exploit the realm of many mental faculties in their art forms. Matters of family, love, affection, sex, society, governance, justice, etc. which form the bulk of media articles, journals, and books, are all explained by faculties of mental functioning.

Most of what has been said or written about the mind is either about how the mind explains everything in life and the world, or how they are influenced by it. But most people have neither dared to attempt nor succeeded in defining what the mind is or detailing how it operates. A few medical doctors and psychologists have made awe-inspiring advances in doing so, and we will deal with their work in this book. This chapter aims to equip the reader with some basic understanding of what has been historically available, in terms of the medical knowledge of the mind.

Challenges In Studying The Mind

Before beginning to understand the mind, let us try to understand the reasons behind the historical failure to study or explain the mind -

The first reason is the absence of an anatomical structure. To understand or define an entity, one must be able to study it. Especially if it has anything to do with medical knowledge or of the human body, it must be isolated from the human body and looked at closely. It must be dissected into smaller parts and analyzed. For example, if one intends to study the heart, the heart is removed from a cadaver, then placed on a table, measured, weighed, photographed, dissected, drawn to scale, examined under the microscope, etc. None of this can be done with the mind.

The mind has no structure. It cannot be isolated from the human body or dissected. It cannot be measured or weighed. One cannot smell or feel the mind. If so, then how do we know it even exists?

We know that the mind exists by witnessing its manifestations; by manifestations, I mean its abilities and activities. Mind is the difference between a living being and a corpse. How do we know that the mind is part of the body? By seeing that it can become diseased and also by seeing that the mind can exist in two states – health and disease, just like every other part of the body. Thus, we can infer that the mind does exist as a part of the human body but without a structure.

Many scholars consider the mind to be the function of the brain. They conceptualize 'mind' as an umbrella term for some of the brain's functions, such as intelligence, emotion, etc. It is not that simplistic either, as plenty of mental faculties do not have any anatomical brain correlate. If the mind has no anatomical structure, then it cannot be concluded as solely a function of the brain.

Instead, the mind is a 'functionalistic' entity. By 'functionalistic' entity, I mean that the mind exists only when functioning. When the mind is not functioning, it does not exist. The mind is not a function of an organ, but the mind is not existent when it is not functioning. In other words, there is no such thing as a 'mind that does not function.'

So, if the mind exists and has no structure, from where does the mind emanate? How do we locate the mind? Is it located in the brain? Several scientific observations have been made in the last few centuries that can help us answer this question. We know that if certain parts of the brain are injured or damaged, the person loses certain mental processes, which means that certain parts of the brain may be attributed to specific mental abilities. Through functional imaging techniques, we can identify areas of the brain that 'light up' when the person feels or experiences a particular emotion, which suggests that 'feelings' and 'emotions' can be attributed to certain functioning parts of the brain. There is strong evidence to link certain neurotransmitters in the brain to certain specific disease states, which in turn means that there are biochemical pathways that are responsible for the healthy state of the mind.

Does all the latter mean that the brain is the structure of the mind? In other words, is there a physical (structural or chemical) correlate in the brain that explains the mind? Not necessarily - because there is a wide variety of mental disorders that exist in people with no identifiable structural abnormalities or disturbances in neurotransmitters. Furthermore, there are mental disorders linked to abnormal functioning of other body systems, with no demonstrable and proven physical or chemical causes. For example, gastrointestinal (GI) symptoms such as nausea, flatulence, and constipation are linked to mental disorders like anxiety. Does the abnormal functioning of the GI system affect the individual's mental state, or vice versa? Or does a single yet unidentified etiology result in the simultaneous malfunctioning of the GI system and the mind? It is well recognized in medical science that 'mental stress' could be related to oral ulcers, skin disorders, allergies, cardiac manifestations such as palpitations, neurological symptoms, etc. Are there demonstrable and proven physical correlates in the brain that could explain the latter manifestations of mental well-being? No. Hence, we cannot reduce the mind to the brain unequivocally, at least with the scientific evidence available. Nevertheless, there is strong evidence in the field of biology for the brain being the predominant seat of faculties attributable to the mind, but it might be premature to conclude that anatomical and chemical characters of the brain alone can explain all that is encompassed by what we term as 'mind.'

So, does that mean that the mind is supernatural? Is the mind eternal, outside the physical body, and attributable to phenomena not amenable to the scientific method of inquiry? No. Not at all – the mind is very much a 'natural' phenomenon, and there is no evidence whatsoever of supernatural phenomena directly or indirectly attributable to the existence or functioning of the mind.

Thus, from what we know thus far, the mind is a natural non-structural entity, a functionalistic entity, a part of the human body that can become diseased, be treated, and be healed well. This is what makes the study of the mind so challenging.

The second reason for the historical failure to understand what the mind is or how it operates is that the studier of the mind is another mind.

When anything is studied, the entity that studies it is the mind. 'Studying' is an activity of the mind. During the study process, the studied entity is kept constant, and the studier (the mind of a person) is trained to be kept steady and is subject to a specific discipline.

For example, suppose an element such as hydrogen is studied. In that case, one can heat it, cool it, boil it, freeze it, force it to react with other chemicals, and multiple people can observe the latter reactions objectively, make judgments, and arbitrate on the findings. The studier's attributes are not expected to affect these measurements, and even if they did, multiple techniques are employable to standardize the studying or observing techniques. We can also train people on how to study chemicals in a standardized fashion and establish a discipline accordingly. This makes studies by various people comparable, increasing the yield of study cumulatively. But, when the mind becomes the object of study, one mind is studying another mind, which allows for several uncertainties, making it incredibly difficult to standardize the observations. It also makes the study's findings unavailable for objective arbitration or judgment. Furthermore, the number of variables to standardize is numerous, and so are methods of standardization. Thus, when it comes to studying the mind, we are constantly concerned if the studier's mind is affecting the observations, and the studier's judgments are called into question on account of mental biases that the studier may possess.

The third reason for the historical failure to study the mind is the difficulty in delineating what is 'normal' when it comes to the mind. The primary yield of the process of studying an entity is to establish what is normal or standard, and then use the latter 'norm' as the yardstick to understand the deviations. The ability to set that objective yardstick is the incentive for further studying, and allows for a consistent system of knowledge to be built over time. With regards to the study of the mind, such a delineation has proved to be extremely difficult, if not impossible due to the first two reasons discussed above.

The final and cementing reason for the inability to make scientific progress in defining the mind is the stigma and controversy associated with any outcome of such a study. The implications of the mind are so extensive, pervasive, and consequential, that any explanation of the mind could have far-reaching effects on the livelihoods of many people. Nearly every study that pertains to the mind is met with opinions, disagreements, or resistance. Sincere attempts to study or reveal facts about the nature of the mind are either censored or subject to deliberate or subversive coercion, thereby making it unattractive for researchers who see public agreeability as a significant bottleneck in translating their hard-earned research findings into policy or clinical practice.

The Freudian School

Despite all these gigantic and formidable obstacles, a Jewish psychiatrist from Austria named Sigmund Schlomo Freud (1856-1939) managed to successfully advance an explanation of the mind (Figure 1). Sigmund suffered a difficult childhood experience at the hands of a sexually abusive father. While this might have prepared him for a deeper understanding of the human mind, it also paved the way for criticism of his work for the reasons mentioned above, especially those citing his 'abnormal' childhood experiences to have unduly influenced his academic work on the mind.

Nevertheless, despite significant resistance and difficulties, including his fleeing the Nazi oppression to London, he worked relentlessly on advancing a model to understand the operation of the mind. He did not define the mind but certainly explained its function. Many historians and scholars have credited Sigmund Freud as one of the few icons who dramatically changed human thought, in rank with the ideas of Copernicus, who claimed the earth was not flat, and Darwin, who claimed evolution through natural selection to explain the living world. In my opinion, Sigmund Freud's most significant contribution was not necessarily his theory to explain

Figure 1: Sigmund Freud

the mind, but the idea that the mind is not beyond the reach of scientific study and that the mind is a physiological entity susceptible to disease states and amenable to medical therapies.

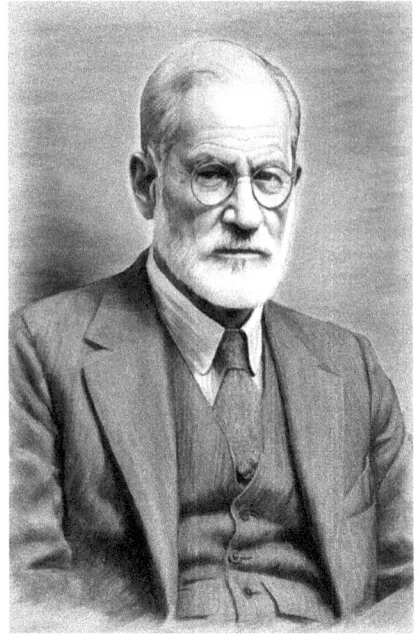

Axioms of the Freudian school

To understand the basis of Sigmund Freud's explanation of the mind, one must know and understand an important principle in physics that dominated scientific thinking immediately preceding Sigmund Freud's time – the law of conservation of energy. According to the latter principle, energy can neither be created nor destroyed but transforms from one form to another. All that exists in the natural world was understood to be one of two entities - matter or energy. The mind was not considered as matter due to the absence of structure; thus, it was understood to be a form of energy. All the functions of the mind are manifested as behavior, and therefore, any behavior must result in a release of energy from the human body that houses the mind, and this released energy results in an impact on the environment or other individuals. Individuals exposed to the energy emanating from the behavior of another individual will be impacted in some way. If the energy of the mind is not expended as behavior, then the mind 'suppresses' the energy, which impacts the mind in some way. These were the basic axioms of the Freudian school of thought.

For example, when the mind functions, it results in words said by the individual or actions performed by the individual. Each word that is spoken and each action that is performed by an individual is the result of the release of energy that has enacted the functioning of the mind. Hence, each word that is spoken influences the individual who spoke the word and every individual who heard the word. It affects the functioning of the mind that spoke the word and the functioning of any other mind that listened to the word. The same is true for any actions performed. This results in a complex network of effects within oneself and others.

Let us consider the incident of a drunk and reckless driver causing a road traffic accident. Due to the crash, traffic flow is affected, and vehicles begin to move slowly. This causes frustration among drivers, who manifest their frustration on nearby drivers. One such driver happens to be an elementary school teacher who becomes frustrated due to the traffic. When he arrives at the school, he continues to feel irritable and ends up yelling for no good reason at one of his students in school. The student, who was yelled at, is now frustrated and upset and goes back home in a bad mood. On the way home, he comes across a neighbor's dog that often barks when he walks by for no apparent reason. Frustrated, he loses his temper and attacks the dog with the stone. The dog, being responded unusually by a vicious stone attack for something it perceives as usual behavior, gets frightened and runs frantically away, and on its run, accidentally enters the street and gets run over and killed by a moving vehicle. The dog's owner is extremely saddened by the unforeseen demise of his beloved pet, ends up consuming more than his usual portion of alcohol at the bar that evening, and on his way back home, ends up wrecking his car due to driving while buzzed... which then results in another traffic jam! As you can see, environmental conditions, including the actions and words spoken around an individual, are the result of energy, which never goes away silently into the dark.

In other words, mental energy never disappears inconsequentially. It transmigrates from one person to another, and keeps moving. Let's imagine the frustrated schoolteacher managed to suppress his emotions and not yell at the students. Maybe the subsequent train of events might be different – the boy would not have thrown the stone on the dog, the dog would not have died, and the dog owner might not have caused another traffic jam. But the schoolteacher who suppressed his anger – the pent-up energy that was never released, what happens to it? What happens to the mind that contains it? What happens to the body that houses that mind? By the principle of conservation of energy, an effect similar in magnitude to that when released by behavior would occur to the mind that suppresses that energy. The impact of such suppression (words or actions) may not produce an immediate effect that is readily apparent. It may seem inconsequential but it only gets pent up in the mind, only to be released later in another form. This is a fundamental underlying principle the Freudian school of thought.

The Basic Drives

So, is the mind a helpless reactant to the environment around it? Are we just played by extrinsic factors in our environment? The answer is a vehement no. There are intrinsic factors that drive the mind. It is the status of these intrinsic factors and stimuli that directly or indirectly determine the mind's response to external factors.

So, what are these intrinsic factors? To understand the nature of these intrinsic factors, one must first understand the purpose of life. To what purpose or end do we live or exist? It may appear to be a pervasive philosophical question with no definitive answer. But it is not. There is a clear and definite purpose for one's physical and biological existence – and that is to live to the maximum, ensure that one's life is survived by progeny, and ensure that the progeny do the same, and typically in that order.

The above claim is not without proof. Instead, every piece of scientific observation about life or any living organism, the study of its anatomy, physiology, and pathological states, would consistently point towards a singular consolidated objective –to survive to the maximum and enable the perpetuation of life through reproduction. Any phenomenon that restricts such functioning is understood to be either disease, disability, or deviance. In other words, any phenomenon that does not satisfy the latter definition of the purpose of life cannot independently exist or continue to exist sustainably. The latter concept may not be readily acceptable to the average person but is a silently understood fact among medical professionals, especially physicians who have had experience and training in the life sciences.

To summarize, the mind, which is the controller of the body's behavior is subject to certain intrinsic factors, the sole purpose of which is to ensure that the body that houses that mind survives to the maximum and brings forth offspring that do the same.

What are these intrinsic factors? They are:

Food
Temperature
Sex

These three are the intrinsic factors that ensure the previously defined purpose of life. Food is required for all metabolic functions of the body; it is the 'fuel' for the body to sustain life. When the body is running low on its fuel, it is manifested by an uncomfortable feeling, i.e., a discomfort felt by the mind, called 'hunger.'

Similarly, the human body (or that of any living organism) could sustain life through its bodily functions only when it can exist in an 'optimal' core body temperature, and this temperature is within a very narrow range for human beings. Outside the optimal range of core body temperature, the chemicals that constitute the body undergo destruction or denaturation, leading to the end of life. Not surprisingly, the study of the scientific literature on the origin of life on planet Earth pivots on the concept of the presence of an 'optimal' temperature to allow the perfect combination of ingredient constituents, catalysts, and chemical reactions necessary for the metabolic processes that enable functioning of a single cell organism. Humans especially have a narrow range of this optimal core temperature, and even a few degrees of temperature variation outside the normal range is considered a severe manifestation of disease. Even within the normal core body temperature range, each person may prefer a different ambient/ room temperature. In standard tradition, the basic needs of life are said to be 'food, clothing and shelter' – and clothing and shelter are essentially a necessity to maintain optimal temperature amidst unfavorable weather conditions.

The third intrinsic factor is the desire for sex, which is a precursor to sexual intercourse, which is a requisite for natural reproduction.

These three factors are 'intrinsic' to the organism – i.e., the need for food, warmth, and sex arises within the organism. These factors represent a particular force or energy that propels the mind, and is called 'libidinal energy'. 'Libidinal' refers to 'libido', often, the psychological term that refers to sexual drive. However, 'libido' is a much broader term, derived from the root word 'libi,' which essentially refers to 'livi,' i.e., to 'live.' In linguistics, the sound 'v-' is often interchanged for 'b-.' Libido essentially refers to the drive to 'live,' and libidinal energy refers to the energy that propels life. Since energy to propel life is wholesomely manifested through the desire to indulge in sexual union, the word 'libido' is popularly used to refer to sexual impulse.

Just like the driver of a vehicle is the person who propels the vehicle and directs where the vehicle needs to go, these intrinsic factors drive the mind, and hence these factors are called 'drives'... and thus the usage of words like 'hunger drive' or 'sexual drive'.

One may wonder if all human behavior and mental faculties could be reduced to just these three intrinsic factors. Does the desire for education, personal recognition, human rights, political freedom, religion, etc., influence the mind strongly, sometimes more emphatically than the desire for food, temperature, and sex? True, there are more sophisticated influences, however, they are simply more complex constructs to indirectly obtain the basic needs, in a more durable and tasteful fashion. In other words, the other drives are meaningless or purposeless if they do not directly or indirectly cater to or augment the gratification of the three intrinsic factors. That is why these three intrinsic factors are referred to as the 'basic' drives.

Furthermore, unlike other more complex needs and desires, such as education, human rights, religion, political freedom, etc., these three drives are present at birth. A newborn baby cries for milk and reaches for the mammary organs without any teaching. It suckles milk without any training. The baby cuddles for warmth and stops crying when swaddled. No one has taught the baby these responses and behaviors. Being present at birth, these drives are called 'innate' drives. A human is born with these innate drives. Sigmund Freud argued that sexual drive is also present at birth. Still, since the physical body is not developed enough to engage in sexual union, the sexual drive is manifest subtly, shaping mental development during infancy and childhood. Freud argued that processes by which the libidinal energy of a baby is 'handled' profoundly influence future behavior or mental health in adulthood. More complex needs and desires that develop as the baby grows into adulthood could all be explained, directly or indirectly, towards a more comprehensive and refined attainment of these innate 'basic' drives. Also, the nature of these innate or basic drives is such that it propels the mind to satisfy these needs 'urgently'. In other words, these drives push the mind to seek instant gratification of the needs, the logical reason for which is obvious – an organism could not survive too long without food or optimal temperature. Furthermore, environmental conditions are constantly changing, so, a lost opportunity to satisfy the drives may never be regained. Thus, postponing the gratification risks the failure of never being able to attain it. For these reasons, the basic drives often compel the mind to seek gratification 'urgently,' which is why these innate drives are also called innate urges.

The phenomenon of life is not a static one. Studies in human physiology reveals that our living body exists in a state of dynamic equilibrium, i.e., the ideal state exists by the perfect interaction of opposing mechanisms. This is because the environment around us constantly changes, thereby disturbing the body's state of equilibrium. Therefore, to sustain life, the human body must possess opposing mechanisms to counter the disturbing forces and restore equilibrium. For example, the human body can function optimally only in a narrow temperature range. But the weather around us is constantly changing – sometimes it is extremely hot outside, and some-times much colder. The body possesses mechanisms to heat itself when the environment is cold and cool itself when it is hot. Ideal body temperature is maintained through a constant battle between these two opposing mech-anisms. The same holds true for blood sugar, blood pressure, hormone levels, etc. For example, if one does not eat for a while or indulges in physical exertion, the blood sugar level falls, which triggers mechanisms in the body to restore the blood glucose level to an acceptable range – a range where other vital organs like the brain could still have access to glucose for continued functioning. Conversely, after a meal, the blood glucose tends to soar, but there are biochemical mechanisms to contain the blood sugar within the normal range, thereby preventing the adverse effects of hyperglycemia. This physiological phenomenon of maintaining a dynamic equilibrium that tends to restore itself to equilibrium when disturbed is called 'homeostasis' ('homeo' means 'one,' and 'stasis' means 'to stay'). When homeostasis exists, the body is in the state of health; when homeostatic mechanisms are defective, the body is in the state of disease.

The Pleasure Principle

In its natural state, the mind is in a state of homeostasis. When the body senses the need for food, sex, or temperature control, the innate drives of hunger, sex, and warmth kick in, disturbing the homeostasis of the mind. When these urges are satisfied, the mind returns to homeostasis, and such a return to equilibrium is marked by the experience of a positive and good feeling– which is called 'pleasure.' Pleasure is that which is experienced when hunger is satisfied, when optimal temperature is achieved, or when sexual orgasm happens. Pleasure serves as a positive reinforcement - as a 'reward' or 'incentive' to inform the mind to keep pursuing the gratification of the innate urges to maximize the probability that the purpose of life is fulfilled. This concept is referred to as 'the pleasure principle'. Sigmund Freud argued that the mind operates through the 'pleasure principle,' propelled by the libidinal energy. While gratification of the innate drives manifests as pleasure (a form of return to homeostasis), non-gratification worsens the scope for restoring homeostasis, and may lead to two down-stream responses – rage and jealousy. Rage represents an affective state of aggression in response to delay or denial of gratification of innate urges. Unfulfilled hunger leads to anger and easy irritability. Unfavorable ambient temperature also results in easy irritability and frustration. Unfulfilled sexual drive leads to rage. Jealousy is a cognitive state of antagonism in response to the perception that another individual is consuming the object of gratification – jealousy is the result of competition for survival (survival being determined by the gratification of innate urges).

The 'It' and 'I'

At this point, we must pause to think about what we have learned so far. The mind brings forth the urges and the mind feels the urges. So, there are at least two identifiable separate components of the mind. One is the component that generates the innate urges and one that feels and responds to those urges. The component of the mind that feels the urges and acts to satisfy them is the conscious self – the 'I' or 'me.' The 'I' feels the urges. Since the 'I' feels driven or under the control of the urges, the urges are felt by the I to be arising from something else apart from the 'I.' In other words, the 'I' perceives the urges as coming from outside the 'I', and hence, the urges could be referred to as 'that' or 'it'.

Sigmund Freud was a German who wrote all his work in his mother tongue, German. He thus referred to the self as 'ich,' which means 'I' or 'me' in the German language and referred to the innate drives as 'es', which means 'it' in the German language. In my opinion, Freud's brilliant choice of words for this nomenclature was a simple, raw, and accurate description of the components of the mind.

The Reality Principle

The 'ich' or 'I' is the conscious self that feels the urges and must act to satisfy the basic urges. For example, when a baby is born, the baby feels hunger drive. It then cries to signal its parents or caretakers, who feed the baby. When the hunger drive is satisfied, it stops crying, smiles, and sleeps. When the baby needs warmth or touch, it cries until it is picked up, hugged, or swaddled. As the baby grows and becomes a child, it develops motor skills of walking and hand movements, allowing it to procure food when hungry. But, as the baby grows and becomes a child, it is increasingly subject to several rules, regulations, and conditions for gratifying its urges. The society is the imposer of these rules and regulations. 'You must not grab another child's food', 'you must eat only at the table', 'you are allowed food only at the designated lunch times' and so on, the society says. Thus, as the child grows into an adult, the 'I' is becoming increasingly subject to more and more limitations. 'You must buy your food', 'you must not beg for food', 'you must share your food', the society says. Based on the geographical, cultural, and religious environment, the 'I' can only eat certain types of food at certain times and cook in specific ways. Similarly, the 'I' is subject to an even more restrictive set of limitations on the gratification of temperature and sexual urges. Essentially, the 'I' faces many obstacles that constantly threaten gratification, and such is the reality of life.'. Essentially, the 'I' cannot satisfy the innate urges based solely on the pursuit of pleasure but has to submit to the reality of what is possible or feasible. Sigmund Freud referred to this concept as the 'reality principle.'

Thus, the 'it' (or basic drives/innate urges) component of the mind operates based on the pleasure principle, and the 'I' (the conscious self) component of the mind responds to the 'it' based on the 'reality principle.'

The Super 'I'

Up to this point in understanding the mind, the concepts are simplistic and straightforward. However, it does not end here. It gets more complex – the 'I' is not only subject to the forces of the 'it' and the limitations of the real world alone. There is another component of the mind, which is also a conscious entity that constantly monitors, evaluates, supervises, advises, and passes judgments on the 'I'. There is another 'I' within us that does not respond to the 'urges' but constantly judges the 'I' that responds to the urges. The mission of this other 'I' is to continually consider if it is the 'better' way to live – is there a better way to go about satisfying the drives? Since the individual sees this part of the mind also as 'I' but a different and 'better' form of 'I', a more noble or 'higher' form of the 'I', Sigmund Freud named it as 'uber-ich,' which in the German language means 'upper-I' or 'higher-I.' The 'uber-ich' is often referred to in lay terms (although not entirely accurate) as the 'conscience' – that which serves as a constant witness of all workings of the mind, evaluating if it is the 'right' way for the 'I' to go about gratifying the 'it'. The 'uber-ich' is the one that judges the 'I' to be good, bad, benevolent, guilty, shameful, remorseless, moral, immoral, etc., In some occasions, the external world praises the' I', but it may end being rebuked by the 'higher I.' Conversely, sometimes, the 'I' is rebuked by the external world, it may be praised by the 'higher I'. Even if the external world approves of the actions of the 'I' in its way of gratifying the innate urges, the 'upper I' may not approve of it. Sometimes, the external world may vehemently deny the actions of the 'I', but the 'upper I' may approve of it as righteous. The eventual state of mind ultimately boils down to how the 'it', 'I', and 'higher I' components of the mind settle scores with one other.

The Id-Ego-Superego Concept

Sigmund Freud explained the mind using the concepts of 'es', 'ich', and 'uber ich', the German words for 'it','I','upper I'. British psychoanalyst, James Strachey and his wife, Alix Strachey who was also a psychoanalyst, together translated Sigmund Freud's writings into English, in which they latinized these words for medical usage, referring to 'es'/ 'it' as 'Id', 'ich'/ 'I' as 'ego' and 'uber ich'/ 'upper I' as 'super ego'. Thus, Sigmund Freud's model of the mind became popular in the Western world as 'Id – Ego – Superego'.

Let us appreciate and understand the implications of the 'Id-Ego-Superego' a bit more. The Id is the source of life on earth, the purest form of the life force. The Id is the force that carries humankind forward in time and allows for the preservation of life. The Id is highly demanding and pushes for instant gratification. The Id puts pressure on the self to meet its demands, and unsatisfied drives lead to disturbance of the homeostasis of the mind. This disturbance is perceived and felt by the self (i.e., the ego). The Ego must investigate the possibilities and feasibilities to fulfill the demands of the Id. The Ego must also work effectively and expeditiously to satisfy the Id. The way each human being is unique arises from the differences in the relative strengths of the Id and the Ego. The Id is strong in some individuals and is less strong in others – it depends on the libidinal energy of the individual. But the latter alone does not decide the outcome. The strength of the Ego, relative to the Id determines the net outcome. If there is a ready supply of the object needed for gratification with no external resistance, then the Ego could simply satisfy the Id. If the Id is relatively more potent than the ego's ability to ward off the Id, it is called 'temptation'. If the Id is weak, or if the Ego is relatively much more potent than the Id, then the person may end up containing the impulses of the Id, or even completely shut the impulses down. In everyday language, this is often referred to as 'self-control'. Here, we need to remind ourselves of the 'law of conservation of energy' as discussed earlier in this chapter. If the Ego ends up successfully shutting down the self from acting upon the impulses propelled by the libidinal energy, then such libidinal energy does not just disappear. It gets suppressed and transformed into something else, which would affect the mind differently.

Furthermore, the superego constantly monitors and oversees the actions of the ego. Even if the ego could readily satisfy the Id, the superego may not approve of the gratification. In such a case, the relative strength of the superego over those of the Id and the Ego determines the net outcome. For example, if there is hunger (Id) and there is food (object for gratification) readily available, then the ego seeks the food and satisfies the hunger, which restores homeostasis, and pleasure happens.

If hunger exists, but food is not readily available, then the ego must find a way to obtain the desired food. If the ego does not have the means to obtain the food 'urgently', then the net outcome is a resultant net of the relative strengths of the Id and the Ego. If the Id is stronger than the ego, then the individual may be 'tempted' to seek gratification through alternative means, such as begging, borrowing, or stealing. But if the ego is stronger than the Id, then the individual may end up suppressing the hunger drive and tolerating the hunger. However, this suppressed drive would influence the functioning of the mind at some point in the future, at some level – the magnitude of the impact of such suppression would be directly proportional to the magnitude of the libidinal energy suppressed.

As mentioned before, the superego becomes an extra component of the equation for the net outcome. The role and impact of the superego increase with the age of the individual. When a baby is born, the effect of the superego is negligible. The baby is in complete submission to the Id. As the child grows and becomes an adult, it develops a superego, the quality and strength of which depends on the environment in which the child is nurtured. The nature of parenting, societal norms, religious inculcation, and individual experiences begin to shape the superego. The superego may disapprove of the ego's attainment of self-gratification even if the object of gratification is readily available for restoring homeostasis. The converse is also true – even if there is no innate urge to drive the ego, the superego may exert pressure on the ego to act, which in turn may be counterproductive to the id and ego, as any resource wasted in pursuit of anything else directly or indirectly related to the objectives of the libidinal energy, is a potential threat to the ability of the individual to restore homeostasis in future. For example, if hunger is present, and food is also available, the gratification may be denied or hindered by the superego – for example, the superego may influence the self to undergo a fast for virtuous reasons. The superego may even go one step further and influence the ego to give away its means and resources such as money or wealth in charity, in the absence of any demands to do so. The superego may exert pressure on the ego in adverse or extreme ways too. For example, it may influence a wealthy man who has all the means in the world to keep himself comfortable and satisfied to forsake all his wealth and become a pauper, risking his entire family's future safety.

Extrinsic Drives

In addition to the two 'intrinsic' sources of influence on the ego (i.e., the id and the superego), there is another 'extrinsic' factor – and that is the external world. The external world demands specific behavior from every individual. The external world's forces could make a person's life comfortable and convenient (by making self-gratification attainable and predictable) or miserable (by punishment or disincentives to make self-gratification non-attainable, uncertain, or impossible). For example, one may choose to live comfortably under an unfair employer or tyrannical government but risk offending the superego which might judge the ego as 'immoral'... or choose to live uncomfortably by antagonizing the unfair employer or tyrannical government thereby becoming unemployed, ending up in poverty, being jailed, or tortured, but satisfying the superego which would judge the ego as 'righteous'.

The impact of the external world, especially that of the society on the Id is extraordinarily complex. Humans, being more sophisticated and complex organisms have more sophisticated Id drives, and the society's reaction and regulation of the Id is also increasingly complex. Let us take for example the innate drive for food - there are a multitude of societal restrictions on satisfying this urge. There are numerous impositions on what constitutes agreeable food. In some parts of the world, there are serious restrictions on meat consumption. Even among communities where meat consumption is allowed, there are serious restrictions on the type of meat permitted to be eaten, which are sometimes more strict than the communities that have altogether restricted meat. There are time restrictions too – there are restrictions on when food is permissible, and when it is not. Throughout the world, people's socioeconomic and 'class' status is reflected in the type of food they eat. The same pattern holds true for the clothing and housing, which also reflects the temperature drive of the Id. Clothing is given great importance, especially in more developed nations, as it is believed that a person's choice and attention to clothing is reflective of their assertion of identity, personality, affluence, and intention. The imposition on clothing also intersects with the sexual Id drive. The impact of the clothing and fashion industry on daily life is tell-tale evidence of the importance and complexity of this drive. Homes, housing, and neighborhoods are also an indirect manifestation of the operation of the temperature factor of the id.

The society restrictions on sex and sexual practices are even more rigid and diverse. There are vast differences between cultures, traditions, and religions as to what constitutes sexual expression, or acceptable man-woman interaction. The age of consent for sex and marital union, the exercise of sexual preferences, the timing of sexual interaction in relation to marriage, etc. are strongly influenced by the society in which an individual resides.

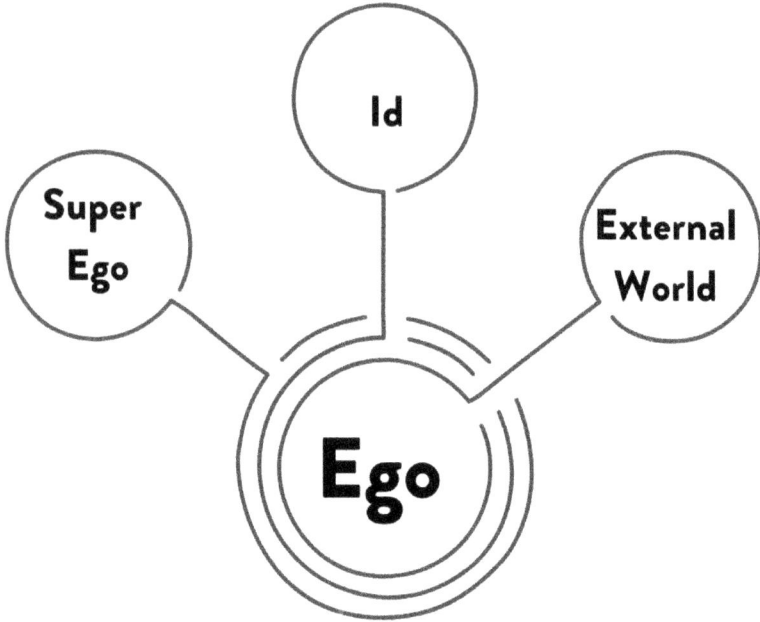

Figure 2: Id – Ego – Superego

The Three Masters

In essence, the ego is subject to multiple influences. Freud argued that the Ego must serve three masters – the Id, the Superego, and the external world (Figure 2). The ego must find ways to satisfy the urges while being judged by the superego as 'worthy', and simultaneously navigating past the obstacles of the external world. If the ego can successfully manage and survive these demands from its masters, then the mind is healthy. If the ego feels that it cannot cope or manage these multiple demands, it undergoes duress – which is often called 'stress' in everyday language. Stress occurs when the demands of the masters of the ego exceed the ability of the ego to fulfill them. In other words, ***'stress' is the result of a supply-demand mismatch experienced by the ego.***

Conflicts

There are situations where each of the three masters commands the ego in different or opposite ways, such that the ego can only serve one of the masters. Such a situation is called *'conflict'*. A conflict represents a situation where at least one of the masters disapproves of how the ego has handled the libidinal energy. For example, a woman may be sexually attracted to a particular male co-worker (an Id signal). But either the superego or the external world may pose obstacles to her gratification. Such a situation is an example of a 'conflict'. Conflict results in stress, which is experienced as an uncomfortable state of mind. The ego must now act in a way to rid this uncomfortable state it is in and return to homeostasis. So, the woman (i.e., her ego) must decide on which master to serve – or more importantly which master to disobey. Based on various factors that account for the relative strength of her Id drive, Superego and the external world, and her body's mental and physical abilities, the woman decides to either satisfy her Id or refrain from doing so. Regardless of which master her ego chooses to serve, the ego will have to face the wrath of the other masters who have been disobeyed. For example, if she manages to satisfy her Id by shunning her Superego, and overcoming the obstacles of the external world, the Superego will evaluate her ego negatively – the outcome being 'guilt'. Or the external world may expose her disobedience to societal norms – the outcome being 'shame'. Conversely, she may shun the Id, and decide not to refrain from gratifying her sexual drive, thereby leading to suppression of libidinal energy, and subjecting her ego to the wrath of her Id – the outcome being 'regret'. Regrets are dangerous – Regrets means the Id has been disobeyed. The suppressed Id drive would then make the mind operate in different ways, so as to relieve her from being in situations where the Id is disobeyed again.

The take-home message is that *conflicts are never inconsequential.* As dictated by the law of conservation of energy, the libidinal energy must be either discharged or transformed into something else. It cannot be destroyed completely. Suppression of the libidinal energy, or the disobedience of the Superego in any form does not disappear silently into the night. It will come back to take its pound of flesh at some point.

Ego-Defense Mechanisms————————————————————

What is the outcome of unresolved conflict? Unresolved conflicts impose punishment on the ego, in the form of painful states of experience. Examples include guilt, shame, regret, sadness, anxiety, etc., The ego must protect itself from such pain, and to do so, it employs certain strategies to either avoid conflict, or divert the libidinal energy, or mitigate the impact of an unavoidable conflict. In the above example, the woman may find herself, for no real reason, disliking her male co-worker. She may find herself behaving passive aggressively towards that male co-worker, for no good reason; or she may find herself unnecessarily disagreeing with him during her interactions with him and rationalizing her actions to antagonize him constantly. Each of these are strategies employed by her mind to 'defend' the ego from the assault of its masters – these strategies are collectively called *'ego defense mechanisms'*. There have been several defense mechanisms described, such as denial, regression, projection, reaction formation, rationalization, sublimation, humor, etc. There is scientific evidence to show that the choice and efficiency of the defense mechanisms correlate with the ability of the individual to adapt and successfully navigate the problems of life. Thus, the defense mechanisms may be either beneficial or detrimental.

The next logical question would be – which part of the mind employs these defense mechanisms to protect the ego? The mind is composed of the id, ego, and superego – if the ego is being protected from the wrath of the id and the superego, which part of the mind is then employing these defense mechanisms? Furthermore, the ego is the 'conscious self' – so if the ego is consciously aware of these mechanisms, then these mechanisms would be ineffective in protecting the ego. In other words, if the ego realizes the existence of defense mechanisms, then the conflict is revealed to the ego thereby nullifying these defense mechanisms. For example, in the case of the woman being sexually attracted to a male co-worker, the strategy of the defense mechanism of passive aggressiveness is to position the male co-worker at an interpersonal status that seems ineligible as a potential mate to the logical mind – in other words, the conscious self (ego) of the woman perceives the specific co-worker as disagreeable or unrelatable, and not 'attractive' as a potential mate, worth her efforts to pursue him. If the ego can understand that her unexplainable aversion to her co-worker is the handiwork of her mind to conceal her potential attraction to him, then those defense mechanisms lose the purpose of their existence. Ego-defense mechanisms are like spies; they are effective only as they are not known to be spies.

Strata of Consciousness

The phenomenon of ego-defense mechanisms inevitably leads to two important questions – What is the part of the mind that employs these defense mechanisms to protect the ego? If the defense mechanisms are altering the perception of reality to the conscious self, is there a mind that is not explorable by the conscious self? The answer to both these questions is a resounding yes. Yes, there are multiple 'strata' or 'levels' of consciousness. The strata of the mind which is available for retrieval of information by the ego is the 'conscious level' – which is why the ego is referred to as the 'conscious self'. There is a deeper stratum of the mind that gathers and stores information that is not retrievable by the ego – a stratum called the *'subconscious mind'*. The ability to retrieve information is called *'memory'*. Thus, information gathered and stored by the subconscious mind cannot be retrieved from memory. The concept of the subconscious mind requires further explanation (Figure 3). Right from birth, an individual begins to have experiences of life. Studies have demonstrated that even prior to birth, the fetus can have experiences – it can experience pleasant and noxious stimuli, hear sounds, etc. All these experiences (by the law of conservation of energy) result in effects on the mind of the baby and get transformed into a form

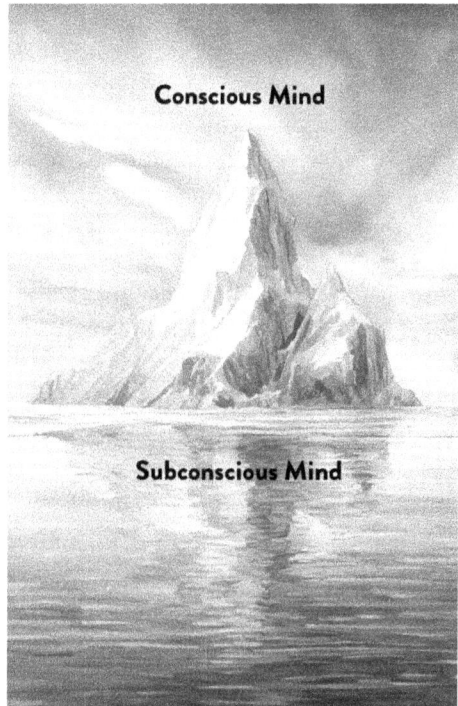

Figure 3:
Subconscious mind

that then gets stored in the subconscious mind. All experiences do not get stored as memories. Only the pleasant ones and a few of the unpleasant ones get stored as memories retrievable by the conscious mind. The most painful of experiences, the ones that are an existential threat to the ego, and the ones that have tremendous potential for unresolved conflict, gets 'put away' in the subconscious mind. The information from these experiences does not get lost, they are stored in the subconscious mind, where they begin to alter the way the Id, Ego, and Superego function. Thus, the mind operates in such a way that it filters and sorts the data from experiences and stores it in either memory accessible to the conscious mind, or as suppressed memories to be handled by the unconscious mind. The mind 'suppresses' unwanted memories to the subconscious level so that the conscious self does not have to deal with them. The subconscious mind sorts the experiences according to its assessment of the strength and capability of the ego based on prior experiences of the individual. It understands what the ego can handle successfully, and what it cannot handle. There is also simultaneous development of the superego during the growth transformation of the baby to the adult. There is also changing circumstances of the external world as well. Considering the strength of the ego, superego, and the external world, and how the ego has handled the challenges of real life, the subconscious mind makes assessments on what the ego can and cannot handle. Based on these assessments, the subconscious mind either keeps information suppressed or reveals it to the ego.

In essence, our mind **sees everything, hears everything**, and **processes everything**, at the subconscious level– but pushes only a fraction of it up to the conscious level. Similarly, the subconscious mind could also conceal or manipulate the information that it pushes to the conscious level. It tries to protect the ego from conflicts by deploying various defense mechanisms as mentioned above. Nevertheless, the strength, quality and sophistication of the subconscious mind also matters – which is why certain defense mechanisms could be detrimental to the ability of the self to cope or adapt with conflicts. These defense mechanisms are called pathological or immature defenses. More sophisticated and capable subconscious minds employ mature and beneficial defenses. In summary, ego defense mechanisms are subconscious processes that are intended by the mind to protect the ego and they are effective only as long as the ego is unaware of them. The ego would try its best to support the propositions of the subconscious mind.

Coming back to the scenario used as an example – the woman's subconscious mind may receive an Id signal of sexual attraction directed towards a certain male co-worker. But based on the nature and capacity of the woman's ego, her Superego, and the circumstances of the real world, the subconscious mind makes an assessment that her ego cannot handle the impulses of the Id, and if allowed to handle such a situation, it would result in a conflict, the eventual outcome might be an unwanted and painful experience (such as shame, guilt, or regret). Hence, her subconscious mind alters or manipulates the conscious mind – to either find him at odds with her, so she would not have to be in a position where she could consciously discover her attraction to him. However, if by some means, it becomes revealed to her, then her ego would have to deal with the conflict – hence, if the defense mechanisms are functioning correctly, she would never feel the sexual attraction towards him, or become aware of the reason for her interaction pattern with him.

The proposition that there is a subconscious mind, and that it influenced or controlled the conscious mind, was one of Sigmund Freud's major contributions to psychology. The effects of the concept of the subconscious mind were far-reaching – it could explain why someone would want to marry someone; or why a father might love one child, and not another one of his children; or why one has a passion for a certain profession, or the expressions of an artist. As impactful as it was, Freud's explanation of the subconscious mind also invited plenty of controversy, mainly because any number of explanations could be given for a person's actions – by what objective evidence could one arbitrate which of these possible explanations could be the real reason behind a person's action? An even more fundamental of question would be – how do we even know that there is a subconscious mind? Can we prove it? If so, how do we explore the subconscious mind? If we cannot explore or witness the subconscious mind, how could we confirm that it exists?

Dreams ————————————————————————————————

Does the mind operate when a person is not conscious? Yes, it does – during sleep. During sleep, a person is not conscious, in the sense that he or she is not aware of the surroundings. So, if mind existed only in the conscious state, then there would be no mental activity during sleep. However, we experience dreams during sleep, and some of these dreams are retrievable in our memories upon waking up from sleep. These dreams are strong perceivable evidence for mental activity at the non-conscious level, i.e., dreams are irrefutable evidence that the mind operates even when one is not conscious during sleep. Modern science has also been able to record objectively the brain activity, and corresponding eye and neuromuscular changes during sleep. Freud proposed that dreams are a 'window' into the subconscious mind. He proposed that by studying and analyzing the dreams, one could get insights into the workings of the mind, which in turn could give the psychiatrist valuable information in being able to untangle the conflicts that may be the source of a person's troubled mental state.

The Stages of Psychological Development————————

Sigmund Freud also developed a model for the development of the mind in early childhood ages, based on how the libidinal energy is channeled within the human body. He described three stages, namely the *oral* phase, the *anal* phase, and the *phallic* phase. He proposed that libidinal energy of the baby is first channeled through its mouth (oral phase), where the baby's source of pleasure (Id gratification) comes from oral activity, initially by suckling milk. Due to such pleasure focus around the mouth, babies tend to place any new object it comes across, in their mouth. Babies also tend to reach objects with their mouths. When the baby is distraught, stimulating the mouth is one easy way of providing pleasure. That is the mechanism behind thumb sucking, or the use of pacifiers to calm a baby.

The next phase of development is when the focus turns to the control of the anus (anal phase) for controlled defecation – The exit of waste material from the body is crucial to maintain health. However, the gastrointestinal waste is much more difficult to excrete than the urinary waste. Feces is extraordinarily unpleasant, and unhealthy to be around. Thus, this may lead to a tendency to avoid or resist defecation. The body focuses pleasurable sensation towards the anus to incentivize defecation. Thus, during this phase of development, libidinal energy gets channelized to the anus. The baby derives pleasure in defecation. Sometimes, children get so enamored with the pleasure, that they begin to utter words related to feces frequently during times of happiness or play. With time, the society imposes strict guidelines for excretion, which becomes apparent during the potty-training phase. During potty-training phase, the child learns that it cannot indulge in defecation at will, but within the constraints imposed by the society. This phase is the first time in life that a human begins to understand competing requirements between trying to respond to the body's demands for pleasure while also being accommodating to the restrictions of society and the environment. The anal phase represents the ego's first real-world attempt to reconcile basic bodily needs with societal restrictions.

The third phase of development is when the child realizes the importance of its biological sexual identity, through awareness of its own genitalia. Sigmund Freud explained that each phase must reach successful completion, and the smooth transition to the next stage is essential for a healthy mental development. He argued that abnormal or deviant behavior in adulthood is the result of stunted, arrested or disturbed developmental phases. Sigmund Freud incorporated many mythological stories in explaining his propositions. He explained several phenomena, which are still given due recognition by many contemporary psychologists, popular among them being Oedipus complex, Electra complex, Penis envy, Castration anxiety and so on. He gave interesting psychopathological explanations for neuroses, and for certain day-to-day occurrences such as 'slip of the tongue'.

Freud's Legacy ——————————————————————————

Sigmund Freud's school of thought focused on the analysis of the mind (i.e., 'psyche') through the interpretation of dreams, and hence is referred to as the 'psychoanalytic' school of psychology. Freud's psychoanalytic school has been both popular and controversial over the years. It has given birth to further modifications over time, the so-called 'Neo-Freudian' psychoanalytic approaches which include sociological and cultural aspects within the psychoanalysis, and 'post-Freudian' approaches which refer to developments in psychology after Freud. Sigmund Freud's contribution and his explanation of the mind are indispensable to the academic study of the mind. He has put forth and pioneered certain concepts in psychology, such as the existence of the subconscious mind, the role of Id/basic urges, the role of Superego, the conflicts experienced by the ego, the role of defense mechanisms, the importance of childhood experiences in shaping adulthood and so on, which cannot be ignored in the field of psychology and psychiatric medicine. The utility of Freud's work is not necessarily about making mentally unhealthy patients normal, or about the cure of mental illnesses. Rather, it was about deep explanations and insights into human behavior, which if unraveled could lead to better mental health – the 'know thyself to make better' kind of approach.

Freud's 'theories' have garnered stiff opposition and valid criticism, especially after his death. The existence of the libidinal energy, Id, Ego, Superego, subconscious mind, or the three phases of development of the mind in childhood are not wholesomely proven. His explanations although extremely useful in understanding the mind, has little utility in mainstream clinical practice. Nevertheless, Sigmund Freud shines like the moon in the dark sky of psychology. American psychologist and a critic of Sigmund Freud, John Kihlstrom admits "More than Einstein or Watson and Crick, more than Hitler or Lenin, Roosevelt or Kennedy, more than Picasso, Eliot, or Stravinsky, more than the Beatles or Bob Dylan, Freud's influence on modern culture has been profound and long-lasting".

Behaviorist School

Freud got the ball rolling first on the academic inquest into the mind, but the impact of his work and the enthusiasm around the criticism of his work paved way for more rigorous study into psychology, often term the 'post-Freudian' era in psychology. Freud explained the inner workings of the mind but did not attempt to explain behavior directly. ***Behavior refers to the observed resultant motor activity of an individual*** - the way an individual conducts him/herself. Behavior is the output of the mind; it is the motor extension of the functional mind. The individual can achieve the goals of the id, ego, and superego, through motor activity of the body (i.e., behavior) . Behavior of an individual is the 'observed' activity of that individual, as observed by another individual. In other words, if a person is not observed in any way, shape or form, behavior cannot be assessed or reported. Since, it is 'observable' and can be witnessed by another individual, behavior is a measurable, reproducible and objective way to study the mind, in contrast to the subjective, non-measurable, non-reproducible dream-based psychoanalytic approach. The latter concept formed the basis for another school of psychology, the 'behaviorist model'.

Behavior is a manifestation of the functioning of the psyche. Individuals behave differently, even when exposed to the same set of circumstances. Each individual's behavior changes depending on the set of circumstances, and within the same set of circumstances. Behavior of a person changes depending on the response the behavior elicits. Behavior has consequences, that may be either positive or negative to the person. Positive or favorable consequences impact the mind in a different way compared to negative or unfavorable consequences. The mind uses the new information gained through the experience of these consequences to modify future behavior. In essence, the mind constantly changes behavior with time based on the information gained from past experiences. This process is called 'learning'. Thus, learning forms the basis for behavior. All minds learn, but at different levels and capacities. Some minds learn fast, while others learn slow. Some minds learn traditionally, while some others through unconventional methods. Some minds can learn everything, while some others learn negligibly. Learning may occur at different speeds in different spheres of knowledge or functioning. The behaviorist model of psychology relies heavily on studying the various aspects of learning.

The behaviorist school of learning was pioneered and advanced by the Russian contemporary to Sigmund Freud – Ian Pavlov (1846 – 1936), one of the most cited physiologist of the 20th century (Figure 4). Ian recognized that by willfully altering the responses to a certain behavior, such behavior could either be reinforced and strengthened, or discouraged and weakened. The event in the environment that incites the behavior is called **'stimulus'** and the resultant behavior is called

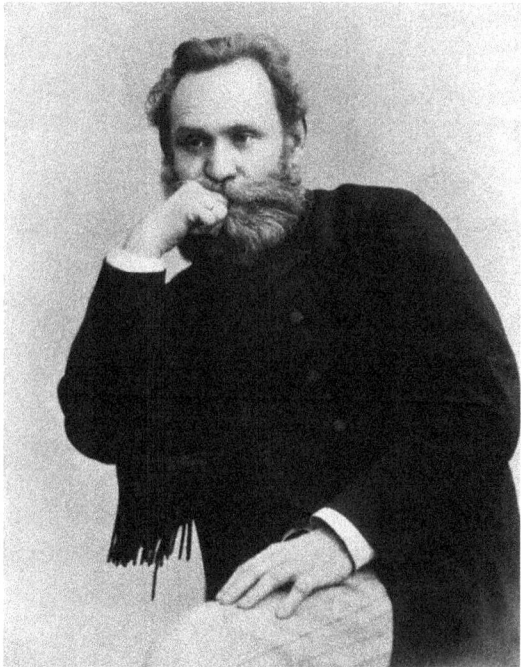

Figure 4: Ian Pavlov

'response'. Through a series of animal experiments, he demonstrated that behavior can be modified by manipulating the stimuli according to desired responses. This phenomenon is called **'conditioning'.**

Conditioning happens through learning – by offering a reward in response to a desired behavior, such behavior could be strengthened, and by delivering a punishment, a certain behavior could be eliminated. Ian Pavlov explained multiple pathways and patterns of learning through concepts such as conventional stimulus, conventional response, conditioned stimulus, conditioned response, unconditional stimulus, unconditional response, classical conditioning, operant conditioning, reward, punishment, reinforcement, extinction and so on. The implications of these studies which were predominantly conducted in animals, began to be extrapolated to human behavior. The word *'shaping'* referring to the process by which human behavior can be modified through planned manipulation of the stimuli in the environment, rewards, and punishment, became popular in public discussion. Behavior modification became a popular intervention in schools, companies, business institutions, law, government, etc., and is still quite popular. Phenomena such as sensitization, desensitization, avoidance, etc can be understood through this school of thought. Undoubtedly, the behaviorist model has more utility in clinical practice and the real world, than Freud's psychoanalytic school. It is notable that Ian Pavlov went on to receive the Nobel Prize in Medicine/Physiology in 1904.

Proponents of the behaviorist school of psychology tend to enthusiastically believe that all problems of the world could be solved by behavior modification and by implementing structured learning programs. But the reality is far from such belief. The behaviorist model is deficient at multiple levels. First, it has utility only in a fraction of the vast array of disorders dealt with in clinical practice, categorized as 'behavior problems." Furthermore, psychiatrists understand that behavior problems are due to other underlying disorders which need to be addressed for a well-rounded clinical improvement of the patient. If the behavior problems are addressed through conditioning of the external environment without dealing with the underlying causative factors, it may solve the problem in the short-term, but may result in some unintended complications in the long-term – which could then be explained only by the Freudian school which would argue that the behavior modification have suppressed the forces of the id-ego-superego complex. The suppressed energy then gets transformed and released at a later time-point. Second, the behaviorist school reduces human behavior to an animalistic or 'subhuman' level. Behavior is approached as a binary function of positive versus negative reinforcement. It is this nature of psychologists to reduce or 'shrink' complex human behavior to simple binary explanations that have led to psychiatrists being referred to as 'shrinks'.

I feel that the most substantial criticism of the behaviorist model is that, unlike animal behavior, human behavior is not merely a response to external stimuli and response patterns. Even in animals, it may not be so. In Tamil, there is an old saying (transliterated to English) that goes... *'pasithaalum puli pullai thingaathu',* which means that a tiger, despite hunger, would not eat grass – implying that, the inherent 'nature' of an organism, has an overriding effect on behavior. Human behaviors are the result of an overly complex set of factors – while external stimuli, reward, and punishment do play an important part, a sophisticated set of internal factors such as personality, character, culture, etc., also play an equally important, if not a more important part in determining behavior. The human psyche is not simple enough to be explained either by an unstandardized dream analysis such as that of Freud or by observable events that could be manipulated in controlled study settings such as that of Ian Pavlov. Humans are much more complex than animals, and each human is unique with a specific set of needs, desires, capabilities, and affinities. The latter understanding led to the next school of thought in psychology that emerged in the post-Freudian and post-Pavlovian era of the 1950s – the 'humanistic school'.

Humanistic School

The humanistic school of thought in psychology incorporated the more nuanced and sophisticated aspect of human life into understanding the human psyche. American psychologists, Abraham Maslow (1908-1970) and Carl Rogers (1902-1987) were two prominent psychologists in this regard. Unlike the Freudian school which studied abnormal individuals and the Pavlovian school which studied animals and humans in controlled settings, the humanistic school studied so-called 'normal' people understand to the functioning of the mind. Humans do have a variety of needs but are prioritized and categorized in a hierarchical manner (Figure 5). The most basic needs are the essentials for living such as food, clothing, and shelter. The latter is similar to Freud's description of the innate drives. The most basic needs are those that require prompt gratification or attention for survival – such as 'do I have food for my next meal? Do I have a place

Maslow's Hierarchy of Needs

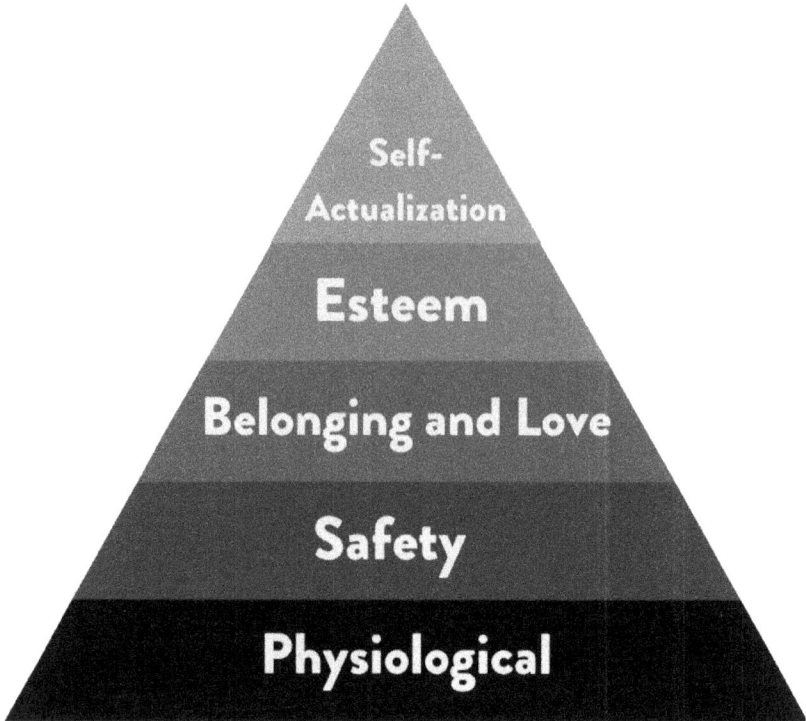

Figure 5: Hierarchy of needs

to shelter tonight?' Once these needs are satisfied, the psyche moves to the next higher level of needs, ensuring the basic needs for the future – 'do I have enough to get me food for next month? Do I have a home of my own forever?' This layer of needs pertains to safety and security. The next higher layer is 'emotional' needs – such as the need for family, friends, close companionships, etc. An extended version is the need to feel part of a larger group of individuals that are similar to them in some way, that may eventually secure personal and generational survival. This is the need for 'identity' – which could be based on their race, ethnicity, religion, color, creed, caste, language, nation, philosophy, ideology, etc. A more sophisticated manifestation of this layer of needs is the desire for 'recognition' in society. The next higher set of needs pertains to self-actualization, which is at the peak of the pyramid of the hierarchy of needs – here is when an individual moves beyond mainstream needs and reaches a point of fulfillment or 'completion'.

For a mentally healthy life, an individual ***must complete each layer of needs in the regular order and move to the next level through a smooth transition.*** While functioning at a certain level, one must simultaneously ensure that the more basic levels continue to be satisfied. Such a life would be a more fruitful, enjoyable, and fulfilling life. However, the real world does not readily permit such progression. A vast proportion of the human population on this planet is born into poverty, where the basic needs for food, clothing, and shelter are not available. They are homeless and may not even have clean food or water access. They live through daily wages that exhaust after feeding themselves. A vast proportion of children in the world go to sleep hungry every night. A vast majority of the poor population continue to complete their entire lives in poverty.

However, many individuals are born or 'thrust' into a level, without having an opportunity to experience the transition. Some are born rich and may never feel the need to transition. Many others are knocked off from their current level to a lower level due to personal or external reasons. Some individuals get 'stuck' in a certain level, and never get the opportunity or the motivation to move to the next higher level. Many people 'skip' one or more levels without satisfying the more basic levels. Some individuals 'sacrifice' fulfillment of certain needs for certain other needs. While there are people who would commit murder for more wealth despite having most of their needs met, some individuals are willing to sacrifice their own lives for their family, nation, caste, language, ideology, etc. Some humans would sacrifice all their needs for the sake of saving underwater animals nearing extinction, which may not be relevant in the next several centuries or millennia. All these extraordinarily diverse variations among human motivations and needs speak to one common theme – the power of human choice on how to conduct life. This power of human choice supports the notion that humans have 'free will', a conscious decision-making capacity that affects their behavior, and that they are not a slave to the conditions that beget and surround them. There has been a plethora of academic and philosophical discussions about the role of 'free will' in psychology.

The humanistic school and the discussion about free will and human choice were profound in psychological academia, which led to several policy and programmatic changes in medical practice and outside of it. The move to consider each human as a free individual impacted society at multiple levels – how children are treated at home and school, how employers treat employees and vice versa, how men and women treat each other, etc., More impactful changes included the development of democratic principles of government, secular principles, acceptance of variations in sexual orientation, deinstitutionalization of sheltered psychiatric patients, etc. Nevertheless, the humanistic school was not perfect either, with its main criticism being the inability to incorporate demonstrable changes in clinical practice or impact the outcome of psychiatric treatments.

The Biochemical School

While the pendulum was swinging quite far in the direction of the humanistic model, momentum was gathering around the study of human biochemistry and neurological sciences. Advancements in laboratory studies and technology such as those involving biochemical analysis like Western blot, ELISA, and PCR, along with the development of genetically altered animal models lead to a tremendous understanding of the biochemical pathways controlling human physiology. Currently, one can study the role of a specific gene, by creating a flock of mice that have that gene removed from their genome, called 'knockout mice'. Further advancements in imaging techniques, such as ultrasound, computed tomography, and functional imaging have led to a deeper micro-level understanding of how the human body functions. The latter improvements have had significant effects on psychology and psychiatric medical practice. We have identified chemicals and neural pathways for each of our emotions, and sensory and motor functions. We have identified parts of the brain and neural networks that affect memory, judgment, anger, motivation, libido, sleep, etc. Electroconvulsive therapy (ECT) has played a major role in the treatment of depression. There is a piling list of ingestible chemicals that can affect mental functioning. These 'psychoactive' chemicals offer a shortcut to alleviating the suffering of psychiatric patients. Psychedelics and other psychoactive medications are also available as 'street drugs' for recreational use. This is the age of the 'biological school' for the mind, which is now the mainstream thought process dominating the discussions and research in the field of psychology and psychiatry.

We now live in the 'biological era' of the mind, which unfortunately is a bit reductionist as well, due to its tendency to understand the mind exclusively in terms of material attributes such as neurochemicals and neuronal pathways. For example, the biological school has contributed to the biochemical understanding of a disease such as depressive disorder to be the deficiency of certain neurotransmitters such as serotonin. Imaging techniques have augmented the tracing of the location of these neurotransmitters to specific parts of the brain. There are also pharmacological substances that can elevate or depress the mood. So, does that mean that mood is entirely 'biochemical'? or that happiness and sadness are merely chemical experiences or biochemical artifacts? No... Mood is an experience of the self, which during homeostasis, gets appropriately changed according to the nature of the stimulus. If one hears good news or receives a benefit, then a positive mood is experienced. If one hears bad news or suffers a loss, then a negative mood is experienced. The time, duration, and intensity of the mood response should be appropriate to the strength of the stimulus. For example, the accidental break of a favorite piece of home décor may elicit sadness, but only for a day. The loss of a home in an accidental fire may elicit sadness for several days, the loss of a pet dog for a few weeks, and the loss of a loved one for months. When the stimulus is removed, then the mood should return to baseline. Such is the normal physiological functioning of the mind. If the nature of the stimulus or duration of the response is disproportionate, then it represents the pathological status of the mind. For example, if sadness from the loss of a piece of home décor lasts for a week, then such sadness is not normal. The underlying mechanism for this interaction between the stimulus and its appropriate mood response is through the fluctuating passage of a particular chemical such as serotonin through a specific neural network in the brain. If this neural network does not function properly, then the mood status of the individual would not be appropriate to the stimulus – for example, one may feel sad despite the absence of any bad news, or loss – such inappropriate mood response (called 'anhedonia') is a pathological state. Although the disorder is in the mood, the rest of the psyche must alter appropriately, resulting in further dysfunction. For example, if one knee joint is diseased through an infection, the body compensates by transferring the weight of the body to the other knee to carry on with walking. So, the otherwise healthy knee begins to bear a disproportionately higher burden and gets injured in due course. Eventually, both knees become diseased, although the mechanism of disease in both knees is different. The initial infection is the etiology, the resultant destruction of the first knee is results is the pathology, and how the normal physiology of even distribution of body weight gets altered to uneven distribution between both joints is 'pathophysiology' and the destruction of the other knee is the 'complication' of this disease process.

These same principles of internal medicine, apply to psychiatric medicine as well. When the mood is in a pathological state, other faculties of the mind such as thought, intellect, motivation, behavior, etc. all bear the burden and begin to get altered. Depression thus may lead to altered thought patterns or may affect intellectual functioning too. A low level of neurotransmitter in a particular area of the brain such as low serotonin availability may be the etiology – and hence depressive disorder may have a biological basis, but the rest of the complex changes that happen with the thought process, intellectual functioning, and behavior may not have an identifiable bio-chemically aberrant basis – they can only be understood by how the mind affects thought, and behavior and vice versa (a psychological explanation). Thus, *happiness or sadness (and other emotions) are not merely biochemical alterations, instead, they are psychological functions enabled through neurochemical transmission.*

In my opinion and understanding, the mind is 'psychological', and is manifested by the interaction of the self and to environment. Certain aspects of the mind have a firm biological basis, i.e., a basis that can be materially represented through anatomical structures and biochemical substances. In simple words, the brain is the seat of the mind, the brain is not the mind.

What is the future direction of psychology? How can the practicing doctor incorporate the wealth of knowledge from all these schools of thought in psychology into everyday clinical practice? It is through a 'hybrid' approach, where the clinician could use Freudian concepts, Pavlovian techniques, humanistic principles, and the biological understanding of the brain and neural networks to comprehend the 'psychopathology' of a disease process and enable the return of the affected mind to gainful functioning to the best possible extent. The latter is achieved through empowering the patient with knowledge of oneself, others, and the world around them – a process called cognitive intervention. Cognitive psychology encompasses the summative approach incorporating all these schools of thought.

'Psychiatry', correctly termed as 'psychiatric medicine' is a field of medicine that deals with mental health and mental illnesses. The word 'psychiatry' must not be used interchangeably with psychology. Psychiatrists are trained and certified medical doctors who treat patients with mental illnesses and consult on enhancement of mental health. A good learning of psychology is essential to the comprehensive clinical practice of psychiatric medicine. The best and most meaningful use of psychology is to contribute to the practice of psychiatric medicine.

There has been significant progress in psychology, but the great challenges to psychiatry still exist. Mental illness continues to have a powerful negative stigma attached to it. Such stigma affects the ability to seek psychiatric care, personal relationships, employment, and public recognition. Many health systems around the world do not have funding or insurance eligibility to compensate for psychiatric medical care. Political ideologies, religious philosophies, and non-medical interferences have disturbed the understanding of the mind in a manner strong enough to impact the understanding of the mind in an academic and utilitarian way.

What we know is a drop, and what remains to be understood and studied is like an ocean. Nevertheless, what have known so far is enough to realize that mental health is of great importance in the practice of medicine and to the overall health of the population at large, and hence the statement of the World Health Organization (WHO), 'There is no health without mental health'.

I often tell my students, *'All specialties of medicine focus on adding years to life except psychiatry which focuses on adding life to the years'.*

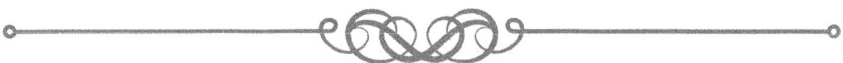

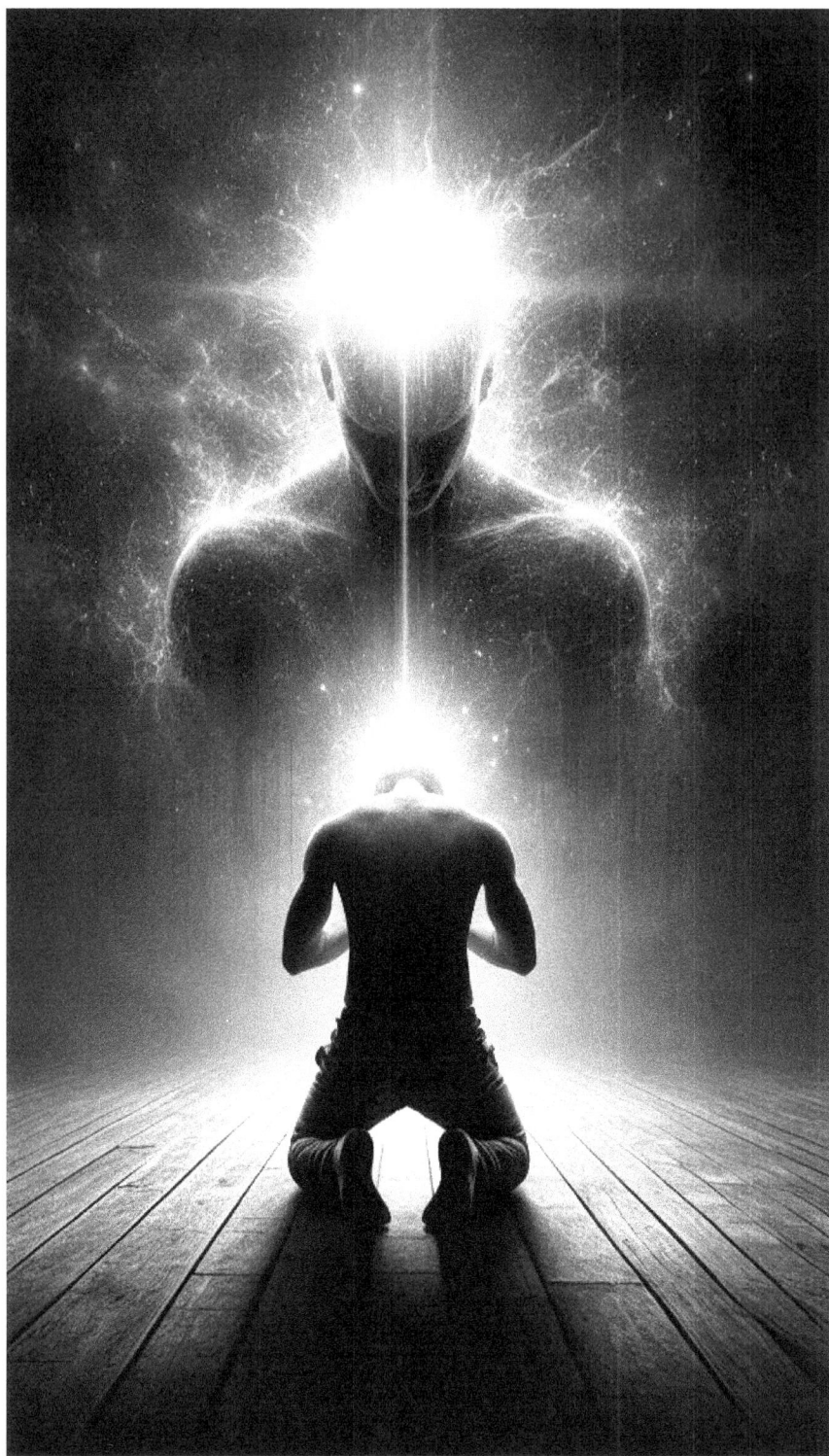

CHAPTER 2

The Million-Dollar Question – What Is The Mind?

Several years ago, while I was finishing inpatient rounds with medical students and residents, a medical student asked me, "Sir, what is diseased in psychiatric illnesses?". His question caught be off-guard in a disapproving manner. He was an astute and diligent medical student, who was nearing the end of his psychiatric rotation. Why would he ask such a silly question, I thought. Nevertheless, my instant answer was "The mind". He remained silent, and we moved on. I could sense he was not satisfied with my answer. A few moments later, I realized I wasn't satisfied with the answer either.

The clinical practice of psychiatry stands out as different from all other medical specialties. For example, in a cardiologist's clinic, there are pictures and models of the heart. The cardiologist could demonstrate the specific location of the heart valve or coronary vessel that is diseased to the patient. He could order specific tests such as an echocardiogram, which renders the heart's beating for visual witnessing. One can auscultate the heart with a stethoscope and hear it beating. A chest X-ray can show if the heart is of the usual size or enlarged. The cardiologist can obtain a 'stress test' where the heart can be forced to function under stress to understand if the patient is at risk for a future heart attack. Similarly, an orthopedic surgeon can show models or even actual skeletal structures for demonstration. One could obtain an X-ray of a bone and see if it is diseased or fractured. Furthermore, samples from the body's organs can be removed (a procedure called 'biopsy') and looked under the microscope by a pathologist, who can 'confirm' the presence or absence of a disease. Thus, the clinical practice of various medical specialties is full of objective measurements which may be simple ones such as the measurement of blood pressure or body temperature, to much more complex methods such as CT scans, MRIs, biopsies, endoscopies, etc. These tests are self-evident and can be easily shared. The interpretation of these tests could be explained in simple terms to the patient. If all tests, turn out to be unremarkable, then the physician concludes that there is no disease and that the patient does not need any further treatment. If any of the tests are abnormal, the physician treats the disease, and repeats the tests after treatment, to see if the treatment has benefited the patient. This is the standard paradigm in all medical specialties.

The practice of psychiatry is not only different from the above paradigm but also unique and complex.   To treat the disorders of the mind, all the principles of internal medicine must be captured and followed, and additionally, the psychiatrist needs special skills to examine the mental status of the patient and more than usual level of common knowledge and intelligence. Psychiatric patients undergo experiences that are outside the realm of usual human experience, and the psychiatrist can access these experiences only through the reports of the patient. No imaging techniques or scans can document what a patient has experienced in his mental state. Altered behavior can be witnessed objectively, but the mental state experienced by the patient during such behavior cannot be witnessed. Thus, we rely entirely on the patient's report, who must present the facts accurately to the psychiatrist. Often, the patient's mental status does not permit such accurate and reliable self-reporting. Therefore, the skill of the psychiatrists matters a lot in collecting information and eliciting signs, thereby leading to significant variation in both diagnosis and treatment between psychiatrists. In the olden days, physicians used to demonstrate physical examination of patients and perform surgeries in public areas to show people how the treatment was performed. In many countries, surgical rooms are still referred to as operating 'theaters'.

A cardiologist could find a murmur in a particular spot in the chest, and by holding the diaphragm of the stethoscope in the same place, could take off the earpieces alone and give it to the student to demonstrate the sign of the murmur. Psychiatric treatment cannot be demonstrated in theaters. The psychiatrist's ability to understand the nuances of the diagnosis and treatment depends not only on the psychiatrist's intelligence and clinical acumen but also on the level of mastery over language, communication skills, persuasion skills, and the overall knowledge about non-medical and worldly matters. Due to such variation in psychiatrists' approach, com-pounded by the lack of objectivity in tests and investigations commonly used in other medical specialties, there is doubt among the public and even among the medical community on whether psychiatry is even a real medical specialty. The habit of deriding mental illnesses and psychiatrists exists even among well-trained and experienced doctors of other specialties. Despite the extraordinary progress that has happened in psychiatry in the last hundred years, there are still significant ever-looming questions plaguing the public and the medical community, such as -

- Are mental illnesses treatable like medical illnesses?
- Are mental illnesses curable?
- What is the bodily organ or entity that is diseased in mental illnesses?
- Where is that entity situated?
- Can the health of the mind be measured or defined?
- And finally, will the medical community agree uniformly on the answers to the above questions?
- Is the mind synonymous with the 'soul'? If not, how is the mind related to the soul?
- Is consciousness a function of the mind? Or is the mind a product of consciousness?

Essentially, there is an intellectual vacuum when addressing these loaded questions, and such a vacuum results from a longstanding reluctance to define the mind. The reluctance has been fueled, at least in part, by the high stakes of concepts related to mental faculties such as the soul, consciousness, human rights, etc. which function as the pivot for religious, political, and philosophical agendas. Thus, a psychiatrist or anyone involved in explaining the mind scientifically or medically might find themselves positioned at the receiving end of criticism and controversy. The stigma has contributed to the historical delay in fulfilling the intellectual vacuum.

'Mind' – A Misused Term

To fill the intellectual vacuum, one must first explain what the mind is, in a way that accommodates the needs of everyday clinical practice of psychiatry. In the last chapter, we reviewed the background historical knowledge about the mind, and that the mind yet needs to be defined or delineated. Any attempt at defining the mind is daunting because of such variations in the use of the word 'mind'. *The use of the term 'mind'*

in academic medicine differs from how the term is used outside medicine.
As explained before, the mind is widely dealt with, in religion, philosophy,
politics, sociology, and human sciences. Even within aspects encompassed
by the scope of the mind, there are a lot of variations in the context of
the use of the word 'mind'. For example, when a person tries to convey
feelings in their most authentic and most sincere form, they say 'from the
bottom of my heart' while simultaneously moving their hand to the left
chest where the heart is anatomically situated – although feelings do not
originate in the heart, but in their head! While one takes the national oath
of allegiance or sings the national anthem, they place their hands to their
heart – although they should be placing it on their head! The latter are just
a few examples to show how deep-seated and ingrained misconceptions
about the mind are.

   Thus, before we attempt to study an entity scientifically, *we need a
standard objective definition of what is being studied or defined.* For
example, let's say we would like to study the physical and chemical properties of water. We would first have to stop using the term 'water', as water
could refer to a wide range of water-like substances. For example, seawater
differs from river water, which differs from tap or bottled water. There
is also mention of 'holy water' in many religions. The composition and
properties of water differs with each of these types of water, and sometimes
vastly so. Therefore, one must come up with a definition – it is called
'formulation' in chemistry. Thus, water is defined as 'H_2O'. Such renaming
through objective delineation serves as a precise platform for communication among scientists and avoids confusion. Scientists worldwide can refer
to the molecule of two hydrogen atoms and one oxygen atom as 'H_2O'. This
allows for a clear separation of the scientific pursuit of knowledge about
water from the other connotation about water. Similarly, doctors have
long used words adopted from relatively less spoken classical languages to
generate terminologies in medical usage to avoid confusion. For example,
the word 'cardiac' is used for the heart, to avoid confusion – cardiac refers
to the anatomic heart, and not the 'heart' that the lay public uses when
they refer to phrases such as 'from the bottom of my heart' or 'my heart
is in love'. Similarly, physicians use the word 'gastric' for the anatomical
stomach, to differentiate it from the layperson who uses the word 'stomach'
to refer to the broad area of the abdomen, as in 'my stomach hurts'.

Manas and Ulan

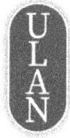

Similarly, the medical community ***needs to avoid using the word 'mind' in medical, scientific, and academic usage.*** Medical doctors must contextually bracket the entity that is diseased in mental illnesses by a novel term and set defining criteria and corollaries to enable a common platform for communication. In one such attempt, in the year 2011, the word ***'manas'*** was introduced at the Indian Psychiatric Society to denote the entity that is diseased in psychiatric illnesses, and its definition was discussed in detail in an adjoining peer-reviewed publication in the Indian Journal of Psychiatry (provided at the end of this chapter). There are reasons for the choice of the word 'manas'. On review of the various words used for the mind across different languages, and cultures, a common theme is noted – the syllables 'm-' and 'n-' have been used together with variations. The word 'mind' also has syllables with 'm-' and 'n-' sounds. During my travel to Hawaii, I witnessed the use of the word 'manas' in common parlance among native Pacific Islanders, to refer to mental faculties, thereby suggestive of an age-old usage of this term. To avoid confusion, the word 'manas' was found to have historical and lin-guistic closeness to the term 'mind' and hence worthy of being introduced to formal medical and academic usage. The word 'psyche' was specifically avoided, as it has also been extensively misused thus far both in medical and non-medical literature. With time, I realized that the word 'manas' has also been used colloquially in multiple societies, interchangeably with the word 'mind'. So, I revised the word again, this time deploying a diligent review of literature, and chose the word 'Ulan', which would be copyrighted to protect its accurate usage in the medical field. 'Ulan' is derived from the word 'ula' meaning 'inside'. 'Ulan' is the one that is inside; inside each human being and is the entity which becomes diseased in psychiatric disorders.

The need to identify and define the diseased entity in mental illnesses is real. Hence, the definition of the manas as that which is the diseased entity in mental illness is a utilitarian one. A utilitarian definition of the mind alone is possible. I find that there is no other definition of the mind that is both possible and practical.

The entire publication is reproduced here at the end of this chapter, and *the readers are strongly recommended to read this paper fully and thoroughly before proceeding to other chapters,* so, as to be able to comprehend the rest of the chapters, where the utilitarian concept of the manas and mental health are repeatedly referenced. It may need to be read multiple times for a well-grounded understanding and its implications discussed with psychiatric experts in peer-reviewed settings to fully realize the scope of this utilitarian definition and its application in clinical practice.

Today, if a medical student asked me the same question 'What is diseased in mental illness', I would answer, 'The Ulan'.

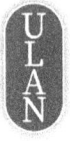

The following is the original publication. Please note, that the word 'manas' in the following publication will be changed to 'Ulan' in the rest of the chapter of this book.

Indian J Psychiatry. 2011 Apr-Jun; 53(2): 99–110;
doi: 10.4103/0019-5545.82532; PMCID: PMC3136034; PMID: 21772641

A Utilitarian Concept of Manas and Mental Health

M. Thirunavukarasu

INTRODUCTION

We, the generation living in the early years of the 21st century, occupy a special position in human history, in that we have witnessed unprecedented and unparalleled growth in the understanding and knowledge about the world around us and life on this planet. While we bask in that glory, let us not forget that there are some important and large questions that remain embarrassingly unanswered. The most conspicuous of those questions is one that is central to the field of psychiatry - "What is the mind?" Nevertheless, psychiatrists have brazenly avoided or ignored this question due to a learned lack of enthusiasm, given the historical inability to achieve a consensus about anything pertaining to the mind. Not to mention the inevitable criticism and/or possible ostracism that relentlessly pursues anyone who takes a stand on this controversial issue. Psychiatrists did not just want to open that can of worms! We simply hoped that if we managed to keep the can closed, the worms would suffocate and die and we would never have to face that uncomfortable question again. We believed that just like we managed to evade the exact definition of mental illness, we would be similarly successful in evading the definition of the mind. However, in the last several decades, human life has transformed so much that we are now faced with a relatively new concept - mental health, which too remains to be defined. The list keeps growing and our silence has been deafening. While our understanding of the human brain, human behavior, and neurosciences has grown exponentially, the task of describing or defining the mind has also become increasingly difficult. Our willful indifference or tactical retreat from confronting these tough questions is not helping us, one bit. Increasingly, we are educating ourselves with an explanation that any definition of mind or mental health is not even a possibility, let alone plausibility. Let me highlight the importance of this issue by discussing the well-known, controversial, yet insightful Rosenhan experiment.

THE ROSENHAN EXPERIMENT

In 1973, American psychologist David L. Rosenhan published the findings of his controversial study, 'On being sane in insane places' in the journal Science, stirring up a lot of reactions and criticisms among the psychiatric community.(1) It was a two-part experiment exploring the consistency and validity of traditional methods of psychiatric diagnoses. For the first experiment, Rosenhan arranged a group of 8 normal individuals called 'pseudopatients' who were known to have no psychological or psychiatric pathology. They included a psychology graduate student, 3 psychologists, a pediatrician, a psychiatrist, a painter and a housewife. Three of them were women and five of them men. Rosenhan was one among them. These pseudopatients appeared at 12 different psychiatric hospitals (11 university or state hospitals and 1 private hospital), reporting a false complaint of repeatedly hearing something such as "thud", or "hollow" or "empty" and gaining secret admission. They used pseudonyms (false names) to feign their real identity. However, other than this fabricated complaint of auditory hallucination, they reported no other problems and behaved completely normal, i.e., as they would usually behave. Rosenhan conducted this experiment to see if psychiatrists could correctly identify the pseudopatients with one fabricated symptom, as sane. To everyone's embarrassment, all these patients were diagnosed with schizophrenia, except the one who appeared at the private institution who was diagnosed with manic-depressive psychosis. All of them were admitted into inpatient wards, with stay ranging between 7 and 52 days and averaging at 19 days. As instructed and planned prior to the study, these pseudopatients stopped complaining of the initial complaint soon after admission. They observed the condition and happenings inside the psychiatric hospitals keenly and took notes diligently. Initially, their note-taking was secretive and discrete, but as soon they realized that no one else was paying attention, they started taking notes openly. They were cooperative, friendly, and pleasant, and were also recorded in the hospital records as being so. Despite all this, none of them were identified as sane during the hospital stay. They were prescribed psychotropic drugs, which they reportedly discarded without the knowledge of the hospital staff. They were released with a discharge diagnosis of 'schizophrenia in remission', after they admitted to being insane but feeling improvement. Some of the results of Rosenhan's experiment came to be known to the staff of a certain teaching psychiatric hospital, which claimed that such errors would not happen at their institution. This claim formed the basis for the second part of the experiment. Rosenhan made an arrangement with this hospital, letting them know that he would send one or more pseudopatients (i.e., sane individuals) to their hospital in the next three month period to gain secret admission. Each staff (including attendants, nurses, psychiatrists, physicians, and psychologists) were asked to rate each patient presenting for admission based on their suspicion of being a pseudopatient and thereby identify the impostors. During the three month period, 193 patients were judged and of these, 41 patients (~21%) were identified as pseudopatients by at least one staff member, while 23 patients (~12%) were identified as pseudopatients by at least one psychiatrist. Nineteen patients (~10%) were identified as pseudopatients by one psychiatrist and one other staff member. The results of this second part of the experiment were more embarrassing than the first – Rosenhan reported that he had sent no pseudopatients to this hospital during that period.

From both these experiments, it can be suggested that traditional methods of diagnosis of mental illness were incapable of identifying, at least uniformly and consistently, even within one nation and one culture, sanity from insanity, and abnormality from normality. In the first experiment, psychiatrists committed a false positive diagnosis of a sane person as insane, i.e., what statisticians would call a Type 2 error. That is to say, the psychiatrists erred on the side of caution by assuming disease in a healthy individual, rather than missing a serious diagnosis such as schizophrenia. This is understandable, given the style of training during medical education where assuming illness in a healthy person (in order to give the benefit of doubt and empiric beneficial treatment) is taught to be more acceptable than missing a diagnosis of a potentially serious illness. In the second part of the experiment, when the staff were consciously alerted of the possibility of faking insanity, they tended to make numerous false negative diagnoses, i.e., Type 1 errors. Due to a significant rate of Type 1 and Type 2 errors, the contemporary diagnostic method for mental illness was unreliable, Rosenhan concluded.

Rosenhan began this article in *Science,* with an open question, "If sanity and insanity exist, how shall we know them?" Its been more than 35 years since this article was published. Do we have an answer for Rosenhan? No. Currently, each mental illness is identified by a set of presenting symptoms or elicited signs. This assembled set of clinical information invariably lends itself to variations arising from culture, language, geography, religion, country, etc. from the view points of both the subject and the psychiatrists; not to mention the wide interpersonal variations and even temporal changes within the same person. Such variations are often resolved by a process of voting or consensus by a select group of experts. Criteria for diagnosis of mental illnesses are then statistically derived, most often by some sort of scoring system on a list of enumerated symptoms for each diagnosis. The lack of these mental illnesses is then understood to be mental health, by principle of diagnostic exclusion. Even the so-called positive definitions of mental health seem to be constructed indirectly from exclusivity of what constitutes mental illness. Mind, on the other hand, is commonly described as a conglomeration or array of a variety of psychological functions such as memory, learning, perception, consciousness, emotions, thought, reasoning, imagination, problem-solving, etc.

In my experience as a clinical and teaching psychiatrist for the last 30 years, I have found these definitions of mind and mental health minimally beneficial in educating medical students, psychiatry residents and fellows, mental health nurses, and paramedics. These definitions are too broad and loose for educating mental health professionals, who are often left without any working definition of mind or mental health necessary for them to understand psychiatric patients and approach them in a comprehensive manner. They are also unable to understand the scientific literature and interpret them properly. Conversely, authors of scientific manuscripts also use terms interchangeably, adding to the confusion. The existing definitions give room for too much interpretation, misunderstanding, and misspeaking of terms. Inevitably, it allows personal bias to creep into science, allowing for exploitation of the field by ideologies operating towards non-medical objectives. Psychiatrists are also unable to explain to patients and the common public alike (especially in popular media) about mind or mental health without confusing the listeners. Worse is that psychiatrists often offer different, sometimes contrasting, and rarely, even contradicting explanations, leaving the public to assume that psychiatrists do not know any more than the others about the mind. Such attitudes are widely prevalent, contributing to the pre-existing stigma in psychiatry. This also stalls progress in the attempts to increase mental health awareness. In essence, our delay in defining the core operating entity of our profession

- the mind or the psyche, has not been beneficial. We have to act, and act now.

IS IT POSSIBLE TO IDENTIFY SANITY FROM INSANITY?

Rosenhan's experiment has left us with a bad taste in the mouth as psychiatrists demonstrated practical inabilities to identify sanity from insanity. If experts themselves were not able to do so, does it not give credence to the philosophical point of view that sanity and insanity are indistinguishable, signaling a dead-end in our road to define mental health? I do not believe so. I see that Rosenhan's experiment could actually constitute proof that sanity can in fact be identified from insanity. At one point, Rosenhan argues that the inability of the staff to correctly identify the pseudopatients could not have been because the pseudopatients did not act sanely enough. To provide evidence for this argument, he states "During the first three hospitalizations, when accurate counts were kept, 35 of a total of 118 patients on the admissions ward voiced their suspicions, some vigorously. "You're not crazy. You're a journalist, or a professor (referring to the continual note-taking). You're checking up on the hospital." While most of the patients were reassured by the pseudopatient's insistence that he had been sick before he came in but was fine now, some continued to believe that the pseudopatient was sane throughout his hospitalization. The fact that the patients often recognized normality when staff did not raises important questions." Clearly, the other inpatients in the psychiatric wards were able to identify these pseudopatients correctly as being sane. While 35 inpatients, i.e., ~30%, of supposedly insane patients could identify a sane individual (i.e., pseudopatient) amongst them, 100% of sane psychiatrists could not do it! In short, Rosenhan's experiment implied that insane laymen could identify sanity more often than sane people who were qualified experts in the field of insanity. While note-taking by the pseudopatients lead other inpatients to suspect sanity, psychiatric staff recorded it as 'writing behavior'. Rosenhan concluded that this was because once a patient was labeled with a psychiatric diagnosis, every behavior is shaded with that label obscuring any possibility of seeing sanity, even if it existed. I would like to extend on Rosenhan's conclusion, while also trying to zero-in on the root cause of this problem. My contention is that the psychiatrist, while evaluating a pseudopatient (or any patient, for that matter) was probably continuously asking him / herself, "Is this patient schizophrenic?" or "Is this patient mentally ill?" The complaint of auditory hallucinations presented by the pseudopatients made the psychiatrist conclude 'yes' to the above questions, thereby arriving at a diagnosis of mental illness. Instead, if the psychiatrists had been asking themselves "Is this person mentally healthy?" or "Does hearing 'thud' make this person not mentally healthy?", they would have chosen to ignore that single complaint or at least become suspicious of it, thereby identifying sanity correctly at some point during the patient-doctor contact – if not during admission, during the stay or at least at the time of discharge. That is, the line of thinking was rooted in identifying mental illness, not mental health. So, it is critically important that clinical evaluation, and hence training and education in psychiatry should start with mental health moving to mental illness and not the other way around.

But to define mental health, we would first have to define mind, which has been a historically daunting undertaking. Before I propose my concept of mind, let us take a look at the history and evolution of the concept of the mind and how it has influenced the present day understanding of the same.

CONCEPT OF THE MIND

Maxwell Bennett's recent review "Development of the concept of the mind"(2) provided an elaborate and comprehensive account of the historical ideologies relating to the mind. Nearly 6000 years ago, man began explaining his experiences of the self, especially intrigued by the experiences during sleep and dreams. He believed them to be wandering, shadow-like entities, which in Shamanism came to be known as 'spirits'. This idea of a wandering spirit capable of ethereal travel into and outside the body continued to exist among cultures, until 8th-5th century BC when in Greece, Homer identified this spirit as the "soul," which he believed was located in the head.(3,4) However, he identified two types of soul. The first type was a sort of a body soul, which in turn was constituted by three entities namely, thymos, noos, and menos. The thymos was considered as the driving force of the body propelling motion and consisted of emotions such as joy, grief, fear, pity, etc. Noos consisted of the rational and intellectual component, responsible for thinking. Menos, on the other hand was to signify an inner rage that is experienced in fierce battle. Menos was considered to be located somewhere in the chest and it is probably the linguistic root for the English word "mind."(4) The second type of soul was an impersonal immortal soul, capable of ethereal travel. This was called as the "psyche," a terminology that is popular till date and becoming the root of several words related to the mind. It is quite interesting to note that Homer was aware of psychological attributes such as emotions, thought, etc. but attributed them to an immortal substance, the soul. During this time, it was believed that the psyche lived in a mystical place called Hades. During the next few centuries, the idea of a personalized immortalized soul for each person began to become consolidated.

Later on, Plato revolutionized the then existing philosophy by now identifying only one soul for each person, called the 'psyche'. This psyche was now constituted of three parts, namely the thymos, the logos, and the pathos. The thymos was similar to the thymos of Homer and was believed to be located somewhere in the chest.(4) The logos was the part concerned with reasoning and it was this part that Plato called the "'mind." Plato believed that the logos (or the mind) existed in the head.(4) The pathos, otherwise called the id, was attributed to bodily appetites of food and drink, and was believed to be located in the liver. It is quite interesting to note that Plato had identified the various psychological attributes of man that he now attributed to the soul, which was located inside the body in multiple places.(4) However, Plato committed that the thymos and the pathos were composed of a corporeal or mortal substance, whereas the logos, i.e., the mind which was concerned with reasoning was incorporeal and immortal, existing even after the death of the individuals. That is, according to Plato, mind (or logos) was the part of the soul (or psyche) that was immortal. Since the capacity to reason was attributed to the soul and considered immortal, morality became to be associated with the soul. Plato's idea, as old as 4th-3rd century BC has dominated Western thought, extending up to this very day. This idea of dualism of the psyche, being composed of a bodily component and an immortal component, i.e. mind was quite attractive for future Christian theology and philosophy, which argued that the bodily mortal components of the soul, namely the emotions (thymos) and appetites (id) existed in all, but the capacity to reason and act (the logos) was immortal and subject to divinity or the supernatural God. Since a part of the soul was immortal, the soul was in general considered to be immortal. Plato, with his concept of dualism made himself and his theory vulnerable to a perennial logical attack of how an incorporeal immortal soul interacted continuously with a mortal corporeal soul! This laid the invisible seeds of what would centuries later transform into the mind-body problem, which is unsolved till date. It is important to note that throughout this time, the soul was continued to be thought of as an "entity" or supernatural "substance," akin to the ghosts or shadows or spirits.

However, Plato's disciple, Aristotle came up with a revolutionary idea departing sharply from his guru's philosophy. He advocated that there were three different types of soul influencing a person – a rational soul (concerned with thinking and analyzing), a sensitive soul (concerned with passions and desires), and a nutritive soul (concerned with appetites and drives). In a way, this classification was similar to the thymos-logos-pathos classification of Plato, but the genius of Aristotle rested in the tenet that none of these were incorporeal substances but merely powers or characteristics or traits of the mortal person. He said that the mind could not be located anywhere inside the body, and was simply an attribute of the body and considered the word "mind" only as a figure of speech. Hence, the recalcitrant problem of solving how the mind interacted with the body (or the brain) became a non-issue.

In Aristotelian terms, interaction of the mind with the body is as absurd as asking how the wood of a table (body) would interact with the shape of the table (mind) or as asking how the pupil of the eye (body) would interact with the vision (mind). Clearly, Aristotle was ahead of his times and in retrospect, I believe that he is still ahead of us too, as this philosophy is not popular in the current system of medicine, which is still dualistic. After Aristotle, the dualism introduced by Plato, adopted and nourished by Christian theology regained momentum as Neoplatonism. However, the central problem of how a mortal corporeal soul could interact with an immortal soul, influencing the life of a mortal man remained painfully unanswered by dualism.

In the 16th century, Rene Descartes introduced a paradigm shift in the philosophy of the mind, by theorizing that emotional soul (or thymos) and the nutritive soul (or the id) were functions of the body, and not of the soul. In essence, Descartes removed thymos and the id from the soul and displaced it to the body. Hence, the logos (or the rational or reasoning entity) came to be the lone constituent of the soul, i.e., the psyche. Descartes maintained that this psyche is immortal and incorporeal. He believed that by doing so, he was solving the problem of dualism, but in essence he merely converted the problem of an incorporeal soul interacting with a corporeal soul, to the problem of a mortal body interacting with an incorporeal psyche. Semantically, one could say that the seeds laid by Platonic dualism blossomed with Cartesian dualism. It is important to note that it is with Descartes, that logos (or mind), which was entrusted with reasoning (and hence morality) came to be synonymous with the immortal soul or psyche. Descartes also introduced the concept of awareness of one's own self, i.e., consciousness to the immortal psyche. This explains why people often conjure up mind, soul, consciousness, morality, and divinity together, using words interchangeably and blurring the differences between them. The current system of medicine and medical education are deeply rooted in the Cartesian doctrine, where the body (identified by a set of physical attributes such as height, weight, locomotion, color, heart rate, blood pressure, etc) is seen as one entity that continuously interacts with another entity called the mind (identified by psychological attributes such as perception, emotions, imagination, etc). The mind is not considered as a part of a body like the heart or lungs, but instead an entity that interacts with the body and vice versa. Since the time of Descartes, there have been several remarkable advances in medicine that not only failed to shake the Cartesian system, but instead became absorbed in it. For example, in the 19th century, Ivan Pavlov demonstrated that learning (which is often regarded as a "mental" capacity) was an involuntary process, suggesting the existence of a machinery in the brain that enables learning. During the same time, Charcot demonstrated that clinical symptomatology in multiple sclerosis patients were correlated to pathological changes in the central nervous system.

Around the same time, Alois Alzheimer showed that the condition called General Paralysis of the Insane (GPI, a complication of tertiary syphilis) was associated with histological changes in the brain, thereby showing that what was termed "insanity" could be related to brain pathology. Despite these advances, which suggested that a change in brain state paralleled a change in the mental state, the Cartesian system remained unquestioned. Instead, this simply formed the basis of explaining the mind-body problem within the Cartesian system, thereby strengthening it.

This paradox became more visible when Alzheimer demonstrated that the loss of memory (which was considered to be a psychological capacity) was shown to be associated with the deposition of amyloid plaques and Nissil's granules in the brain. This was the first time that a mental disorder was shown to be associated with a neurological pathology. The Cartesian system assimilated the paradox by shifting the disease of Alzheimer's dementia from the arena of psychiatry to neurology. This forms the central issue of the problem - if changes in brain states are understood to be causal in the mental states, then psychiatry is no different than neurology. The Cartesian system will continue to see psychiatry and neurology as different, as its doctrine dictates that mind and body are different yet interacting entities. Steven D Edwards in his article, 'The body as object versus the body as subject: The case of disability'(3) highlights this problem as follows, "....... more recent theorists can be charged with Cartesianism of a related kind in which the brain plays the role of Descartes[] disembodied soul. From either of these perspectives, the self is to be defined in ways which make no reference to the body. The traditional Cartesian recruits mental properties which are detachable from the body. The modern Cartesian also recruits mental properties but typically claims these to be identical with brain states." However, this unnoticed problem of the Cartesian system unearthed by Alzheimer's findings received serious attention when Emil Kraepelin suggested that mental illness has a biological basis, rooted in both environmental and genetic factors. By doing so, Kraepelin was able to explain the biological basis of psychiatric illness using neurosciences, while at the same time maintaining psychiatric illness distinct from neurological illness, thereby introducing "neuropsychiatry." Nevertheless, the Cartesian system of dualistic approach to the mind and body is still widely prevalent among the medical community, medical education system and the common public alike. It is important to come to the realization that the mind-body problem and the concomitant burden of explaining how the psyche (regardless of how it is defined) interacts with the body (or brain) is simply an artificial by-product of the Cartesian system of medicine, which we have chosen to accept by default. Hence, it is not incumbent upon me to explain mind-body interaction, if I choose to discard the Cartesian system, and adopt an Aristotelian-like method of thinking.

All the above refer only to the ideas prevalent in the Western world. The Eastern world ideas of the soul are quite different, although there have been strikingly similar parallels. The soul is called the "aatman" in Sanskrit (like "atmen" in German, signifying a common Indo-Germanic origin). There is a school of thought that distinguished a mortal personal life-soul called the jeevatma, which interacts with an immortal divine impersonal soul called the paramatma. This ideology called the Dvaita (meaning "two") philosophy is akin to the Platonic-Cartesian dualism of the Western world. However, unlike the western world the non-dualistic schools of philosophy that mortal personal soul is simply the manifestation of the supreme all-pervading immortal soul such as the Advaita (meaning "non-dual") and Vishistadvaita (meaning "non-duality with uniqueness") and hence cannot be distinguished apart from each other (akin to Aristotelian philosophy) constitute a much more popular stream of thought than the Dvaita philosophy in India. Interestingly, these Indian philosophies do not commonly regard the soul with psychological attributes such as emotions, memory, learning, etc unlike the Western systems. The Indian systems of medicine do refer to abnormalities in the body (as the irregularities of the humors) to underlie the mechanistic explanation of mental illness, while maintaining mental illnesses as a separate discipline, akin to the line of thought prevalent in the current post-Kraepelin era. However, since modern mainstream medicine is largely the contribution and extension of Western thought, dualism is more popular in modern medicine than Aristotelian ideas.

THE LIABILITIES OF PSYCHIATRY

Why has it been so hard to define the mind? Why has there been no consensus with any concept? And why is this issue so controversial? There are several reasons. First, there are no animal models for studying the human mind or mental illnesses. Secondly, stringent research about the human mind has several human rights related and ethical limitations. Thirdly, the study of the human mind is invariably done by another human mind, and hence an unbiased objective interpretation of findings becomes difficult.(5) There is another very important reason too - any concept of the mind has far-reaching implications not just in medicine, but also outside it. This can be well understood by looking into the history of mental illnesses. Man has been concerned, bothered, and disturbed by deviant phenomena and human behavior, such as crime, violence, sexual deviations, mental illnesses, etc. Man has been trying to control, contain, and manipulate such deviant phenomena to his own ends. Such deviant phenomena have far reaching implications in multiple spheres of life. Initially, such deviant phenomena were thought to be an issue of morality and sin. Hence, it was historically dealt with by religions and faith systems which have come to dominate contemporary thinking. In due course, such deviant phenomena were also thought to be an issue of law and crime with legal implications, and hence law makers and law enforcement authorities have also come to influence concepts pertaining to these deviant phenomena. People of medicine, whose primary duty was to relieve human suffering have obviously been interested in these deviant human phenomena. Physicians tried to study that part of the self that was the reason for such deviant phenomena, and that study lead to the discipline of psychiatry. Over the course of the last few centuries, medicine has become streamlined by scientific methods. We live in the era of science, where faith- and religion-based claims are relentlessly contested by science. Drafting of legal policies also seem to need the support of science to move ahead without controversy. Hence, there is a huge incentive for non-scientific interests to influence scientific approach to such deviant phenomena, which is the title job of psychiatry and its allied disciplines. Scientists in this field are consciously and unconsciously influenced by personal and non-personal sources of bias and conflict, while investigating the nature of the mind. Today, all ideological battles and conflicts are fought in the proxy of science, and hence any definition of the mind by people of science is going to cost somebody a lot. Therefore, it is important to make clear that the proposed concept of mind is only meant to be a medical conceptualization of what appears to be the subject of interest and study in the field of psychiatry. Being physicians, in principle, we are interested in studying the mind only for the purpose of relieving human suffering, just like any other specialty. Our primary purpose is not to influence law or morality in a society by any means. Hence, I am apprehensive of using the word "mind" or "psyche" anymore to describe the subject of study in the field of psychiatry, as these words derive themselves from those which we would like to consciously distance ourselves from, such as divinity, immortality, soul, morality, etc. Through centuries of indoctrination and linguistic idiosyncrasies, we are hard-wired to think in a certain way when the words "mind" or "psyche" are used, consciously or unconsciously. Therefore, I would like to deliberately avoid using the terms "mind" or "psyche." If so, then what am I trying to conceptualize? Let me paraphrase my objective - I am not trying to conceptualize the mind or the psyche, as the world has known it. Instead, I am trying to conceptualize that part of the human self that is the subject of interest in the scientific study triggered by deviant human phenomena, only for the purpose of providing medical relief to human suffering. That is to say, I have identified what I am conceptualizing by the very purpose for which it is being scientifically studied by a health professional. I would baptize what I am conceptualizing by a term unused in contemporary western literature, in order to sever any connections or relations to what has already been philosophized for the mind/psyche and to willfully exclude any pre-existing assumptions about it. I chose to use the word "manas" for this purpose. Hence, I would hereby attempt to conceptualize the "manas," not the mind or the psyche so as to stay away from the liabilities incumbent on conceptualizing an entity that has been philosophized in multiple different ways, without even being defined. In other words, manas is that part of the mind or psyche that we are concerned about as doctors, and nothing else.

SCOPE OF CONCEPTUALIZING THE MANAS

In the last few decades, there have been remarkable advances made in the fields of psychology, evolutionary biology, genetics, cognitive neurosciences, psychopharmacology, and behavioral sciences. There are new psychological phenomena and brain mechanisms that are being uncovered continuously, most of which are still being studied in detail. The proposed concept of the manas is not intended to accommodate all existing ideas in these fields pertaining to it.

Instead, it would only include the core ideas in the field, essential for formulating a working definition. Let me explain what I mean by 'core' ideas. James Trefil has explained the dynamics in the arena of scientific knowledge by using three concentric circles (Figure 1).(6) The innermost circle is the "core," which consists of time-tested ideas, which are no longer disputed within the scientific community. They are ideas that are considered to be beyond reasonable doubt. For example, the idea that the earth is a globe, the idea that sun is at the center of the universe and evolution of man are some of the core ideas in science. It is possible that core ideas may be disproved in the future, but the likelihood of that happening is exceedingly rare. The next circle is the "frontier," which consists of current scientific research and new ideas. The scientific frontier is actively populated by new ideas, which continue to be debated and tested repeatedly. Most ideas in the frontier are expelled after repeated testing, while few

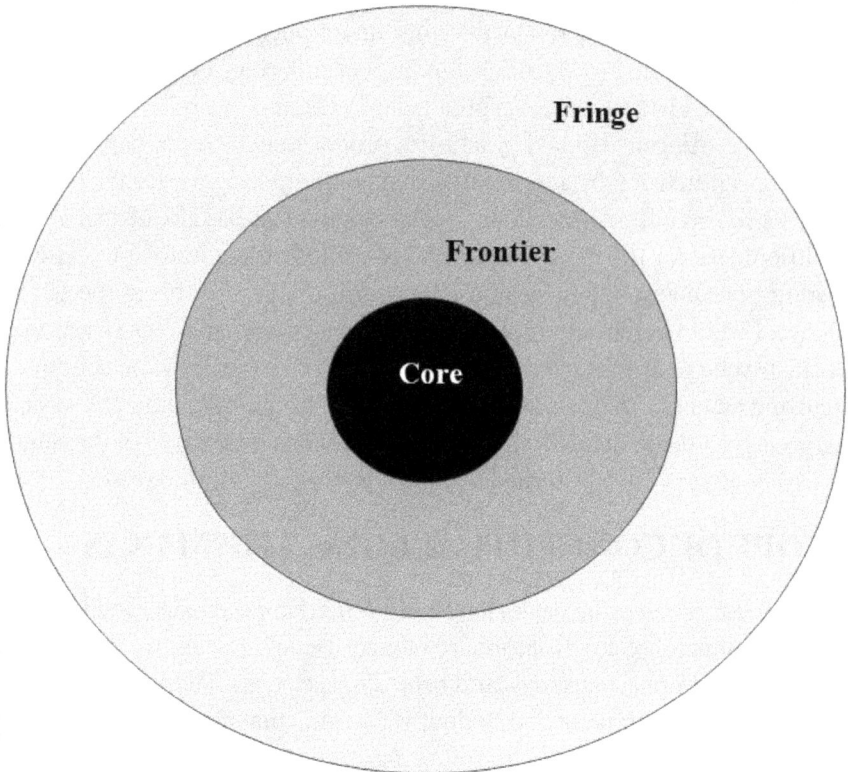

Figure 1: Scientific knowledge and areas: The three concentric circles
(Reproduced with permission from James Trefil)

which survive intense scientific inquiry are internalized into the core. The outermost circle of scientific knowledge, which is farthest from the core, is called the "fringe," which is populated by ideas that often make the average scientist uncomfortable about its claims. A lot of what is called pseudo-science, such as the claim that flying objects such as the UFOs exist are considered to be fringe ideas. A lot more evidence would be needed before they are internalized further. I would like to extrapolate Trefil's description to our conceptualization of the manas - the part of the human self that is the subject of interest to the scientific study triggered by human deviant phenomena and behavior. I would try to include only those ideas that have been internalized by the psychiatric scientific community as core ideas. This way, the concept is open to be modified further by the internalization of new ideas in the future.

OBJECTIVE OF CONCEPTUALIZING THE MANAS

The supreme objective of conceptualizing the manas is to provide a simple, working concept to medical students, psychiatry residents, nurses, paramedics, psychiatrists, students and professionals of all allied clinical disciplines, to enable them to understand mental illness and mental health in a uniform and consistent way so that they can navigate the health system better and provide more comprehensive care for those seeking psychiatric help. This would enable all mental health professionals to speak the same language, without room for personal bias or interpretation. The other objective is to enable the common public to understand the implications of mental health and illness without confusion, which would go a long way in avoiding unnecessary miscommunication and misconceptions and in reducing the stigma attached to mental illness and the seeking of psychiatric help. That is to say, I am attempting to model a utilitarian concept, using core ideas for medical purposes only.

MANAS - A UTILITARIAN MEDICAL CONCEPT

Considering all of what has been said before, I would like to describe the concept of the manas as follows:

- Every human being has one, and only one personal indivisible manas
- Manas is not a substance or matter of any nature; nor is it an energy or force
- Manas is a neither an attribute nor a part of the body. Instead, manas is an attribute or part of the self, just as the body is an attribute or part of the self
- Manas is a utilitarian medical concept
- Manas is a functional concept, i.e., manas is evident only as long as the self functions
- Manas ceases to exist if the self ceases to function or exist. Manas is not immortal
- Manas has at least one basis that is biological, and hence can be affected by biological processes
- There is nothing supernatural about the manas; nor does it communicate or interact with anything that is supernatural
- Manas is not in anyway related to the soul

- Manas cannot travel outside the self or the body; nor does it have any powers, whatsoever
- Manas has no direct effect on anything else other than the self of which it forms a part
- Nothing can have a direct effect on the manas, except through the self of which it forms a part
- Manas can exist in a state of health or disease
- Manas is that part of the self that is primarily diseased in mental illness
- Manas is what that is healthy in mental health

Manas is defined as the single indivisible amalgamation of three substituents namely:

1. Mood
2. Thought and
3. Intellect

- Mood, thought, and intellect always exists in a manas. There is no manas that has only one or two of these substituents
- A change in any one of these substituents produces congruent changes in the others
- The interface between the manas and the self is a bodily function of awareness called consciousness
- Without manas, there is no behavior
- If the manas is not affected, then the condition is no longer psychiatric.

Now, let me explain the above in further detail. Manas is a personal entity that is indivisible into further components that can independently exist. Here, manas is not considered as part of the body, as the body can exist without the manas. However, the manas cannot exist without the body. Body is an integral component of the self, and a functional concept of the self is the manas. In Aristotelian-like terms, the retina of the eye (body) can exist without sight (manas), but sight cannot exist without the retina. Nor can the sight exist if the retina is not functioning. The retina and the sight together constitute the visual system (self). Also, when the visual system ceases to exist (as in death or coma), sight ceases to exist, even if the retina exists. Another example is the analogy of a computational system or computer (self). The operating system software (manas) such as Windows, Macintosh, or Linux is an integral part of the computer (self), without which a computer is useless. This software cannot exist without a hardware (body) i.e., hard disk, RAM, CD-ROM, etc. However, the hardware can exist without the software. The operating system can then perform several functions like running a movie, playing or song, editing a photo, calculating a mathematical problem, etc (psychological attributes like learning, memory, emotions, etc). The operating software (manas) and its attributes are evident only as long as the computer system is functioning. For the operating system software (manas) to run on the computer system (self), electricity is needed by the hardware (body). Electricity does not power the system software, it powers the hardware - but that enables the software to run on the hardware, hence enabling the proper functioning of the computer system. That is, electricity (consciousness) enables the hardware to realize the software loaded into it, and at this point an assembly of hardware parts now becomes a computer. Similarly, consciousness is the bodily function of awareness that serves as the interface between the manas and the self. Consciousness is not the manas, and manas is not the consciousness, but consciousness is what that allows manas to make a body into the self. I hope that this clarifies the idea of a functional concept. Also, consciousness has a purely biological basis and anything that affects consciousness can affect the manas.

It is important that this functional concept of the manas is not to be misunderstood to be the same as the popular philosophical concept of the mind, called "functionalism." The latter philosophy(7) understands mental states to have a functional role in converting inputs received by the brain into outputs (i.e., behavior). My concept differs from functionalism in two major ways.

First, my concept pertains to manas, whereas functionalism pertains to the mind which philosophers have defined variably. Second, manas does not exist primarily by virtue of having a function of performing a task for the self, instead manas itself is a function of the self, or the result of a functioning self. Also, I have mentioned that manas has at least one basis that is biological. This means that manas can be explained mechanistically by biological processes, such as neurochemistry and neural networks. In turn, the manas can be manipulated by the use of biologically active substances such as drugs. However, this basis is a mechanistic explanation for the manas, and does not imply causality. For example, electricity can be explained by the flow of electrons. This does not mean that flow of electrons causes electricity; it simply means that flow of electron is electricity. Similarly, biological processes such as the altered flow of neurotransmitters across a neural circuit are mental illness, and may not necessarily be the cause of mental illness. From literature, we do know that psychotherapy is beneficial in the clinical setting.(8–11) Hence, manas in turn may affect the biological functioning too, which in turn may affect mental states. The latter, although strictly speaking biological, is not typically biological. Hence, the idea that manas has at least one basis that is biological is not to be interpreted that there is another supernatural or unscientific non biological basis. It simply means that the manas may in situations be the basis for other typical biological processes. Hence, the other basis for the manas if any is an atypical biological basis. Again, such convoluted explanation has become necessary only because in the Cartesian system, biological theory pertains to processes of the "body" and not the self. If we discarded the Cartesian system and think of biological theory as pertaining to the "self," then I could simply say that manas has a biological basis.

In the manas concept, the mood is all that constitutes "feeling." This includes what is traditionally considered as affect in psychiatric literature. It includes joy, sorrow, grief, jealousy, pity, fear, anger, anxiety, etc. The thought is all that constitutes "thinking." It includes beliefs, faiths, ideas, imagination, etc. The intellect is all that constitutes "analyzing" or "problem solving." The intellect does not merely refer to what is often called "higher functions." Rather, intellect encompasses all computational processes of the self, i.e., receiving information from the environment and from within the self, processing that information and delivering outputs. Such intellect is basic for survival. For example, if an organism receives input that it is in need of food or water (from internal sources like serum glucose or sodium concentration or from outside sources likewise), it is processed in a certain way and results in procuring of food. This is in essence a problem solving function, and can be attributed to the intellect.

In this concept of manas, it is important to note that although there are three identifiable substituents, none of them can exist alone and they never disappear. Mood, thought and intellect always exist in any manas. There is no manas that has only one or two of these substituents. They are identifiable in the manas, but not separable. Here is a good example - consider a wheel made of polished steel that is spinning fast. When it spins fast and steady, you will begin to see two or three different colors. But these colors, although identifiable separately, cannot be extracted separately from the spinning wheel. When the wheel stops spinning, none of these colors will be visible.

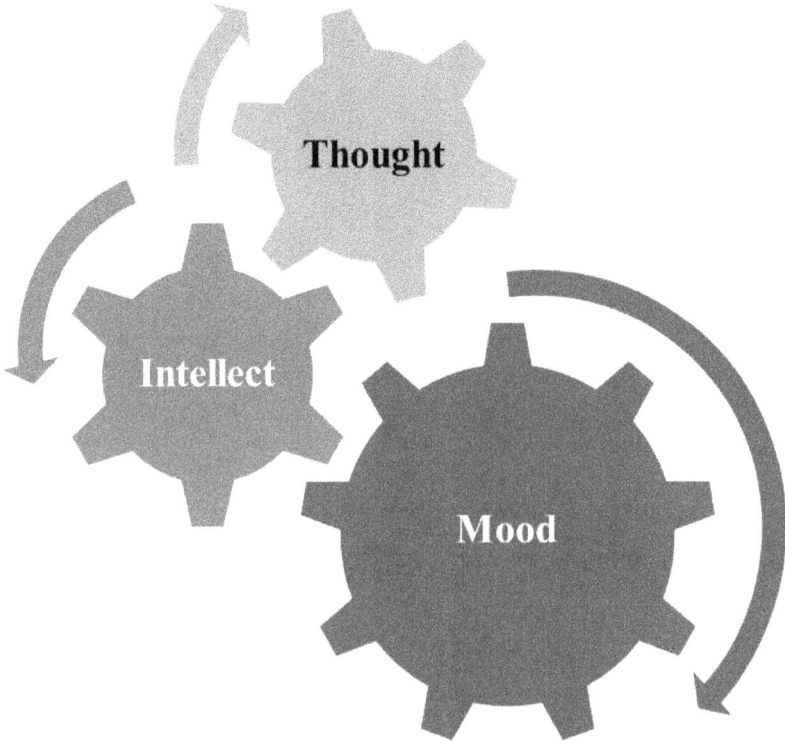

Figure 2: Three constituents of the manas, operating simultaneously, synchronously and harmoniously.

At any given point, there is a certain mood, certain thought, and a certain intellect - continuously functioning and occurring (Figure 2). All these function congruently, i.e., a change in one by an external or internal stimulus affects a change in the remaining two. For example, if I hear a good news (positive stimulus), such as winning a lottery ticket I feel happy (mood), have congruent thoughts such as buying a fancy car or a flat-screen TV (thought) and how I can allocate the money to make those purchases (intellect). Happy feelings beget positive thoughts and vice versa.

On the other hand, if I hear a bad news (negative stimulus) such as the death of a loved one, I feel sad (mood), have congruent thoughts such as thoughts of being with the loved ones and how life would be without them (thought) and also decide how I would have to inform relatives and friends and arrange a funeral (intellect). All three components are intimately and inseparably intertwined and act synchronously, harmoniously, simultaneously and congruently - which is why I have used the words "single indivisible amalgamation." If this congruency or synchrony were to be affected, then the manas has become adversely affected, signaling abnormality. There may not be isolated abnormalities in any of the three substituents such as mood, thought or intellect but there may be abnormalities in the way they become amalgamated, thus affecting behavior, conduct, personality, preferences, orientation, etc. For all practical clinical purposes of psychiatric evaluation, diagnosis and treatment, everything pertaining to our field can be accommodated by this concept of manas and its substituents. Every psychological capacity or attribute has some extension or implication in all three substituents, although it may have more connections to one particular substituent, under which it can be classified for practical purposes. For example, learning is primarily an intellectual capacity, i.e., a computation capacity of the brain. However, learning is always associated with a mood and thought at some level. Similarly, emotions such as grief or rage are primarily mood, but they are associated with congruent thoughts at some level.

CONCEPT OF MENTAL HEALTH

As mentioned above, manas is a medical concept, which automatically implies that the manas can be in one of two states - health or disease. Hence, it becomes important to conceptualize a healthy manas, i.e., mental health from a diseased manas. Mental health is a relatively new concept in Western systems of medicine. It has its origins in scientific literature only within the last century and its importance has not yet been recognized fully in mainstream psychiatry. But mental health has been a well recognized concept in Indian literature. In classical Tamil literature more than 2000 years ago, there is specific mention of the word "mana nalam," which literally means "mental health." In the Tamil literary work Thirukkural, Thiruvalluvar notes "mana nalam man uyir akkam", which means that mental health is the root source for a better world and better life. It is anything but stunning to see that the importance of mental health has been recognized a couple of millennia ago. Mental health professionals of the present day need to concentrate more on promoting mental health, rather than merely treating mental illness. As with any branch of medicine, prevention is better than cure and promoting well-being could be the first step in reducing the burden of illness. But to promote mental health, one must first define it. But does mental health even exist? Was Freud right when he said that mental health, i.e., a normal ego (in his language) is "an ideal fiction"? I think Freud was partly right and partly wrong. He was right in calling it an ideal state, but wrong in calling it fiction. Mental health can only be an ideal state, as health by itself is an ideal or utopian state. But the reason why Freud called it fiction was probably because it is commonly understood that mind, as interpreted by behavior is subject to a lot of variation at several levels - interpersonal, cultural, geographical, national, racial or ethnic, linguistic, religious, etc. The idea that parameters of mental health cannot be generalized across the entire population is almost ubiquitous. I think this is one place where there is a consensus about mental health - that no consensus is possible!

But, I beg to differ. I believe we are right in understanding that there are a lot of variations in mental health. But, we are too naive to assume that such variations cannot be accommodated into a unitary concept. The world is becoming increasingly globalized and nearly every society is pluralistic in one way or the other. Even societies that are not pluralistic are witnessing pluralism and living in it through the media. People of various religions, cultures, races, ethnicities, languages, nations, ideologies, etc have all learned to live with each other harmoniously for the most part. When people have learnt to resolve their mental differences and find common ground to live, why cannot we as doctors, find a common ground for identifying parameters for health? I believe that barring exceptions and extremes, we can for the most part find practical solutions to overcome this limitation in conceptualizing mental health. One way of conceptualizing mental health is as the absence of any of the mental illnesses listed in the Diagnostic and Statistical Manual of Mental disorders or any diagnostic manual, for that matter. This is probably the easiest solution, but it is undoubtedly useless. Mental health cannot be a diagnosis of exclusion, because such a concept defeats the whole purpose of conceptualizing it. The purpose is to promote mental health – not treat mental illness. That is to say, the clinical strategy to promote health is distinct from the strategy to treat illness. For example, the clinical approach to promote cardiac health and prevent coronary artery disease is completely different from the approach needed to treat angina or myocardial infarction. Hence, cardiac health cannot be diagnosed as an absence of myocardial infarction. Let us make one point clear - The presence of mental illness implies the absence of mental health, but the absence of mental illness does not imply the presence of mental health. This is why, in the Rosenhan experiment the pseudopatients were incorrectly identified as insane, as the diagnosis of sanity and insanity were both clinically approached with the same strategy.

Based on the concept of the manas, I would like to propose a concept of mental health as follows:

- The object of health in mental health is the manas (as delineated by the manas concept)
- Mental health is a medical and utilitarian concept
- The health status of the manas is a two-dimensional spectrum (Figure 3)

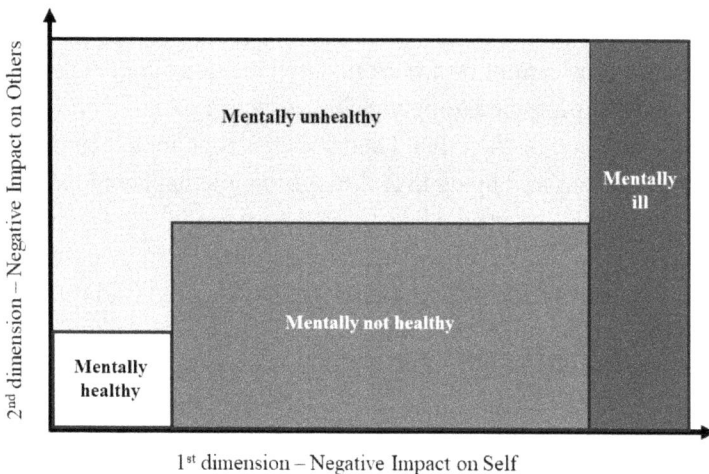

Figure 3: Two-dimensional spectrum model of mental health

- The first dimension is a continuum of the negative impact of the health status of the manas on the self
- The second dimension is a continuum of the negative impact of the health status of the manas on others

- The entire space of the spectrum may be divided into four mental health statuses, namely
  a. Mentally healthy
  b. Mentally not healthy
  c. Mentally unhealthy
  d. Mentally ill
- "Mentally healthy" is a mental health status that occupies a rather narrow space in the spectrum, with the least negative impact in both dimensions. Mentally healthy can be identified by the presence of all three of the following criteria (Figure 4).
  a. Awareness of one's own self
  b. Ability to relate well with others
  c. All of one's own actions are useful, or at least not detrimental to one's own self and others

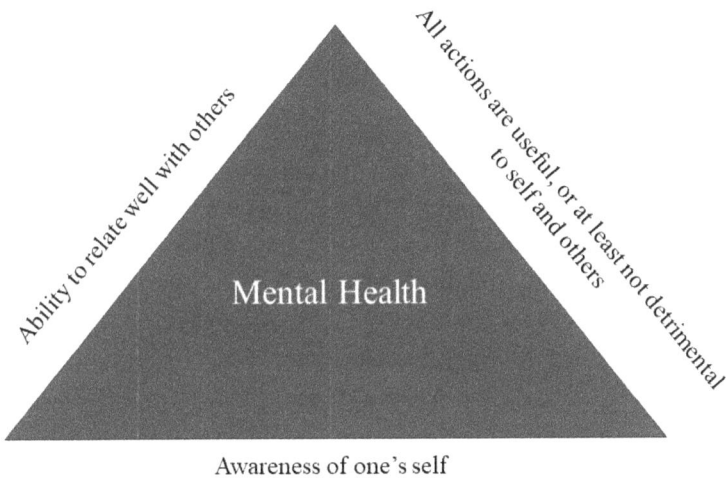

Awareness of one's self

Figure 4: Triangular model of mental health

- "Mentally not healthy" is a mental health status that occupies a space defined by intermediate to high negative impact in the first dimension and least to intermediate impact in the second dimension. That is to say, mentally not healthy individuals suffer due to the condition of the manas, but others are affected relatively less
- "Mentally unhealthy" is a mental health status that occupies

a space defined by variable impact in the first dimension but moderate to high impact in the second dimension. That is to say, mentally unhealthy individuals cause suffering to others due to the condition of the manas, but the self may or may not suffer seriously.

- "Mentally ill" is a mental health status that occupies a space defined by maximal or most severe impact in the first dimension, with a variable impact in the second dimension. Depending on the environmental conditions such as access to medical care, response to management, social support system and awareness of mental illness, the second dimension becomes variable.

- The above mental health concept is applicable only in the assessment of individual people at clinical setting; it is not applicable in the non-clinical setting and not for any group of people identified by a certain denominating factor (such as religion, culture, geography, ethnicity, nation, etc)

Let me expand on the above ideas. First of all, let me reiterate that the object of health in the mental health concept is not the mind or psyche, as the world has known it before. It is the manas, as conceptualized earlier. Mental health is understood as a two dimensional spectrum, as a one-dimensional spectrum would imply that there is a gradual slope between mental health and mental illness. Rather, extensive clinical experience and evidence-based literature suggests otherwise. For example, obsession (a thought) may play a role of a trait, a personality disorder or as serious mental illness such as obsessive-compulsive disorder (OCD), i.e., in a wide spectrum of disorders.(12) However, if mental health is understood to be a unidirectional spectrum, then it could be misunderstood that obsessive personality is simply a midway in the pathophysiological process from obsessive trait to OCD. But evidence-based literature suggests that obsessive traits and obsessive personality disorders can be standalone conditions as well. It is to avoid such misconceptions from plaguing the concept that the mental health spectrum is understood as being two-dimensional. Next, the dimensions are chosen based on how the manas handles a certain insult to health. If the manas shields the self from the suffering using a compensatory mechanism, the suffering is often passed on to others. This is probably what happens with mentally unhealthy individuals. The manas has no insight of the abnormality, while there is a deviant behavior that causes suffering to others. Hence, the suffering to one's own self is minimal or variable. Personality disorders are the best example for this category. Other examples would be certain paraphilias (sexual disorders) such as voyeurism, pedophilia, etc and conduct disorders. On the other hand, when the manas has a ready insight into the abnormality, there is significant suffering to the self. In such cases, subjects try to contain their problems adjusting their lifestyles to accommodate their problems, which may or may not indirectly affect others. Regardless, the suffering is relatively more to the self than to others. This seems to be the case with mentally not healthy individuals. Best examples include alcoholism and drug abuse, deliberate self-harm, anxiety, phobia, and certain sexual disorders like fetishism.

Mental health is a spectrum - which implies that the exact borders between the four mental health states could be blurry continuum. Clinical acumen is critical in such rare ambiguous situations. It is important to note that a certain disorder may exist in one or more mental health states. The best example would be sexual disorders, i.e., paraphilias. There are various sexual disorders, some in which the subject's action results in more suffering to others such as rape, pedophilia, voyeurism, and frotteurism. The subject himself may feel no suffering or remorse. Such sexual disorders need to be identified from other conditions in which there is no suffering directly intended or delivered to others, such as fetishism. However, the subjects may (or may not be) distressed and suffering from their conditions. I prefer to call the latter, sexual deviations and the former, sexual perversions; and place sexual deviations under the mentally not healthy category, while placing sexual perversions under the mentally unhealthy category. Thereby, the approach to sexual deviations would be distinct from the approach to sexual perversions. The latter is just one example of how a single group of disorders may be classified in a clinical utilitarian way.

The rationale underlying the two-dimensional spectral model of mental health is to emphasize that the clinical approach to promote mental health differs according to the mental health status of the manas. The algorithm (Figure 5) to navigate through the spectrum would be as follows –

First, it is identified if the subject is mentally healthy by analyzing the three criteria as mentioned above. If the criteria are satisfied, then the approach

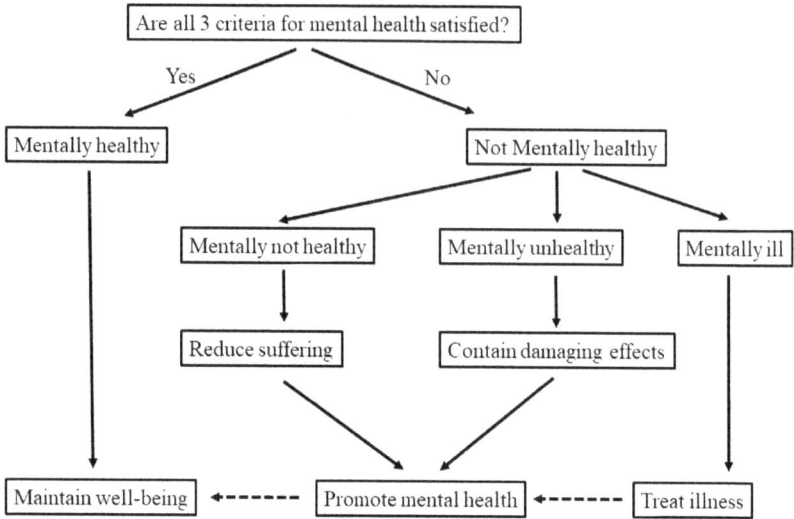

Figure 5: Algorithm for the clinical strategy for managing mental health problems using the mental health concept

to a mentally healthy person would be to promote the existing wellbeing. If these criteria are not reasonably satisfied, then the subject is "not mentally healthy". The approach now completely differs - the next step would be to identify if the subject is mentally unhealthy or mentally not healthy or mentally ill, using the above mentioned two-dimensional approach. If the subject is mentally ill, the usual recommended treatment is pursued with the intention to treat mental illness. If the subject is mentally not healthy, the approach would be to minimize his or her suffering with the intention to promote mental health. Instead, if the subject is mentally unhealthy, the approach would be to first contain the suffering delivered to others, with an intention to promote mental health. Most importantly, this concept of mental health is applicable only to individual person in the clinical setting. It is not applicable to groups identified by any denomination. For example, this concept of mental health cannot be used to assess if Nazis were mentally healthy or not; or if people of a certain religion or culture are more mentally healthy than others. Such an application is unscientific as mental health pertains to the manas. Groups of people do not have a manas.

CONCLUSION

"Psyche" has been the name for a disembodied soul since the time of Descartes and even before. The Cartesian doctrine has deeply penetrated modern thought, which is the reason why disorders for which an organic biological (i.e., typically biological) cause could not be identified are often referred to psychiatrists. This is because, as mental health professionals, we have not filled the big gap of what constitutes the target of psychiatric practice. We have also not identified what constitutes the healthy state of that target - something that almost every other medical discipline has been able to achieve. Unless we identify the target of our practice and identify its healthy state, psychiatrists will continue to be called "shrinks," and skeptic meaningless anti-psychiatry propaganda will continue to find ground. In order to identify that target of our practice, we need to deliberately eliminate all pre-existing misconceptions attached to the words "mind", "psyche", "soul", etc. Also, psychiatrists are people of medicine and people of science. Hence, scientific methods of inquiry should be rigorously adopted to deliver progress. How can such scientific methods be adopted if we have not identified the target of our practice and the healthy state of that target?

As a first step, I have made an attempt to conceptualize the target as the manas - a concept that is quite different from other major theories of the mind philosophized before. Which of these concepts of the mind is the right one? I do not know. More importantly, I do not care! I do not care what the mind is; I only care about that part of the self that I am medically and scientifically concerned about. To differentiate what I am concerned about from what may or may not exist, I have used a different name, unused in western mainstream psychiatric literature before. Mind could be anything, for what it is worth but, I am only concerned about the manas!

A condition, medical or non-medical that does not have an identifiable biological cause cannot be, by default, placed under the jurisdiction of psychiatry. If there is no detectable problem with the manas (i.e., its substituents or its amalgamation) in that condition, it can safely be considered non-psychiatric, for all practical purposes. But regardless of whether a subject has a psychiatric condition or not, every person in the population can be individually assessed for his/her mental health status, and thereby public health measures to promote mental health can be undertaken. This will also allow us to study mental health (not just mental illness alone) from an epidemiological standpoint, which I believe is very important for expanding our idea of mental health. Most controversies around psychiatry are because we have practically only one diagnosis, at least from the standpoint of the common public. And that diagnosis is "mental illness" - a label that has humongous consequences for the subject in all spheres of life. This is the reason for the stigma in psychiatry and Rosenhan has pointed it out clearly. Placing all mental health states under this one label is what that invites controversy, skepticism, and dissent. Such dissent is understandable. For example, there is no reason why fetishism and schizophrenia should both be given the label "mental illness." There is also no reason why anxiety and pedophilia are both given the same label "mental illness." It is important to identify not just mental health, but the varying shades of it by the type of clinical strategy needed. Several disorders in diagnostic manuals of psychiatry may not be mental illnesses but merely mentally unhealthy or mentally not healthy states. This will allow for the elimination of stigma attached to psychiatry. Clearly, the above concepts are infantile and need to be fine-tuned further. These concepts are open to modification, given the appropriate reasons. Future directions would include reassembling all diagnostic categories in the Diagnostic and Statistical Manual (DSM) and/or International Classification of Diseases (ICD), according to mental health states of the manas. Another important future direction would be to conduct population-based epidemiological studies of the mental health states and their distributions. So manas can be defined as a functional concept constituted by mood, thought, and intellect, which are nicely amalgamated and synchronized and cannot function in isolation. They always function in unison. Mental health can be defined as the fulfillment of the following three characteristics: (a) awareness about one's own self, (b) ability to relate well with fellow human beings, and (c) all his or her deeds and activities are useful to one' own self as well as others, at least not detrimental to self as well as others.

Acknowledgments

I acknowledge the extensive contributions of Dr. Pragatheeshwar Thirunavukarasu, MD (Resident, General Surgery, University of Pittsburgh) in formulating the above concepts and drafting the script.

Footnotes

Presidential address delivered at ANCIPS-2011, New Delhi
Source of Support: *Nil*
Conflict of Interest: *None declared.*

References

1. Rosenhan DL. On being sane in insane places. Science. 1973;179:250–8.
2. Bennett, Maxwell R. 'Development of the concept of mind', Australian and New Zealand Journal of Psychiatry. 2007;41(12):943–956.
3. Edwards SD. The body as object versus the body as subject: The case of disability. Med Health Care Philos. 1998;1:47–56.
4. Santoro G, Wood MD, Merlo L, Anastasi GP, Tomasello F, Germano A. The anatomic location of the soul from the heart, through the brain, to the whole body, and beyond: A journey through Western history, science, and philosophy. Neurosurgery. 2009;65:633–43.
5. "Anti-psychitray" and "History of anti-psychiatry" (Last cited on 2011 Feb 22). Available from: http://www.wikipedia.org.
6. Scott EC. 1st ed. Greenwood Press; 2009. Evolution vs Creationism. ISBN 0-313-32122-1.
7. Kendler KS. A psychiatric dialogue on the mind-body problem. Am J Psychiatry. 2001;158:989–1000.
8. Cape J, Whittington C, Buszewicz M, Wallace P, Underwood L. Brief psychological therapies for anxiety and depression in primary care: Meta-analysis and meta-regression. BMC Med. 2010;8:38.
9. Roder V, Mueller DR, Mueser KT, Brenner HD. Integrated psychological therapy (IPT) for schizophrenia: Is it effective? Schizophr Bull. 2006;32:S81–93.
10. Svartberg M, Stiles TC, Seltzer MH. Randomized, controlled trial of the effectiveness of short-term dynamic psychotherapy and cognitive therapy for cluster C personality disorders. Am J Psychiatry. 2004;161:810–7.
11. Tai S, Turkington D. The evolution of cognitive behavior therapy for schizophrenia: current practice and recent developments. Schizophr Bull. 2009;35:865–73.
12. Fineberg NA, Sharma P, Sivakumaran T, Sahakian B, Chamberlain SR. Does obsessive-compulsive personality disorder belong within the obsessive-compulsive spectrum? CNS Spectr. 2007;12:467–82.

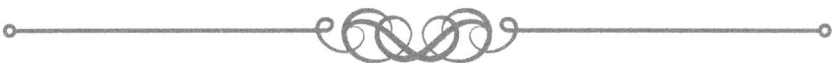

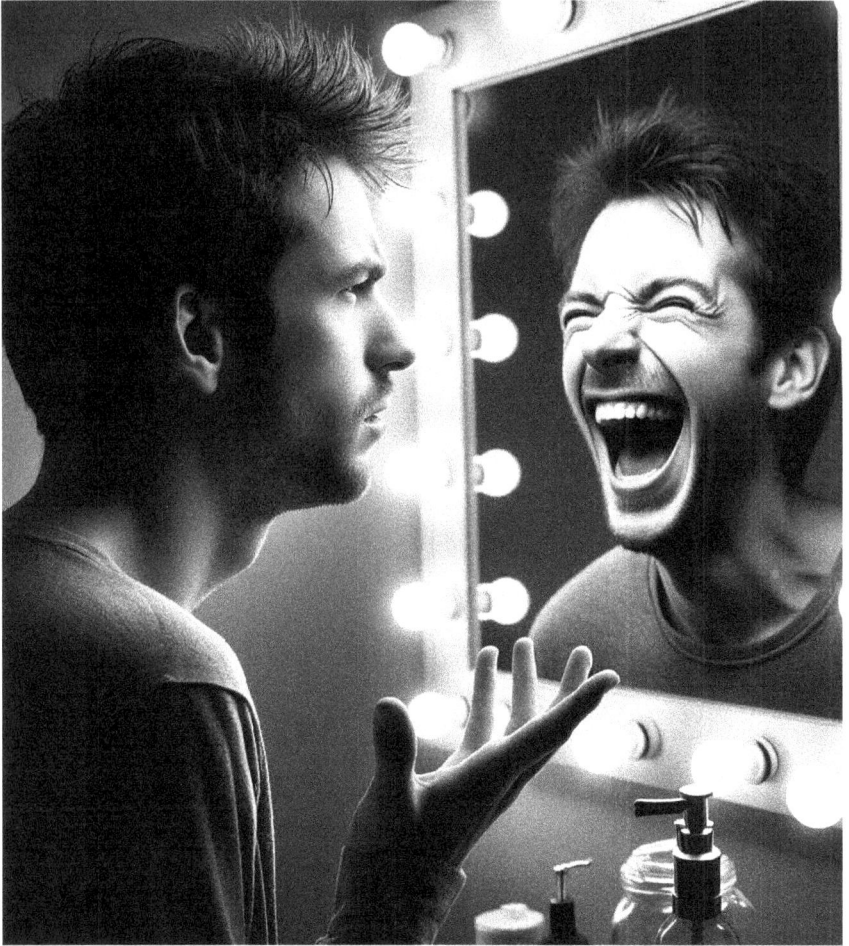

*"O Magic Mirror! Tell me, tell me!
What is normal?"*

CHAPTER 3

The Billion-Dollar Question - What Is 'Normal'?

The word 'normal' is ubiquitous in the medical world. Medical professionals and the common man use it widely, broadly, and loosely. The word 'normal' is used as the dividing line between that which is 'right' and 'wrong', between 'healthy' and 'diseased', and between 'acceptable' and 'not acceptable'. The word 'abnormal' is considered an undesired and unwanted state. In popular culture, even negative descriptions such as 'evil', 'devil', 'Satan', etc are sometimes treated with positive euphemisms in specific contexts. Still, the word 'abnormal' is considered undesired in every context.

In clinical psychiatry, the words 'normal' and 'abnormal' have far-reaching and extraordinary consequences for the patients, compared to other contexts of usage.

So, let us explore what the word 'normal' means, and its utility in the field of psychiatry.

The word 'normal' has changed in its usage over the last few centuries. Etymologically, the root word 'nor-' refers to 'not'; and 'mal-' refers to 'bad', 'wrong' or 'ill'. In essence, 'normal' refers to 'not bad', or 'not ill', and in due course came to be used interchangeably for 'good', 'correct', 'typical', 'standard', etc. The predominant use of the word 'normal' is in the field of geometry and mathematics. In geometry, the word 'norma' meant 'upright', i.e., at right angles (90 degrees). Therefore, the word 'norma' was also used for the carpenter's square, an instrument that is used to measure right angles. Even in everyday language, when a person acts upright and morally, he is said to 'square his actions'.

In mathematics, the word 'normal' is used to describe the distribution pattern of a group of numbers. For example, let us take a group of numbers, such as the heights of the children in a classroom. Let us say, we would like to see how the heights of the children in the classroom are

Normal Distribution Bell Curve

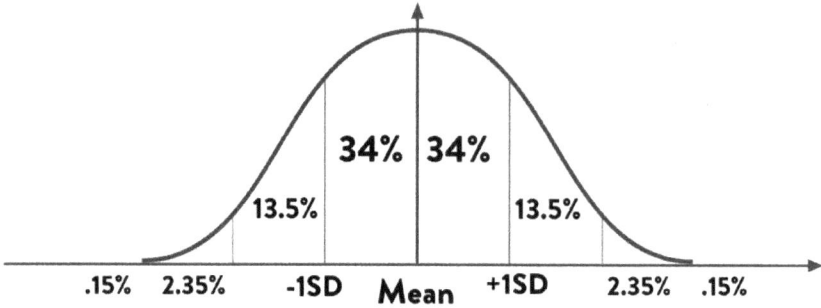

Figure 1 – Normal distribution curve

distributed. To do so, first, the average height is calculated by dividing the sum of all heights by the number of students. This will allow us to calculate the difference between each student's height and the average. The latter measure is called 'deviation', i.e., a measure of how much each student's height has deviated from the group's average height. Next, we can calculate the deviations of each student, and then calculate a measure of the average deviation for this set of numbers. Such a measure is called 'standard deviation'. Usually, most students are of a similar height and therefore the average height is closer to the height of most students. Fewer students are shorter or taller than the average. The number of people deviating far from the average, i.e., the extremely short and the extremely tall students is very small. Therefore, if we plot a graph with the height along the x-axis, and the number of students along the y-axis, the resultant graph will look like the one shown in Figure 1 – essentially a 'bell-shaped' curve, with the top of the bell closer to the average height of the students. The top of the bell is at right angles with the x-axis, and hence such a bell-shaped distribution of numbers is called a 'normal' distribution. Thus, a normal distribution refers to the pattern of distribution of a group of numbers, where most of the numbers are closer to the average number, and there is a smooth and even deviation of the numbers on both sides of the average. Most groups of numbers in nature could be understood as being under the normal distribution pattern. For example, height, weight, IQ, etc. of the general population could all be understood as being distributed normally in nature. In due course, the 'average' number came to be understood as the 'typical' or 'standard' number. Hence, the word 'normal' came to be used inter-changeably for 'standard' or 'typical', which is rather unfortunate, because ***'normal' is a word originally used to describe the pattern of distribution of a group of numbers, not describe the position of an individual number.***

For example, let us take a college classroom of adults – If their heights are distributed such that few of them are short, many are of average height, and few are tall, then such a group is 'normal' in terms of height. Similarly, if their IQs or test scores are distributed such that few of them score bad, with most in the average range, and few of them score excellently well. Such a group is also 'normal' regarding their mental ability or performance. Instead, if there is a classroom, where half of them is very short (let's say, 4 feet in height), and the rest half is exceptionally tall (let's say 6 foot tall), then there will be no one in the average height (i.e., no one who is 5 feet tall)! Such a distribution will not be 'bell shaped'. Similarly, if 90% of students are more than 6 feet tall, and the rest are extremely short with heights less than 4 feet, such distribution will also not be bell-shaped. Thus, one can describe these classroom groups as not being 'normal' classrooms. Such is the correct usage of the term 'normal'. ***The word 'normal' is not to be used to describe any single data point or person. Such usage of the word would be an inaccurate use of language.***

Unfortunately, the word 'normal' is now being used synonymously with 'standard', and 'typical', which then begins to have different connotations and implications in different contexts. For example, in the field of educa-tion, if a child behaves or performs outside the typical or 'norm', the child is labeled as 'abnormal', which then begins to have profound implications – other children's parents are now concerned about their child being with an abnormal child. There are high-functioning children that are also labeled as 'abnormal'. Furthermore, children who are capable of performing better with the right support and guidance end up not getting such help because of the stigma of being labeled 'abnormal'.

In the field of medicine, 'normal' is synonymous with 'health/healthy', and 'abnormal' refers to 'unhealthy' or 'diseased'. In medical usage, the word 'normal' is chosen and deployed variably, three of which are worthy of mention. The first is ***'normality as average'*** – i.e., normal is that which is the 'middle' of extremes, observed in the general population. A classic example is the height of a person. Normal height is often the average height of the general population. The disadvantage of such a usage if that there is no underpinning of the usage of the term 'normal' to health implications. It is to circumvent the latter disadvantage, another variation is employed, which is **'*normality as ideal*'.** For example, the overall trends in a population's weight or body mass index (BMI) may rise to unhealthy levels due to improper diet or lifestyle. Hence, the average weight or BMI of the population may be higher than desired, and hence, it may not be appropriate to denote the average weight of the population as the normal weight. Instead, the ideal body weight or BMI, which through research studies is found to be associated with the best health outcomes could be referred to as 'normal weight'. The disadvantage of such a usage of the term normal is that it cannot accommodate a vast array of parameters, where the ideal number cannot be assigned as 'normal'. Take for example, intelligence quotient (IQ) – it is impossible to assign any level of IQ as the 'ideal IQ', and even if it were possible, it would not be rational or practical to assign the ideal IQ as the 'normal IQ'. The third variation in the term is **'*normal as biologically appropriate*'.** A fit example for this type of usage would be sexual orientation, such as heterosexuality vs homosexuality. Sexual orientation towards the opposite sex serves the purpose of reproduction and perpetuating one's genetic imprint in the world, while homosexuality is counterproductive to such purpose, and hence could be termed 'abnormal'. In essence, the third variation of normality hinges on a teleological explanation. However, the disadvantage of such a definition is that it does not fit the extremes of the so-called normal behavior. For example, the attraction between an extremely old man and a woman who cannot procreate or reproduce to bring forth offspring would also be considered abnormal, through this method of approach. In summary, no single principle to designate normality is universally applicable or utilitarian in clinical medicine. Normality is a misnomer at best. As a clinician, I am more concerned about what is 'healthy', rather than 'normal'. In other words, as a physician, I am more concerned about enabling my patient to function better and be healthier, rather than trying to achieve a 'target normal' parameter. I aim to make my patients function better than average, better than normal, which is what patients also prefer.

Often, a patient with complaints feels relieved if all the tests are reported as 'normal'. But, as a doctor, I would be more worried if the tests were normal, as now I have an unidentified cause for the patient's suffering.

In the field of psychiatry, describing an individual as 'abnormal' has far-reaching consequences in employment, interpersonal relationships, ability to borrow or loan money, marriage, etc. Furthermore, most if not all the symptoms of mental illness could be caused by non-psychiatric disorders, which would need to be ruled out first. For example, depressed mood, fatigue, loss of appetite, loss of interest, muscle aches, body aches, headaches, palpitations, weight gain, weight loss, dizziness, numbness, weakness, nausea, abdominal pain, diarrhea, constipation, loss of consciousness, memory disturbances, shortness of breath, cough, etc. – all of which are manifestations of common psychiatric diagnoses including depression and anxiety, are also manifestations of a wide variety of non-psychiatric diagnosis extending across multiple specialties. Often, psychiatric diagnoses co-exist with one or more non-psychiatric diagnoses and complicate the presentation and pathophysiology. Notwithstanding these intricacies, non-psychiatric specialists tend to 'push away' any non-typical presentation of common problems of their specialty as 'mind-related', which becomes a burden for the psychiatrist to carefully tease psychiatric diagnosis from concurring non-psychiatric diagnosis. As a side note, for the latter reasons, I often assert (contrary to common thinking) that it is paramount *for a clinical psychiatrist to possess a thorough knowledge of internal medicine and bridging knowledge of the fundamentals of other specialties.* Hence, it is common practice for psychiatrists to obtain many tests to reach an accurate diagnosis (or diagnoses). Consequently, it is not uncommon for most if not all these tests to be reported as 'normal'. Most doctors lean towards a psychiatric diagnosis to explain the patients' symptoms when the tests for bodily functions are reported as negative/usual. The common man often does not understand the above-mentioned nuances. He hence is startled when the psychiatrist goes on to establish the need for ongoing psychiatric care after the tests are reported as 'normal'.

In my daily practice, I am often faced with questions from the patient's family members on whether their loved one is 'normal'. A wife asks if her depressed husband if he is 'normal'. A husband asks if his wife who has trouble going to sleep, is 'normal'. Teachers ask if their autistic and dyslexic students are 'normal'. An employer wants a psychiatric opinion if an employee's constant late to work is 'normal'. The judicial court would like to know if the plaintiff who committed murder is mentally 'normal'. These questions are loaded, often posed preposterously, and do not lend themselves to a straightforward yes/no response.

The point I am trying to drive home to the readers is that *'normal' is not the optimal term for medical usage.* It is fraught with unintended and counter-productive consequences, that amplify stigma, affect treatment, and sometimes do so irreversibly. I encourage my colleagues and trainees to use more specific language to describe mental health parameters. I instruct my patients and their families to use different terms while enquiring about their loved ones, such as 'Is my husband doing fine?', 'is my wife getting better?', etc.

As much as I prefer that the word 'normal' be avoided in clinical medicine, it is imperative to recognize the vacuum that its disappearance creates. There is a need for a word to describe the position of what is desirable at the minimum, and a word to describe the deviation from the desired position.

For example, in the previous chapter, I described the components of the Ulan to be mood, thought, and intellect. It then becomes essential to identify the so-called normal mood and how to differentiate it from the abnormal mood. The same logic also applies to the other components of the Ulan (thought and intellect).

Thus, each component must be described in desirable and deviant positions. Below, I shall discuss the appropriate clinical terms to be used in each of the three components of the Ulan.

Normal Mood

Etymologically, the word 'mood' is an alteration of the word 'mode'. A 'mode' refers to a certain theme of functioning. For example, a car has several driving modes, such as sporty mode, economy mode, comfort mode, etc. The car's functioning principles remain the same in all the modes. What differs is the driver's 'experience' or 'feel' while driving the car. The driver feels racy, sportive, accelerant, and thrilled in a sporty mode. In the smooth mode, the driver feels like the car is transitioning smoothly between speeds, without any bumps or jerks. Each mode has a role in fully experiencing the car and is acceptable, but in the right setting, and for the right intensity. 'Mood' of the mind can also be understood similarly. The mood is determined by what happens around an individual and is a consequence – which is why it is referred to as 'affect' in medical language. In other words, mood is the manifestation of the mind that has been 'affected', and mood disorders are referred to as 'affective disorders'.

For example, an unfortunate event such as the loss of property or the life of a loved one causes the individual to be sad or depressed. In contrast, a fortunate event like winning a lottery prize causes the individual to be happy or elated. Similarly, the mood must be appropriate in intensity. For example, the death of the nation's president or a favorite actor may bring sadness but should be mild and not last long. The death of a loved one may bring forth sadness for several weeks or months. Similarly, happiness or elation should also be proportionate in intensity. An inappropriate intensity also signifies a deviation from the so-called 'normal'.

In other words, mood or affect is 'congruent' to the presence, nature, and intensity of the stimuli or happenings around the individual. If the mood is incongruent – i.e., if sadness or elation occurs in the absence of an appropriate stimulus, or if the intensity is disproportionate to the intensity of the stimulus, then such a mood is 'incongruent', and thus needs medical attention for treatment. Thus, rather than categorizing mood as 'normal' vs 'abnormal', it would be more appropriate to identify mood as 'congruent' or 'incongruent'. Such congruence should not be decided based on simplistic information or criteria, but only after a thorough mental status examination and psychiatric history taking.

Normal Thought

Unlike mood, which is a consequence (i.e., 'affect' of) a stimulus in the environment, thoughts are autonomous and spontaneous. Thoughts can arise 'out of the blue'. Thoughts result from cortical activity of the brain, and the mere presence of consciousness triggers thoughts. The occurrence of thoughts and consciousness are so synchronous, that they are practically inseparable in time, and hence, the widespread and never-ending debate in philosophical circles 'I think therefore I am' vs 'I am therefore I think'. Any person can have any type of thought at any time. Hence, ***there is no such thing as an 'abnormal' vs 'normal' thought.*** The nature, timing, or pervasiveness of the thought cannot be used to assess if the thought component

ULAN of the Ulan is functioning correctly.

For example, when I give lectures to the public about thought disorders, there is a frequent question from the people – 'If a common man says that he is thinking of God, or has a thought that he is God or a messenger of God, we could call him crazy or insane or as having a mental illness? But isn't that what religious icons have also claimed? If so, how do we tell the difference between what mental illness is and what is not? Other examples – is a thought to harm others normal or abnormal? Are thoughts about sex normal or abnormal? Are thoughts about communicating with God or supernatural forces, normal or abnormal? The people who are often considered great men and women, scientists, philosophers, reformers, religious icons, etc., have often been those with thoughts that are vastly different and far-fetched from those of the common man.

The difference between what is acceptable thought functioning and what is considered a medical disorder of thought is the ability of the individual to dismiss or dispose of the thought. No thought is abnormal if it is under the will and ability of the individual to dismiss. An individual must be able to dispose of a thought at will. If that is the case, there is no reason to consider an individual having an 'abnormal' or unhealthy thought. If an individual is not able to ward off or dispose of a thought, then such a condition is unhealthy and needs medical attention. When an individual is not able to dismiss thoughts at will, then the self becomes a slave to the thoughts – which is what happens in obsession, paranoia, etc. Thus, *rather than categorizing thought as 'normal' vs 'abnormal', it would be more appropriate to identify thought as 'dismissible' or 'indismissible'.* Such dismissibleness of thought should not be decided based on simplistic information or criteria, but only after a thorough mental status examination and psychiatric history taking.

Normal Intellect

The intellect component of the Ulan refers to computation, problem-solving, logic, and reason. Intellect is a complex multifaceted component of the Ulan. Although highly capable intellect is desirable, measuring one's intellect alone cannot be a helpful determinant in the macro aspects of life and health. In other words, many individuals with a more capable intellect experience less health, happiness, or financial success in practical life than those with a less capable intellect. Furthermore, the overall capability of the intellect, if measured, would be plottable on a scale from very low to very high, with no clear identification of what is normal or abnormal. A more practical and medically utilitarian benchmark would be 'adequacy'; here I mean adequacy for independent functioning and living. An individual's intellect must be capable of functioning at a level that allows independent functioning and living of the person. If so, it would be considered 'adequate', and if not, 'inadequate'. Thus, ***rather than categorizing intellect as 'normal' vs 'abnormal', it would be more appropriate to identify intellect as 'adequate' or 'inadequate'.*** Such adequacy of intellect should not be decided based on simplistic information or criteria, but only after a thorough mental status examination and psychiatric history taking.

Normal Behavior

Behavior is a sum manifestation and output of the functioning of the amalgamated components of the Ulan, namely mood, thought, and intellect. Since neither of these components can be understood as abnormal vs normal, ***it is impossible to classify behavior as normal vs abnormal.*** Such a classification would be an oversimplification and inaccurate. As mentioned earlier in this book, behavior is the 'observed' activity of an individual, and hence assessment of the acceptability of behavior depends on the observer. Furthermore, the acceptability of behavior is based on three factors – namely place, context, and timing. Thus, the observer of a person's behavior determines the acceptability of the behavior from the standpoint of the observer himself, based on its utility relative to the place, context, and timing of the behavior. The individual must understand this concept and modify his or her behavior by his or her own intention, in the presence of being observed to one's own benefit – in which case it can be safely considered as 'normal'. Suppose an individual cannot consider the reports of his behavior or is unable to modify behavior despite having the intention to do so, or both. In that case, such behavior can be considered 'abnormal'. In other words, 'responsiveness' to reports of behavior is healthy, and non-responsiveness to reports of behavior requires medical attention. ***Thus, rather than categorizing behavior as 'normal' vs 'abnormal', it would be more appropriate to identify behavior as 'responsive' or 'irresponsive'.*** Such responsiveness of

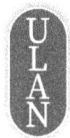

behavior should not be decided based on simplistic information or criteria, but only after a thorough mental status examination and psychiatric history taking.

Summary

Thus, I would like to conclude this chapter with this message – 'Normal' is a term most appropriate to describe the distribution pattern of a group of numbers, or collection of data, and is best avoided while describing a person or a single parameter. It is best to avoid the term 'normal' and use more specific and clinically utilitarian terms in psychiatry or medicine. The most appropriate clinical terms are listed in the table next –

Table 1: Appropriate clinical terminology to replace usage of 'normal' vs 'abnormal' (Mananalam Clinic Experience)		
Mood	Congruent vs Incongruent. Congruence refers to the appropriateness of the affect to the stimulus (the presence, nature, intensity, and duration).
Thought	Dismissible vs Undismissible. Dismissibility refers to the ability of the self to dispose off any thought at will.
Intellect	Adequate vs Inadequate. Adequacy refers to the sufficiency of the intellect to conduct independent life, and engage in learning.
Note: The above parameters can be assessed only after thorough psychiatric history taking and mental status examination	

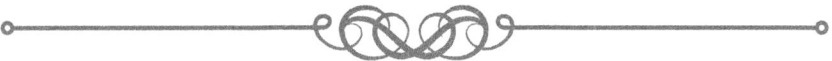

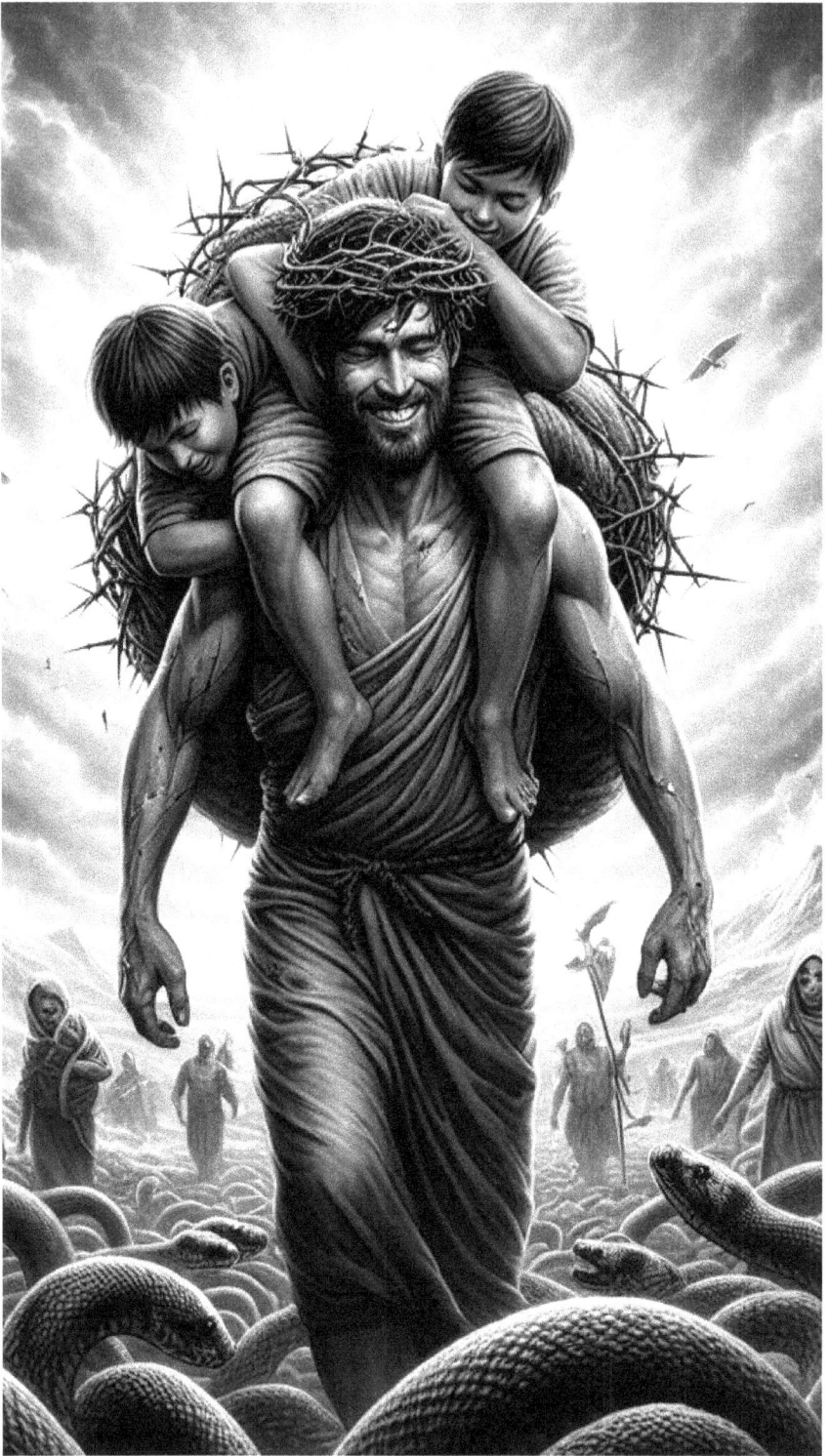

CHAPTER 4

The Trillion-Dollar Question - What is Mental health?

Other Contributors: Priyanka Ramesh MBBS, Aimee Dubin DO

Mental health is both an ancient and a modern concept. Humans have recognized the importance of mental health for thousands of years. For example, the Thirukkural, which is regarded as an ancient scripture of two-line sayings of wisdom nearly 2000 years ago in the classical language of Tamil, has at least one verse that directly references mental health –'***Mananalam mannuyirk kaakkam***.' The latter translates as 'mental health is needed for gainful sustenance of life'.

The above verse demonstrates that the importance of mental health was well-recognized as early as 2,000 years ago. However, Thirukkural is a classical work of literature, not of medicine. In the academic works of medicine, little has been mentioned about mental health. The well-known academic resource for medical students, psychiatry trainees, and psychiatrists, the 'Comprehensive Textbook of Psychiatry', initially published in 1967, did not discuss mental health or normality in the mental state until its eighth edition in 2004. Nevertheless, the latest edition has an entire chapter dedicated to 'mental health'. Thus, mental health is a relatively newer concept in academic medicine.

For most of its time, discussions in academic psychiatry have focused on mental illnesses and disorders rather than mental health. Mental health was considered to be the absence of mental illnesses. It reflected the attitude that existed in other fields of medicine, too. Somatic/physical health was considered existent if identifiable diagnoses were absent. Essentially, health was a diagnosis of exclusion through the absence of diagnosis of illnesses. However, with time, doctors have begun to recognize 'health' as a standalone phenomenon and that health can be 'enhanced' or 'promoted.' Doctors also began to understand that promoting health could reduce disease or its occurrence in society in the long term. Parallel thought processes occurred in the field of psychiatry as well. In a way, the problem of identifying mental health as the absence of mental illnesses was recognized as a logical fallacy needing rectification, even as early as the time of Dr. Rosenhan (refer to the publications reprinted in Chapter 2 for the Rosenhan experiment).

It is not that mental health experts cared less or willfully ignored the task of defining mental health. It was simply too difficult! Stigma and controversial afflictions surrounding mental illnesses in the yester-era were prohibitive to such work. For example, Sigmund Freud readily dismissed mental health as an ideal fiction. Dr. Frederick Redlich, the Dean of Yale School of Medicine in 1957, said, "We do not possess any general definition of normality and mental health from either a statistical or clinical point" and Sir Aubrey Lewis, the first Professor of Psychiatry at what is now the King's College London wrote in 1958 that mental health was an 'invincibly obscure concept'.

However, the last few decades have seen a rapidly increasing discussion about mental health. Several psychologists have come forth with models and explanations of mental health. We shall discuss each important model in detail in this chapter. However, I do not wish to leave any surprise to the reader until the end of this chapter. None of these models are clinically applicable to the practicing psychiatrist, and they have one common theme of deficiency, which shall become apparent to the reader at the end of the latter discussion.

Over the last several decades of my practice in psychiatry, I have come across numerous studies, articles, and presentations about mental health. It would be beyond the scope of this book to be able to enumerate each such study. However, I could broadly group the approaches to the concept of mental health into the following schools of thought –

- Mental health as 'above normal' or 'above average'
- Mental health as 'positive psychology'
- Mental health as 'maturity'
- Mental health as 'resilience'
- Mental health as 'socio-emotional intelligence'
- Mental health as a 'subjective sense of well-being'
- Mental health as 'positive spiritual emotions'

Now, let's discuss each of these approaches to mental health in some detail.

Mental Health as 'Above Normal' or 'Above Average'

As discussed in an earlier chapter, the yardstick used to differentiate diseased individuals from the non-diseased was the concept of 'normality'. Falling short of the yardstick of normality was considered a disease. As an extension of the latter school of thought, mental health was understood to surpass the normal into a super state of being 'above-normal' or 'above-average'. This model of mental health was one of the oldest forerunners in the previous century.

Austrian-British social psychologist Marie Jahoda (1907-2001) was famous for her work 'Ideal Mental Health' in the 1950s, which aligns with this school of thought. She identified characteristics in most people regarded as 'normal': efficient self-perception, realistic self-esteem and acceptance, voluntary control of behavior, accurate perception of the world, sustaining relationships and giving affection, self-direction, and productivity.

The limitation of this model is that we revert to the inherently defective binary way of viewing the mental state as 'normal vs abnormal'. Also, the above-mentioned criteria are overlapping, redundant, and too subjective for clinical practice.

Mental Health as 'Positive Psychology'

This school of thought is probably the most popular and widely talked-about model of mental health, especially among the lay public. Psychologists largely propelled this school of thought.

This model identifies characteristics or aspects considered to be 'positive' aspects of individuals who are considered to be mentally healthy and then focuses on promoting such aspects with the presumption that the latter would enhance mental health. An example of the line of thinking of this model would be like this – When a person is depressed, the cognition of the individual is found to be pessimistic. As a corollary, mentally healthy people are considered to be optimistic. Thus, it is considered, by inference, that by promoting optimism, individuals could be made mentally healthy. Another example – anxiety is a manifestation of mental disorder, and mentally healthy people are found to be relaxed without anxiety. Thus, it is considered by inference that mental health could be brought about by promoting relaxation (by meditation, yoga, etc.) in an individual. Such is the logic of this school of thought of mental health.

Based on this logic, several psychological models have been proposed. Martin E. Seligman, an American psychologist at the University of Pennsylvania, is quite famous for this positive psychology model and has focused on promoting positive traits such as optimism and hope.

There have been models of an individual's personality development, and hence, an explanation of the mind based on such concepts. The most well-known such model is that of the German-immigrant American psychologist Erik Erikson, who explained the entire span of the psychosocial life of an individual in 8 stages, which involved the ability to develop trust vs mistrust, autonomy vs doubt, initiative vs guilt, industry vs inferiority, identity vs role confusion, intimacy vs isolation, generativity vs stagnation, and ego integrity vs despair. For example, he proposed that in the first stage of life (birth to 18 months), if a child's needs are cared for promptly and fulfilled predictably, then the personality develops to incorporate trust as a trait. If the child's needs are left unfulfilled or unpredictably fulfilled, then the personality develops to incorporate mistrust and anxiety. He went on to explain all the eight stages through similar logic. Essentially, mental health could be understood through positive traits or characteristics, and by working to promote such characteristics, mental health could be achieved. Dr George Vaillant, a psychiatrist at Harvard Medical School, based on his famous 'Grant Study' (a longitudinal study of more than 700 individuals), added two more stages to Erikson's model, namely 'career consolidation' (after the stage of intimacy vs isolation), and 'keeper of meaning' (after generativity vs stagnation).

All these developments from this school of thought are often called 'positivism' in psychology. Offshoots of this philosophy have allowed entire industries to thrive, including self-help books, motivational speeches, literature, music, art, yoga, meditation, architecture, interior design, aroma therapies, counseling, cognitive approaches, behavior modification, biofeedback techniques, etc.

The disadvantages of this school of thought are, however, apparent. First, the list of 'positive' attributes, including hope, courage, wisdom, love, trust, inspiration, optimism, etc., is long and practically endless. Second, they are overlapping and redundant. Third, they are unreasonably subjective and non-measurable. Even if measured, the contributions of each of these attributes to mental health are not calculable. Finally, such a pervasive model of understanding cannot be applied in a standardized way in the clinical setting of a practicing psychiatrist.

Mental Health as 'Maturity'

The brain is unique in its anatomic and physiological development. Unlike the other parts of the body, which reach a peak anatomic development relatively early in the life span, after which the effects of aging begin to set in, the brain continues to exhibit plasticity well into the later decades of life. For example, the lungs of a 15-year-old individual are more likely to function efficaciously and optimally than the lungs of a 60-year-old individual. The ability of the mind to function seldom reaches a peak and continues to improve as long as the anatomical and physical health of the brain is protected from the insults of disease or drugs. For example, physically healthy 70-year-old individuals are likely to be more mentally healthy than physically healthy 30-year-old individuals. Prospective studies by American psychologist Laura Carstensen suggest that individuals are less depressed and show more emotional modulation at 70 years than at 30.

The above understanding shines light on a unique aspect of mental functioning and mental health – that mental functioning improves with age and that life may be a journey to an ever-nearing walk to the target of ideal mental health and not a static target that can be achieved at all ages. If this is indeed true, then it could be inferred that adolescents are mentally healthier than children, middle-aged individuals are mentally healthier than adolescents, and geriatric individuals are mentally healthier than the rest of the people. This could be an oversimplification, but it does appear that human societies have long recognized this pattern to some extent, as reflected in the nearly universal tradition in most long-established societies of 'respecting the elderly' or the hierarchies of privileges with increasing age. In Asian societies, for example, seniority or age is a criterion for promotion to more critical professional and societal positions.

There is more to be said about the importance of maturity in mental health. Each attribute discussed in Erikson's model, such as identity, intimacy, generativity, and career consolidation, are not concrete targets but a continuum. For example, identity issues in adolescence are different and less complex than identity issues after age 50. The pursuit and object of intimacy evolves with age, as it is different at 40 years compared to what it was at 20 years of age. The viewpoint of consolidating a career and its place in life differs for a 25-year-old and a 50-year-old. Intelligence is static, but wisdom grows with age.

However, there is one major limitation to accepting this model of mental health as a mainstream paradigm – it is inapplicable in the clinical setting, as all these age-based assumptions are acceptable only as long as the neurological status of the central nervous system is healthy and free of influences from disease and drugs, which is rare in the clinical setting. Nevertheless, this model teaches us essential principles in mental health – that it depends on the body's physical health and can be constantly enhanced with age, unlike physical health. Efforts to maintain physical health are crucial to the most optimal performance and improvement of mental health with age.

Mental Health as 'Resilience'

The word 'resilience' refers to the quality of recovering from injury or stress and returning to a pre-injury state. In the field of psychology, it refers to the ability of the individual to 'bounce back' after suffering damage or stress. Loosely termed, it means a 'tough' individual.

As I have explained in a previous chapter, the mind, like any other physiological entity of the human body, exists in a state of homeostasis. It is constantly exposed to stress and damaging forces that disturb homeostasis. Resilience is its ability to restore homeostasis.

In other fields of medicine, there is a school of thought that disease is the result of the improper ability of the body to recover from forces of illnesses and that health can be promoted by enhancing the ability to recover. An easy example is the concept of 'immunity'. Infections occur due to infec-tion-producing microorganisms. While one school of thought promotes health by preventing exposure to such infections or pursuing treatments to eradicate such organisms that have entered the body, another school of thought conceptualizes infectious disorders as the result of the failure or inability of the immune system to thwart the organism. Essentially, the latter approach assumes that the 'ideal state of health' is when the immune system should be able to thwart any disease-producing organism and that any disease is nothing but a result of a failed defense system. This model entirely shifts the responsibility of health to the individual. Some people firmly believe all cancer is due to a defective immune system and that therapies to battle cancer should be immune-based. Such people chase immunity-enhancing supplements, and an entire industry works to cater to the needs of such individuals. A parallel line of logic in psychiatry is the concept of 'resilience', akin to the concept of 'immunity'.

A lot has been written in psychology about resilience as the measure of mental health. Many strategies have been proposed to build or develop re-silience, such as coping strategies and mechanisms, hoping that enhanced resilience could promote mental health.

Resilience is indeed an important factor in the overall understanding of mental health, but seeing resilience as the root of mental health is like placing the carriage before the horse. I see resilience as a measure and manifestation of mental health and not as a building block or component of mental health. That is, mentally healthy individuals are often resilient, and mentally unhealthy/ill individuals are often not resilient, but the converse is not necessarily true. A good artist could express his art and talent in painting and may produce a good painting. But teaching someone how to paint cannot make them a good artist.

Mental Health as 'Socio-Emotional Intelligence'

The most recent generations of humankind have begun to place more emphasis on other's emotions during social interaction. Understanding the nuances of other's emotional states in the social setting has become an important skill and factor in success in nearly all spheres of life. Intelligence has been traditionally measured based on computational and linguistic performance. Focus has shifted from the latter to 'emotional' intelligence in the social realm.

The importance of exploiting socio-emotional intelligence is not an entirely novel development. Greek philosopher Aristotle (384 – 322BC) is known to have said, *"Anybody can become angry – that is easy, but to be angry with the right person and to the right degree and at the right time and for the right purpose, and in the right way – that is not within everybody's power and is not easy."* All emotions, including anger, fear, excitement, surprise, disgust, hate, etc., have a biological reason to exist and emanate from the human brain. These emotions are signals sent by the deeper parts of the Ulan to educate the conscious self on how to deal with the outside world. Emotions can be used strategically to one's benefit.

On experiencing a particular emotion, one must look inward and interrogate logically the cause and rationale for such emotion and learn from the signals sent by the deeper Ulan on how to act in the future to our benefit. The latter principle is also helpful in cognitive therapy as well.

A growing body of literature focuses on this aspect alone and morphs it to explain the larger concept of mental health. In my opinion, the socio-emotional intelligence aspects of an individual is a component of mental health. Still, it is not a wholesome explanation, as we shall see in the later parts of this chapter.

Mental Health as a 'Subjective Sense of Well-Being'

Another proposed measure of mental health is the subjective or self-reported sense of well-being. In contrast to other measures often clinically determined by a mental health professional, the individual's subjective sense of well-being is self-reported. For example, the subjective sense of happiness in life could be used to determine mental health. As expected, a wide range of qualities could be potential candidates for this measure. The eight foremost positive emotions prioritized in this model have been gratitude, love, joy, compassion, forgiveness, trust, hope, and awe. The advantage of this model of understanding mental health is that it bears some seemingly obvious validation. For example, there have been several studies that seem to suggest that happy people were less likely (even as much as half as likely) to die at an early age or become disabled as unhappy people after controlling for other factors such as income, education, body weight, smoking, drinking, and disease states. The disadvantage of this model is that the issues involved in measuring or studying a sense of well-being are complicated and clouded by historical relativism and value judgment.

In my opinion, attributes of a sense of well-being are valid surrogate markers for mental health but not actionable components of mental health. In other words, mentally healthy individuals experience happiness and joy, but all those who experience joy and happiness are not necessarily mentally healthy. Most importantly, these attributes of a sense of well-being are not actionable targets – for example, one cannot achieve mental health by trying to achieve 'happiness' – that would be an elusive and endless search.

Mental Health as 'Positive Spiritual Emotions'

More recently, attributes such as 'good character', 'morality', and 'spiri-tuality' have been introduced into the discussion of mental health. Such attributes are inevitably associated with the pro-social nature of individuals and societal well-being. Advances in laboratory and animal research, neurochemical imaging, and functional scanning of the brain have augmented neuroscientific explanations for certain behaviors attributed to such moral and spiritual qualities, which may be exclusive of other essential functions. For example, mother hamsters whose brains have the cortex removed cannot do mazes but can still perform the maternal functions of caring for their pups. In contrast, mother hamsters whose brains have the limbic system regions removed can do mazes but cannot perform maternal functions for their pups. However, positive parental behavior can also be understood as a learned function from society, hence attributable to the neocortex. Being a good parent is a combination of unselfish, inborn parental love (a prosocial mammalian capacity attributable to the limbic system) and learned behavior from social modeling attributable to the cortical functions of the brain. Similarly, prosocial attributes that may constitute good character, spirituality, or morality are a complex combina-tion of emotional drives and learned behavior.

A model of mental health called 'Model G' defined mental and spiritual health as the amalgam of the positive emotions that bond humans to each other. This model included eight positive and moral emotions: love, hope, joy, forgiveness, compassion, faith, awe, and gratitude. One must note that the common thread for all these emotions pertains to how a human being relates or bonds with others. These emotions are common denominators in all significant religions or faiths. None of these eight emotions listed are just about the self. Self-indulgent positive emotions, such as contentment/happiness, interest, excitement, humor, and a sense of mastery over self – emotions that one might need even when on a deserted island or in a situation that requires competence and performance, have been omitted from this model. From advances in neuroscientific research, we learn that such positive emotions have a biological basis identifiable in the brain and hence imply that these motions have evolved through natural selection to enhance the survival of the individual and society. Such pro-social emotions might also reflect behavioral adaptations that permitted the survival of the relatively defenseless individuals and their extremely defenseless children in the wild environment a million years ago. In the last few decades, neuroscientists such as John Allman and Giacomo Rizzolatti have studied parts of the brain, such as the limbic spindle (Von Economo) cells and mirror cells that could explain prosocial human mentation, that may underlie those positive mental emotions mentioned above.

Another area of the brain crucial to positive mental health attributes is the prefrontal cortex, which oversees the estimation of rewards and punishments and plays a critical role in adapting and regulating emotional responses to new situations. Thus, the prefrontal lobes are deeply involved in our emotional, moral, and spiritual lives. We are also aware of 'mirror neurons' located in the insula and anterior cingulate of the brain, which are more developed in humans than in primates and appear to mediate empathy, i.e., the ability to feel the emotions of another. These mirror neurons may form the fundamental biological basis for more complex empathy-based emotions embodied in morality or spirituality.

Several studies suggest that religion has a positive effect on happiness in life and sometimes may also serve as a determinant of happiness. Psychological explanations include the ability of religion to provide meaning or purpose in life. However, religion offers a supportive social infrastructure during distress and despair. Tenets of mainstream religions inculcate pro-social emotions and behavior, which are, in turn, related to reducing anxiety about coping with stressful situations. Churches and mosques, for instance, are the source of emotional, social, and economic support for most families in Western communities. Furthermore, religious beliefs help shift the degree to which an individual believes they control their life from internal to external forces, thereby freeing the ego from guilt for failures, shortcomings, and irresponsible behavior. Ideas of fate, luck, and destiny provide solace and comfort at times of misery and despair. In my opinion, religion offers a tempting alternative to the inevitable truth about uncertainty in all aspects of life, the heightened awareness of which could be understood to be the root cause of anxiety, by unapologetically advancing the idea that everything about life is controlled by an all-powerful, all-knowing entity who always acts in your interest. Spirituality and religion advance the idea of hope that undesirable and unpleasant, horrible, and adverse events will decrease over time and promote the idea that ordinary events are sufficient to incite wonder and joy. Whatever the explanation, it is indisputable that religion positively affects happiness and a sense of well-being. Increasingly sophisticated neurological research on such positive emotions by investigators such as Jan Panskepp, Marco Iacoboni, Barbara Fredrickson, and Andrew Newberg has made the consideration of religion, spirituality, and moral character indispensable to the wholesome understanding of mental health.

However, the role of religion and spirituality is too value-laden to serve as a comprehensive model of mental health. Like the other models of mental health discussed above, this spiritual model of mental health suffers from the same limitation – happiness and positive spiritual emotions are often found in those with mental health but do not form an actionable component of the mental health paradigm.

Mental Health - What Have we Learned so Far?

So, what have we learned from the various models of mental health discussed above? Firstly, it is evident that mental health has been recognized as an existent entity to be contended with and is not just the mere absence of mental illnesses. Secondly, we have neither defined nor identified the elemental components of mental health. Thirdly, it would be a terrible mistake to assume or consider any of the above models as comprehensive or superior to the other models. From different vantage points, these models all speak of the same markers or manifestations of mental health. In other words, various researchers have identified various manifestations of mental health. They have seen various attributes displayed by those who are mentally healthy, with an incremental effect. To some extent, they are all credible.

But the elephant in the room that we have not contended with is – what is the common theme that underscores all these models of mental health? Can vague attributes such as happiness, joy, gratitude, compassion, empathy, trust, etc., be broken down into more fundamental elements? Can the inexhaustible list of such attributes be consolidated by a few finite elements that are clinically applicable? Can the subjectiveness of such attributes be reduced to the maximum to reduce interobserver variability and bias? And more importantly, can we identify a model of mental health that is globally applicable to all humans on earth, beyond cultural, racial, and ethnic differences?

My answer is a solid yes for all the above questions. Mental health is not beyond reasonable clinical understanding and applicability. It is not an elusive and uncapturable concept. Any truth can be conceptualized in multiple models that may be credible and valid. But what matters in the real world is if it can be applied to the everyday clinical practice of psychiatry and clinical psychology. Throughout my nearly 40-year clinical experience in psychiatry, I have worked on developing such a model of mental health, a 'utilitarian' model that can be used in the clinical setting.

A Utilitarian Model of Mental Health

The utilitarian model identifies 'Ulan' as that which is healthy in mental health. For more information on the Ulan, please refer to Chapter 2. The utilitarian model is based on identifying the 'elemental components' of mental health. Elemental components refer to the basic operational units (i.e., 'building blocks'), which cannot be further broken down into practically applicable simpler components. These basic operational units interact in more complex ways depending on the context and manifest as many attributes, traits, or qualities. The Ulan being a functionalistic concept, the elemental components of mental health are functional aspects of the Ulan. Three elemental components are identified in this model, namely –

1. Awareness of one's own self.
2. Ability to relate well with others.
3. Act in ways that are beneficial to self and non-detrimental to others.

This model being utilitarian, all three elemental mental health components are 'actionable' in nature, meaning these three components can be clinically intervened for improvement.

Now, let us examine the role of each of these elemental components.

The First Component - Awareness of One's Own Self

As discussed in the previous chapters, Ulan is a single indivisible unit, and each person (or self) has only one Ulan. The ability of the self to be aware of its Ulan is referred to as 'insight' in clinical medicine. Insight is an indispensable aspect of an optimally functioning Ulan. It is used to describe if a person has an awareness of the issues related to their mental illness or affliction. However, the utilitarian model asserts that even in the absence of mental illness, an individual requires an accurate awareness of one's own self for the purpose of being mentally healthy. Awareness here refers to conscious knowledge of the self's needs, capabilities, and limitations. Some examples include -

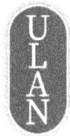

> What do I know? And what do I not know?
> What do I not know for sure?
> What makes me miserable?
> What can I tolerate?
> What am I unable to tolerate?
> What is achievable by me?
> What is beyond my scope of accomplishment?
> What are my strengths? And my weakness?
> What are my insecurities?

An accurate awareness of such limitations allows one to set realistic goals and tasks that can be completed. Completion of a task is termed 'success'. Thus, accurate awareness of one's own self is essential for reaching success. Repeated successes promote confidence, optimism, and resilience at times when failures happen. The components of the Ulan, namely mood, thought, and intellect, are then able to function better, and the cycle of success perpetuates itself. Such repeated successes allow for more complex attributes such as happiness, hope, joy, etc.

On the other hand, lack of awareness or inaccurate awareness of one's own self leads to non-completion of tasks, termed 'failures'. Repeated failures promote frustration, pessimism, and hopelessness, reducing resilience during distress. The components of the Ulan, namely mood, thought, and intellect, adjust accordingly to the failure pattern, and the cycle of failures perpetuates itself.

The awareness of one's own self is thus the most fundamental of the three elemental components of the utilitarian model of mental health.

The Second Component - The Ability to Relate Well With Others

The ability of an individual to survive and succeed in society depends on his interaction with other fellow human beings. Interaction with others constitutes what we call in psychiatry 'behavior'. Relating with other human beings is inevitable and easy. But relating well with others is a skill. By relating 'well', I mean relating in a way that maximizes one's and others' well-being.

Each relationship has two aspects –

- Purpose – the purpose of the relationship can be derived from the context and nature of the circumstance that brings two people together. These are not under the control of any individual. 'Why am I relating with this person?'
- Goal – the goal of a relationship can be decided by the individuals involved. 'What can I achieve through this relationship?'

In general, there are two types of relationships, and an individual should be able to identify the purpose and goals in both settings appropriately. The two types of relationships are –

- Dispensable
- Indispensable

Dispensable relationships include those that an individual can do without, those that last for a short term, and those that do not have long-term effects on one's life unless interfered with. The context of the relationship is often societal convenience; its nature is reversible or exchangeable and often short-lived. The goal of these relationships is to successfully pass the time spent in the best possible way without incurring any damage to oneself. Examples of dispensable relationships are the association with a fellow traveler in an aircraft or public transport or the person ahead while waiting in line at the grocery store. These associations last a few minutes, if not hours, and occur due to societal arrangements to maximize everyone's convenience. Unless interfered with, these relationships do not have any long-term effects. A valuable attribute to be successful in these relationships is tolerance. The less communication, the better.

Indispensable relationships include those that an individual cannot do without, potentially long-term, and will have long-term effects on one's life. The context of the relationship is either by sanguinity (blood-related or by birth), law, marriage, or contract. The goal should be to reduce the occurrence and frequency of bitter events in the long run so that these relationships are tolerable throughout one's lifetime. Indispensable relationships include relationships with parents, spouses, children, colleagues, employers, employees, classmates, etc. These associations last for our lifetime, and even if they don't, the effects of these relationships can last for our lifetime. So, active care and intervention are needed to avoid conflicts and bitterness in the long term. Short-term niceties could be sacrificed for long-term conflict avoidance. A valuable attribute to be successful in these relationships is honesty. The more communication, the better.

The above constitutes fundamental knowledge about relationships. An individual must be able to differentiate relationships as dispensable and indispensable and successfully attain the goals of each relationship depending on the type, context, and circumstance of each relationship. Under-relating and over-relating can both result in problems. Communication is critical, and less or more than the required amount of communication can also result in problems.

Note – the ability to relate well with others (second component of mental health) depends on accurate awareness of one's self (first component of mental health). The latter principle is essential in the clinical setting, as most problems arising from relationships are due to inaccurate awareness of one's own self.

The Third Component - Act in Ways That Are Beneficial to Self and Non-Detrimental to Others

As discussed in the earlier chapters, the purpose of life for a human being is to live to the maximum and ensure one's progeny is perpetuated. Hence, all actions of an individual must be in ways that benefit one's own self. Any behavior detrimental or harmful to the self, directly or indirectly, physically or emotionally, or in social spheres of life is a potential sign of mental health problems. Deliberate self-harm, neglect of one's health, willful consumption of toxic and addictive substances, suicide, and high-risk behavior are all often dismissed by the general public as 'foolish', 'poor judgment', or 'reckless' behavior. But these are all indeed signs of problems with mental health. Nevertheless, it does not mean that an individual can pursue self-benefit with no regard for others or indulge in activities that are detrimental to others and society. Societal well-being is integral for everyone's well-being in the long term. Hence, everyone should be able to act in a way that is beneficial to themselves but also non-detrimental to society.

This elemental mental health component has the most potential for actionability, relative to the other components. There is ample room and scope for behavior modification to promote the efficacy of this component, and great benefit can be achieved through even minor but durable modifications in an individual's actions.

States of Mental Health

Mental health status is a spectrum of various states, the boundaries of which are discernible but not very conspicuous. The tools for discernibility between the various states could be identifiable through the effect of one's mental health status on the self and the others.

To establish the status of the mental health of an individual, the following criteria should be satisfied –

1. The individual must be evaluated through a comprehensive clinical examination.
2. Such clinical examination should include both a physical examination of health and a mental health status examination.

3. The examination should be performed by a physician trained in mental health status examination, preferably a trained psychiatrist.
4. All three components of mental health status should be assessed through a comprehensive and detailed history taking and examination.

Once the above criteria are satisfied, the individual could be classified as 'mentally healthy' if,

1. There is absence of any psychiatric diagnosis.
2. All three elemental components of the above-described utilitarian model of mental health, namely awareness of one's own self, ability to relate well with others, and the actions of the individual are beneficial to self and non-detrimental to others, are fulfilled.

If the above two criteria are unmet, the individual cannot be classified as mentally healthy. Those individuals that cannot be classified as mentally healthy can then be further designated into one of the following three groups, arranged in order of increasing severity as follows –

1. Mentally not healthy (mNH)
2. Mentally unhealthy (mUH)
3. Mentally ill (mI)

These three groups are not identifiable through variations in the elemental components but instead based on the impact of their mental health status on themselves and others.

'Mentally not healthy' (mNH) individuals are often those individuals who are not mentally healthy (because they either have a known psychiatric diagnosis or failed to satisfy acceptability on the three elemental components of the utilitarian model of mental health, or both), but the nature of their mental health status is such that, the impact of their mental health state negatively impacts the self, but not others – in other words, the bearer of the suffering as a result of the imperfect mental health state is the self and not others. Some examples are deliberate self-harm, substance abuse problems, anxiety disorders, somatoform disorders, transvestitism, and mental retardation. mNH individuals often have some level of retained insight into their disorder and suffering. They are amenable to potentially beneficial psychiatric therapy but often refrain from seeking help due to the stigma attached to seeking help from a psychiatrist. Often, psychological intervention is needed, with little need for pharmacological intervention.

'Mentally unhealthy' (mUH) individuals are often those individuals who are not mentally healthy, but the nature of their mental health status is such that the impact of their mental health state negatively impacts others relatively more than the self – in other words, the bearer(s) of the suffering because of the imperfect health state is/are others and not much of the self. Anti-social personality disorder, voyeurism, frotteurism, sadism, sexual assault/perversions, and pedophilia arise out of mental health states, where the primary bearer of suffering because of these disorders is others rather than the self. The individual not only lacks insight but also remorse. It is not uncommon for the individual to derive pleasure from others' suffering. Due to the adverse impact on others' lives, these individuals are at threat of legal complications, because of which they often refrain from seeking medical help. The disorders within this region of the mental health spectrum can be subject successfully to clinical intervention and behavior modification to control the negative impact of their mental health state, but the challenge is often unearthing the presence of these disorders that are kept concealed by the individuals and those dearest to him due to fear of legal implications.

'Mentally ill' (mI) individuals are often those individuals who are not mentally healthy, and the nature of their mental health status is such that the impact of their mental health state negatively impacts themselves (relatively more than the other two states), and also others – in other words, the bearer of the suffering because of the imperfect health state is the self, and the degree of suffering is high, or the potential to suffer severely is high. Schizophrenia and major depressive disorder are typical examples. Often, these individuals are questioned by society about their ability to perform well in society again. Although excellent treatment options exist, the patient or their loved ones are reluctant to seek medical/psychiatric help because of the stigma attached to mental illnesses.

Summary

The utilitarian model of mental health is the only clinically applicable model for the practicing psychiatrist. The three components of mental health are awareness of one's self, ability to relate well with others, and acting in a way that is beneficial to oneself and non-detrimental to others. If all three criteria are satisfied, in the absence of a known psychiatric diagnosis, the individual can be considered 'mentally healthy'. Those who do not fulfill the 'mentally healthy' criteria could be either 'mentally not healthy' (i.e., the primary bearer of the suffering is self, more than others) or 'mentally unhealthy' (i.e., the primary bearer of the suffering is others more than self), or 'mentally ill' (i.e., the primary bearer of the suffering is the self, and the others, but extremely high suffering for the self). Categorizing a patient's mental state under the utilitarian model allows for precise and effective treatment planning and improving patient outcomes.

We have compiled the list of psychiatric diagnoses with corresponding the Ulan component that is primarily affected as well as the typical mental health state resulting from it.

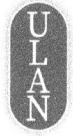

U
L
A
N

DSM Disorders	ICD-9	ICD-10	Mental Status	Ulan component primarily affected
Neurodevelopmental disorders				
Intellectual disability (Intellectual developmental disorder/ global developmental delay/ unspecified), Communication disorders (Language, speech sound, stuttering, social, unspecified), Autism spectrum disorder, Attention-deficit hyperactivity disorder (combined/inattentive/hyperactive/unspecified/others), Specific learning disorder (impairment in reading/writing/mathematics), Motor disorders (coordination/ stereotypic movement/ tic disorders), Other neurodevelopmental disorders (Other/unspecified)	299, 307.2, 307.21- 307.23, 307.3, 307.9, 314, 314.01, 315, 315.1, 315.2, 315.32, 315.35, 315.39, 315.4, 315.8, 315.9, 317, 318.1, 318.2, 319	F70-F73, F79, F80, F80.2, F80.81, F80.89, F80.9, F81, F81.2, F81.81, F82, F84, F88-F90, F90.1, F90.2, F90.8, F95, F95.1, F95.2, F95.8, F95.9, F98.4	Mentally Not-healthy	Intellect
Schizophrenia spectrum and other psychotic disorders				
Schizotypal (Personality) Disorder, Delusional Disorder, Brief Psychotic Disorder, Schizophreniform Disorder, Schizophrenia, Schizoaffective Disorder (Bipolar/ Depressive type), Substance/Medication-Induced Psychotic Disorder, Psychotic Disorder due to Another Medical Condition (With delusions/With hallucinations), Catatonia Associated with Another Mental Disorder, Catatonia Disorder due to Another Mental Disorder, Unspecified Catatonia, Other Specific Schizophrenia Spectrum and Other Psychotic Disorder, Unspecified Schizophrenia Spectrum and Other Psychotic Disorder	293.81, 293.82, 293.89, 295.4, 295.7, 295.9, 297.1, 298.8, 298.9, 301.22	F06.0, F06.10, F06.20, F20.81, F20.9, F21-F23, F25, F25.1, F28, F29	Mentally Ill	Thought

DSM Disorders	ICD-9	ICD-10	Mental Status	Ulan component primarily affected
Bipolar and related disorder				
Bipolar I Disorder (manic, hypomanic, depressed, unspecified), Bipolar II Disorder, Cyclothymic Disorder, Substance/Medication-Induced Bipolar and Related Disorder, Bipolar and Related Disorder Due to Another Medical Condition (manic, hypomanic, mixed), Other Specified Bipolar and Related Disorder, Unspecified Bipolar and Related Disorder	293.83, 296.40-296.46, 296.50-296.56, 296.7, 296.8, 296.89, 301.13	F06.33, F06.34, F31.0, F31.11-31.13, F31.2, F31.4, F31.5, F31.73-31.76, F31.81, F31.89, F31.9, F34	Mentally Ill	Affect
Depressive Disorders				
Disruptive Mood Dysregulation Disorder, Major Depressive Disorder (single or recurrent episode), Persistent Depressive Disorder (Dysthymia), Premenstrual Dysphoric Disorder, Substance/Medication-Induced Depressive Disorder, Depressive Disorder Due to Another Medical Condition (with depressive features, major depressive-like episode, mixed), Other Specific Depressive Disorder, Unspecified Depressive Disorder	294.83, 296.20-296.26, 296.30-296.36, 296.99, 300.4, 311, 625.4	F06.31, F06.32, F06.34, F32.0-32.5, F32.9, F33.0-33.3, F33.41-33.42, F33.9, F34.1, F34.8, N94.3	Mentally Ill	Mood
Anxiety Disorders				
Separation Anxiety Disorder, Selective Mutism, Specific Phobia (animal, natural environment, blood-injection-injury, situational, other), Social Anxiety Disorder (Social Phobia), Panic Disorder, Panic Attack Specifier, Agoraphobia, Generalized Anxiety Disorder, Substance/Medication-Induced Anxiety Disorder, Anxiety Disorder Due to Another Medical Condition, Other Specified Anxiety Disorder, Unspecified Anxiety Disorder	293.84, 300.00-300.02, 300.09, 300.22, 300.23, 300.29, 309.21, 313.23	F93, F94, F40.218, F40.228, F40.230-40.233, F40.248, F40.298, F40.1, F40, F41.1, F06.4, F41.8, F41.9	Mentally Not-healthy	Mood

DSM Disorders	ICD-9	ICD-10	Mental Status	Ulan component primarily affected
Obsessive-Compulsive and Related Disorders				
Obsessive-Compulsive Disorder, Body Dysmorphic Disorder, Hoarding Disorder, Trichotillomania (Hair-Pulling Disorder), Excoriation (Skin-Picking) Disorder, Substance/Medication-Induced Obsessive-Compulsive and Related Disorder, Obsessive-Compulsive and Related Disorder Due to Another Medical Condition, Other Specified Obsessive-Compulsive and Related Disorder, Other Specified Obsessive-Compulsive and Related Disorder, Unspecified Obsessive-Compulsive and Related Disorder	294.8, 300.3, 300.7, 312.39, 698.4	F06.8, F42, F45.22, F63.3, L98.1	Mentally Not-healthy	Thought
Trauma- and Stressor-Related Disorders				
Attachment Disorder, Disinhibited Social Engagement Disorder, Posttraumatic Stress Disorder (includes Post-traumatic Stress Disorder for Children 6 Years and Younger), Acute Stress Disorder, Adjustment Disorders (with depressed mood, anxiety, mixed, disturbance of conduct+/-emotions, unspecified), Other Specified Trauma- and Stressor-Related Disorder, Unspecified Trauma- and Stressor-Related Disorder	308.3, 309.0, 309.24, 309.28, 309.3, 309.4, 309.81, 309.89, 309.9, 313.89	F43.1, F43.20-43.25, F43.8, F43.9, F94.1, F94.2	Mentally Not-healthy	Mood
Dissociative Disorders				
Dissociative Identity Disorder, Dissociative Amnesia (with dissociative fugue), Depersonalization/Derealization Disorder, Other Specified Dissociative Disorder, Unspecified Dissociative Disorder	300.12-300.15, 300.6	F44.0, F44.1, F44.81, F44.89, F44.9, F48.1	Mentally Not-healthy	Thought

DSM Disorders	ICD-9	ICD-10	Mental Status	Ulan component primarily affected
Somatic Symptom and Related Disorders				
Somatic Symptom Disorder, Illness Anxiety Disorder, Conversion Disorder (Functional Neurological Symptom Disorder) (with weakness/paralysis, abnormal movement, swallowing or speech symptoms, attacks or seizures, anesthesia or sensory loss, special sensory symptoms, mixed), Psychological Factors Affecting Other Medical Conditions, Factitious Disorder (includes Factitious Disorder Imposed on Self, Factitious Disorder Imposed on Another), Other Specified Somatic Symptom and Related Disorder, Unspecified Somatic Symptom and Related Disorder	300.11, 300.19, 300.7, 300.82, 300.82, 300.89, 316	F44.4-44.7, F45.1, F45.21, F45.8, F45.9, F54, F68.1	Mentally Not-healthy	Thought (Cognition)
Feeding and Eating Disorders				
Pica (children or adults), Rumination Disorder, Avoidant/Restrictive Food Intake Disorder, Anorexia Nervosa (restricting type or binge-eating/purging type), Bulimia Nervosa, Binge-Eating Disorder, Other Specified Feeding or Eating Disorder, Unspecified Feeding or Eating Disorder	307.1, 307.50-307.53, 307.59, 307.89	F50.01, F50.02, F50.2, F50.8, F50.9, F98.21, F98.3	Mentally Not-healthy	Thought (Behavior)
Elimination Disorders				
Enuresis, Encopresis, Other Specified Elimination Disorder (with urinary or fecal symptoms), Unspecified Elimination Disorder (with urinary or fecal symptoms)	307.6, 307.7, 787.60, 788.39, 788.30	F98.0, F98.1, N39.498, R15.9, R32, R15.9	Mentally Not-healthy	Thought (Cognition)
Sleep-Wake Disorders				
Insomnia Disorder, Hypersomnolence Disorder, Narcolepsy (with cataplexy +/- hypocretin deficiency or autosomal dominant cerebellar ataxia, deafness, and narcolepsy or autosomal dominant narcolepsy, obesity, and DMII, or narcolepsy secondary to another medical condition)	307.42, 307.44, 347.00, 347.01	F51.01, F51.11, G47.411, G47.419, G47.429	Mentally Not-healthy	Thought (Cognition)

DSM Disorders	ICD-9	ICD-10	Mental Status	Ulan component primarily affected
Breathing-Related Sleep disorders				
Obstructive Sleep Apnea Hypopnea (Idiopathic central sleep apnea, Cheyne-Stokes breathing, Central sleep apnea comorbid with opioid use), Sleep-Related Hypoventilation (Idiopathic hypoventilation, Congenital central alveolar hypoventilation, Comorbid sleep-related hypoventilation), Circadian Rhythm Sleep-Wake Disorders (Delayed sleep phase type, Advanced sleep phase type, Irregular sleep-wake type, Non-24-hour sleep-wake type, Shift work type, Unspecified type)	327.21, 327.23-327.26, 786.04, 780.57, 307.45	G47.20-G47.24, G47.26, G47.31, G47.33-G47.37, R06.3	Mentally Not-healthy	Thought (Cognition)
Parasomnias				
Non–Rapid Eye Movement Sleep Arousal Disorders (Sleepwalking type, Sleep terror type), Nightmare Disorder, Rapid Eye Movement Sleep Behavior Disorder, Restless Legs Syndrome, Substance/Medication-Induced Sleep Disorder, Other Specified Insomnia Disorder, Unspecified Insomnia Disorder, Other Specified Hypersomnolence Disorder, Unspecified Hypersomnolence Disorder, Other Specified Sleep-Wake Disorder, Unspecified Sleep-Wake Disorder	307.46, 307.47, 327.42, 333.94, 780.52, 780.54, 780.59	F51.3-F51.5, G47.00, G47.09, G47.10, G47.8, G47.9, G47.52, G25.81	Mentally Not-healthy	Thought (Cognition)
Sexual Dysfunctions				
Delayed Ejaculation, Erectile Disorder, Female Orgasmic Disorder, Female Sexual Interest/Arousal Disorder, Genito-Pelvic Pain/Penetration Disorder, Male Hypoactive Sexual Desire Disorder, Premature (Early) Ejaculation, Substance/Medication-Induced Sexual Dysfunction, Other Specified Sexual Dysfunction, Unspecified Sexual Dysfunction	302.70-302.76, 302.79	F52.0, F52.21, F52.22, F52.31, F52.4, F52.6, F52.8, F52.9	Mentally Not healthy	Thought (Cognition)

DSM Disorders	ICD-9	ICD-10	Mental Status	Ulan component primarily affected
Gender Dysphoria				
Gender Dysphoria (in children or adolescents and adults), Other Specified Gender Dysphoria, Unspecified Gender Dysphoria	302.6, 302.85	F64.1, F64.2, F64.8, F64.9	Mentally Not-healthy	Thought (Cognition)
Disruptive, Impulse-Control, and Conduct Disorders				
Oppositional Defiant Disorder, Intermittent Explosive Disorder, Intermittent Explosive Disorder, Conduct Disorder (Childhood-onset type, Adolescent-onset type, Unspecified onset), Antisocial Personality Disorder, Pyromania, Kleptomania, Other Specified Disruptive, Impulse-Control, and Conduct Disorder, Unspecified Disruptive, Impulse-Control, and Conduct Disorder	301.7, 312.32- 312.34, 312.81, 312.82, 312.89, 312.9	F91.1- F91.3, F91.8, F91.9, F60.2, F63.1, F63.2, F63.81	Mentally Not-healthy	Thought (Behavior)
Substance-Related and Addictive Disorders				
Alcohol-Related Disorders Alcohol Use Disorder (Mild, Moderate, Severe), Alcohol Intoxication (With use disorder mild, moderate, or severe or without use disorder), Alcohol Withdrawal (with/without perceptual disturbances), Other Alcohol-Induced Disorders, Unspecified Alcohol-Related Disorder	291.81, 291.9, 303.00, 303.90, 305.00	F10.10, F10.129, F10.20, F10.229, F10.232, F10.239, F10.929, F10.99	Mentally Ill	Thought (cognition)
Caffeine-Related Disorders Caffeine Intoxication, Caffeine Withdrawal, Other Caffeine-Induced Disorders, Unspecified Caffeine-Related Disorder	292.0, 292.9, 305.90	F15.929, F15.93, F15.99	Mentally Ill	Thought (cognition)
Cannabis-Related Disorders Cannabis Use Disorder (Mild, Moderate, Severe), Cannabis Intoxication (with/without perceptual disturbances), Cannabis Withdrawal, Other Cannabis-Induced Disorders, Unspecified Cannabis-Related Disorder	292.0, 292.89, 292.9, 304.20, 305.20, 305.90	F15.10, F12.122, F12.129, F12.20, F12.222, F12.229, F12.922, F12.929	Mentally Ill	Thought (cognition)

DSM Disorders	ICD-9	ICD-10	Mental Status	Ulan component primarily affected
Hallucinogen-Related Disorders Phencyclidine Intoxication (With use disorder mild, moderate, or severe or without use disorder), Other Hallucinogen Intoxication (With use disorder mild, moderate, or severe or without use disorder), Hallucinogen Persisting Perception Disorder, Other Phencyclidine-Induced Disorders, Other Hallucinogen-Induced Disorders, Unspecified Phencyclidine-Related Disorder, Unspecified Hallucinogen-Related Disorder	292.89, 292.9, 304.50, 304.60, 305.30, 305.90	F16.10, F16.129, F16.20, F16.229, F16.929, F16.983, F16.99	Mentally Ill	Thought (cognition)
Inhalant-Related Disorders Inhalant Use Disorder (Mild, Moderate, Severe), Inhalant Intoxication (With use disorder mild, moderate, or severe or without use disorder), Unspecified Inhalant-Related Disorder	292.89, 292.9, 304.60, 305.9	F18.10, F18.129, F18.20, F18.229, F18.929, F18.99	Mentally Ill	Thought (cognition)
Opioid-Related Disorders Opioid Use Disorder (Mild, Moderate, Severe), Opioid Intoxication (with/without perceptual disturbances), Opioid Withdrawal, Other Opioid-Induced Disorders, Unspecified Opioid-Related Disorder	292.0, 292.89, 292.9, 304.00, 305.50	F11.10, F11.122, F11.123, F11.129, F11.229, F11.929, F11.99	Mentally Ill	Thought (cognition)
Sedative-, Hypnotic-, or Anxiolytic-Related Disorders Sedative, Hypnotic, or Anxiolytic Use Disorder (Mild, Moderate, Severe), Intoxication (With use disorder mild, moderate, or severe or without use disorder), Withdrawal (With/without perceptual disturbances), Other Sedative-, Hypnotic-, or Anxiolytic-Induced Disorders, Unspecified Sedative-, Hypnotic-, or Anxiolytic-Related Disorder	292.0, 292.89, 292.9, 304.10, 305.40	F13.10, F13.129, F13.20, F13.229, F13.232, F13.239, F13.929, F13.99	Mentally Ill	Thought (cognition)

DSM Disorders	ICD-9	ICD-10	Mental Status	Ulan component primarily affected
Stimulant-Related Disorders Stimulant Use Disorder (Mild, Moderate, Severe), Stimulant Intoxication, Cocaine, Without perceptual disturbances, Amphetamine or other stimulant, With perceptual, Cocaine, With perceptual disturbances, Stimulant Withdrawal, Other Stimulant-Induced Disorders, Unspecified Stimulant-Related Disorder	292.0, 292.89, 292.9, 304.20, 304.40, 305.60, 305.70	F14.10, F14.129, F14.20, F14.122, F14.23, F14.229, F14.922, F14.929, F14.99, F15.10, F15.122, F15.23, F15.129, F15.20, F15.229, F15.929, F15.99	Mentally Ill	Thought (cognition)
Tobacco-Related Disorders Tobacco Use Disorder (Mild, Moderate, Severe), Tobacco Withdrawal, Other Tobacco-Induced Disorders, Unspecified Tobacco-Related Disorder	292.0, 292.9, 305.1	F17.200, F17.203, F17.209, Z72.0	Mentally Ill	Thought (cognition)
Other (or Unknown) Substance-Related Disorders Other (or Unknown) Substance Use Disorder (Mild, Moderate, Severe), Other (or Unknown) Substance Intoxication, Other (or Unknown) Substance Withdrawal, Other (or Unknown) Substance-Induced Disorders, Unspecified Other (or Unknown) Substance-Related Disorder	292.0, 292.89, 292.9, 304.90, 305.90	F19.10, F19.129, F19.20, F19.239, F19.929, F19.99	Mentally Ill	Thought (cognition)
Non-Substance-Related Disorders Gambling Disorder	312.31	F63.0	Mentally Ill	Thought (cognition)
Neurocognitive Disorders				
Delirium (intoxication, withdrawal, medication-induced, due to other medical condition), Delirium due to multiple etiologies, Other Specified Delirium, Unspecified Delirium	292.81, 293.0, 780.09	F05, R41.0	Mentally Ill	Thought

DSM Disorders	ICD-9	ICD-10	Mental Status	Ulan component primarily affected
Probable Major Neurocognitive Disorder Due to Alzheimer's Disease (With/without behavioral disturbance), Possible Major, or Mild, Probable Major Neurocognitive Disorder Due to Frontotemporal Lobar Degeneration (With/without behavioral disturbance), Possible Major, or Mild, Probable Major Neurocognitive Disorder With Lewy Bodies (With/without behavioral disturbance), Possible Major, or Mild, Probable Major Vascular Neurocognitive Disorder (With/without behavioral disturbance), Possible Major, or Mild, Major Neurocognitive Disorder Due to Traumatic Brain Injury (With/without behavioral disturbance), or Mild, Major Neurocognitive Disorder Due to HIV Infection (With/without behavioral disturbance), or Mild, Major Neurocognitive Disorder Due to Prion Disease (With/without behavioral disturbance), or Mild, Major Neurocognitive Disorder Probably Due to Parkinson's Disease (With/without behavioral disturbance), or Mild, Major Neurocognitive Disorder Due to Huntington's Disease (With/without behavioral disturbance), or Mild, Major Neurocognitive Disorder Due to Another Medical Condition (With/without behavioral disturbance), or Mild, Major Neurocognitive Disorder Due to Multiple Etiologies (With/without behavioral disturbance), or Mild, Unspecified Neurocognitive Disorder	294.10, 294.11, 331.83, 331.9	F02.80, F02.81, G31.84, G31.9	Mentally Not-healthy	Intellect
Probable Major Neurocognitive Disorder Due to Frontotemporal Lobar Degeneration (With/without behavioral disturbance), Possible Major, or Mild	294.10, 294.11, 331.83, 331.9, 799.59	F02.80, F02.81, G31.84, G31.9, R41.9	Mentally Not-healthy	Intellect

DSM Disorders	ICD-9	ICD-10	Mental Status	Ulan component primarily affected
Personality Disorders				
Cluster A Personality Disorders Paranoid Personality Disorder, Schizoid Personality Disorder, Schizotypal Personality Disorder	301.0, 301.20, 301.33	F60.0, F60.1, F21	Mentally Unhealthy	Thought (Cognition)
Cluster B Personality Disorders Antisocial Personality Disorder, Borderline Personality Disorder, Histrionic Personality Disorder, Narcissistic Personality Disorder	301.50, 301.7, 301.81, 301.83	F60.2-60.4, F60.81	Mentally Unhealthy	Thought (Cognition)
Cluster C Personality Disorders Avoidant Personality Disorder, Dependent Personality Disorder, Obsessive-Compulsive Personality Disorder	301.4, 301.6, 301.82	F60.5-60.7	Mentally Unhealthy	Thought (Cognition)
Other Personality Disorders Personality Change Due to Another Medical Condition, Other Specified Personality Disorder, Unspecified Personality Disorder	301.89, 301.9, 310.1	F60.89, F60.9, F07.0	Mentally Unhealthy	Thought (Cognition)
Paraphilic Disorders				
Voyeuristic Disorder, Exhibitionistic Disorder, Frotteuristic Disorder, Sexual Masochism Disorder, Sexual Sadism Disorder, Pedophilic Disorder, Fetishistic Disorder, Transvestic Disorder, Other Specified Paraphilic Disorder, Unspecified Paraphilic Disorder	302.2-302.4, 302.81, 302.83, 302.84, 302.89, 302.9	F65.0-F65.4, F65.51, F65.52, F65.81, F65.89, F65.9	Mentally Unhealthy	Thought (Behavior)
Other Mental Disorders				
Other Specified Mental Disorder Due to Another Medical Condition, Unspecified Mental Disorder Due to Another Medical Condition, Other Specified Mental Disorder	294.8, 294.9, 300.9	F06.8, F09, F99	Needs MSE	Needs MSE

DSM Disorders	ICD-9	ICD-10	Mental Status	Ulan component primarily affected
Medication-Induced Movement Disorders and Other Adverse Effects of Medication				
Neuroleptic-Induced Parkinsonism, Other Medication-Induced Parkinsonism, Neuroleptic Malignant Syndrome, Medication-Induced Acute Dystonia, Medication-Induced Acute Akathisia, Tardive Dyskinesia, Tardive Dystonia, Tardive Akathisia, Medication-Induced Postural Tremor, Other Medication-Induced Movement Disorder, Antidepressant Discontinuation Syndrome, Other Adverse Effect of Medication	332.1, 333.92, 333.72, 333.72, 333.99, 333.85, 333.72, 333.99, 333.1, 333.99, 995.20, 995.29	G21.11, G21.19, G21.0, G24.02, G25.71, G24.01, G25.1, G25.79, T43.205A, T43.205D, T42.205S, T50.905A, T50.905D, T50.905S	Needs MSE	Needs MSE
Relational Problems				
Parent-Child Relational Problem, Sibling Relational Problem, Upbringing Away From Parents, Child Affected by Parental Relationship Distress	V61.20, V61.29, V61.8	Z62.29, V62.820, V62.891, Z62.898	Mentally Not-healthy	Needs MSE
Relationship Distress With Spouse or Intimate Partner, Disruption of Family by Separation or Divorce, High Expressed Emotion Level Within Family, Uncomplicated Bereavement	V61.03, V61.10. V61.8. V62.82	Z62.0, Z63.4, Z63.5, Z63.8	Mentally Not- healthy	Needs MSE
Abuse and Neglect				

DSM Disorders	ICD-9	ICD-10	Mental Status	Ulan component primarily affected
Child Physical Abuse, Confirmed or Suspected, Other Circumstances Related to Child Physical Abuse, Child Sexual Abuse, Confirmed or Suspected, Other Circumstances Related to Child Sexual Abuse, Child Neglect, Confirmed or Suspected, Other Circumstances Related to Child Neglect, Child Psychological Abuse, Confirmed or Suspected, Other Circumstances Related to Child Psychological Abuse	995.51-995.54, V15.41, V15.42, V61.21, V61.22, V62.83,	T74.02XA, T74.02XD, T76.02XA, T76.02XD, T74.12XA, T74.12XD, T76.12XA, T76.12XD, T74.22XA, T74.22XD, T76.22XA, T76.22XD, T74.32XA, T74.32XD, T7632XA, T76.32XD, Z69.010, Z69.020-Z69.021, Z62.810-Z62.812, Z69.011	Mentally Not-healthy	Needs MSE
Adult Maltreatment and Neglect Problems				
Spouse or Partner Violence, Physical, Confirmed or Suspected, Other Circumstances Related to Spouse or Partner Violence, Physical; Spouse or Partner Violence, Sexual, Confirmed or Suspected, Other Circumstances Related to Spouse or Partner Violence, Sexual; Spouse or Partner Neglect, Confirmed or Suspected, Other Circumstances Related to Spouse or Partner Neglect; Spouse or Partner Abuse, Psychological, Confirmed or Suspected, Other Circumstances Related to Spouse or Partner Abuse, Psychological; Adult (Physical, Sexual, Psychological) Abuse by Non-spouse or Non-partner, Confirmed or Suspected, Other Circumstances Related to Adult Abuse by Non-spouse or Non-partner	995.81-995.83, 995.85, V15.41, V15.42, V61.11-V61.12, V62.83, V65.49	T74.01XA, 74.01XD, T74.11XA, T74.11XD, T76.11XA, T76.11XD, T74.21XA, T74.21XD, T76.21XA, T76.21XD, T74.31X, T74.31XD, T76.31XA, T75.31XD, Z69.11, Z69.12, Z69.81, Z69.82, Z91.410, Z91.411	Needs MSE	Needs MSE

DSM Disorders	ICD-9	ICD-10	Mental Status	Ulan component primarily affected
Educational and Occupational Problems				
Academic or Educational Problem, Problem Related to Current Military Deployment Status, Other Problem Related to Employment	V62.3, V62.21, V62.29	Z55.9, Z56.82, Z56.9	Needs MSE	Needs MSE
Housing and Economic Problems				
Homelessness, Inadequate Housing, Discord With Neighbor, Lodger, or Landlord, Problem Related to Living in a Residential Institution, Lack of Adequate Food or Safe Drinking Water, Extreme Poverty, Low Income, Insufficient Social Insurance or Welfare Support, Unspecified Housing or Economic Problem	V60.0-V60.2, V60.6, V60.89, V60.9	Z59.4,-Z59.7, Z59.9	Needs MSE	Needs MSE
Other Problems Related to the Social Environment				
Phase of Life Problem, Problem Related to Living Alone, Acculturation Difficulty, Social Exclusion or Rejection, Target of (Perceived) Adverse Discrimination or Persecution, Unspecified Problem Related to Social Environment	V60.3, V62.4, V62.89, V62.9	Z60.0, Z60.2-Z60.5, Z60.9	Needs MSE	Needs MSE
Problems Related to Crime or Interaction With the Legal System				
Victim of Crime, Conviction in Civil or Criminal Proceedings Without Imprisonment, Imprisonment or Other Incarceration, Problems Related to Release From Prison, Problems Related to Other Legal Circumstances	V62.5, V62.89	Z65.0-Z65.4	Needs MSE	Needs MSE
Other Health Service Encounters for Counseling and Medical Advice				
Sex Counseling, Other Counseling or Consultation	V65.40, V65.49	Z70.9, Z71.9	Needs MSE	Needs MSE

DSM Disorders	ICD-9	ICD-10	Mental Status	Ulan component primarily affected
Problems Related to Other Psychosocial, Personal, and Environmental Circumstances				
Religious or Spiritual Problem, Problems Related to Unwanted Pregnancy, Problems Related to Multiparity, Discord With Social Service Provider, Including Probation Officer, Case Manager, or Social Services Worker, Victim of Terrorism or Torture, Exposure to Disaster, War, or Other Hostilities, Other Problem Related to Psychosocial Circumstances, Unspecified Problem Related to Unspecified Psychosocial Circumstances	V61.5, V61.7, V62.22, V62.89, V62.9	Z64.9, Z64.1, Z64.4, Z65.4, Z65.5, Z65.8, Z65.9	Needs MSE	Needs MSE
Other Circumstances of Personal History				
Other Personal History of Psychological Trauma, Personal History of Self-Harm, Personal History of Military Deployment, Other Personal Risk Factors, Problem Related to Lifestyle, Adult Antisocial Behavior, Child or Adolescent Antisocial Behavior	V15.49, V15.59, V15.89, V62.22, V69.9, V71.01, V71.02	Z72.810, Z72.811, Z72.9, Z91.49, Z91.5, Z91.82, Z91.89	Needs MSE	Needs MSE
Problems Related to Access to Medical and Other Health Care				
Unavailability or Inaccessibility of Health Care Facilities, Unavailability or Inaccessibility of Other Helping Agencies	V63.8, V63.9	Z75.3, Z75.4	Needs MSE	Needs MSE
Nonadherence to Medical Treatment				
Nonadherence to Medical Treatment, Overweight or Obesity, Malingering, Wandering Associated With a Mental Disorder, Borderline Intellectual Functioning	278.00, V15.81, V40.31, V62.89, V65.2	E66.9, R41.83, Z76.5, Z91.19, Z91.83	Needs MSE	Needs MSE

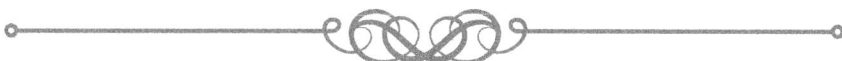

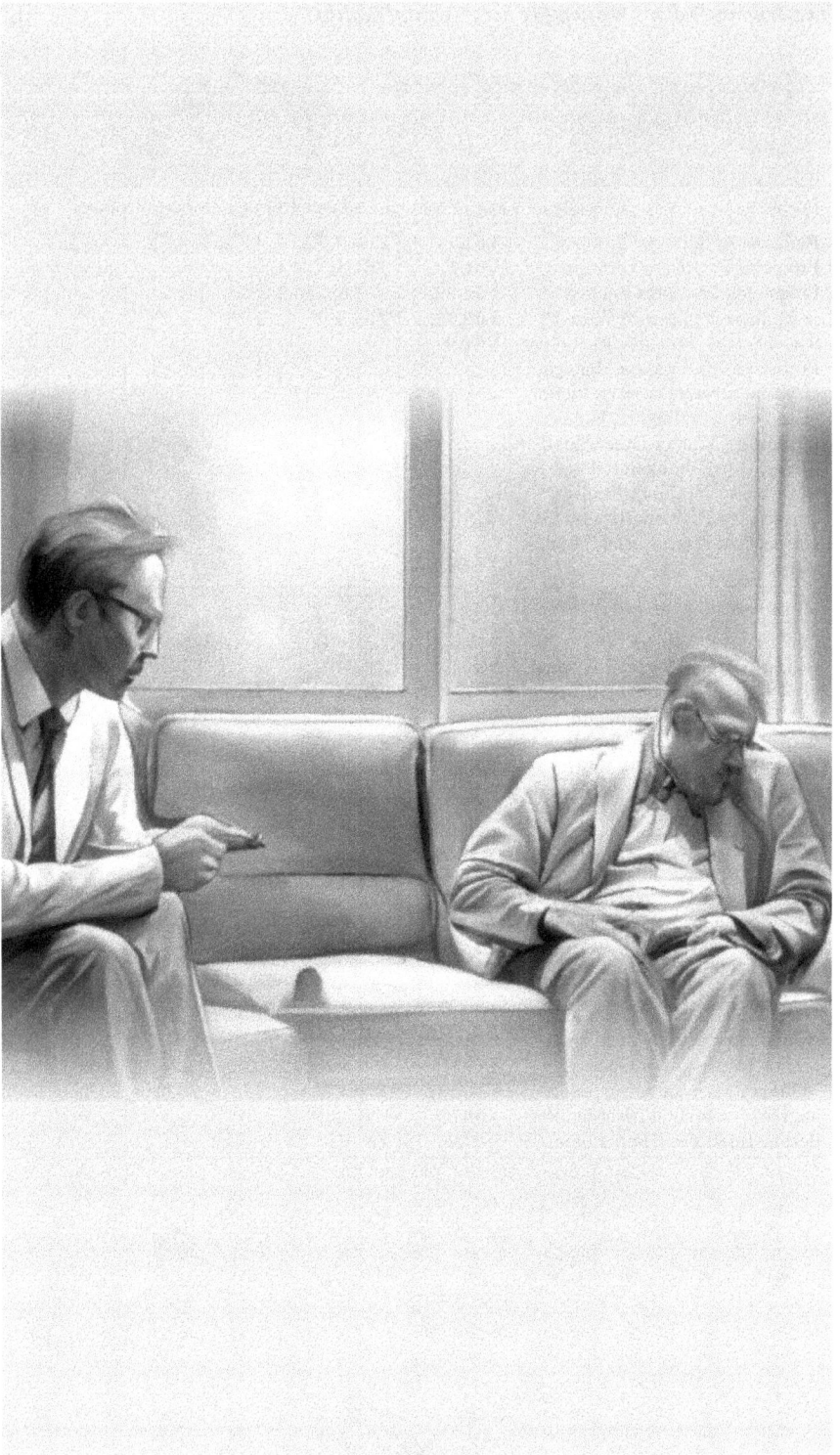

CHAPTER 5

The Toolbox - Psychiatric Clinical Examination

Other Contributors: Stalin R Subramanian, MD, Moses Evbuoman, MD

Psychiatry is a specialized branch of internal medicine. By being a branch of medicine, the principles governing psychiatric history-taking and examination follow similar lines as that of a traditional history-taking and clinical examination in Internal Medicine. A solid foundational knowledge of basic sciences, and clinical examination skills in Internal Medicine is a prerequisite and complement to psychiatric history taking and examination.

A student of psychiatry must diligently observe the interviewing and examination techniques employed by experienced and skilled psychiatrists repeatedly over several years, while simultaneously practicing those skills in the clinical setting, to gain proficiency.

The topic of psychiatric history-taking and examination is extraordinarily vast compared to other specialties of medicine, and a comprehensive review of the same is beyond the scope of this book. However, I would like to highlight various vital aspects that would be necessary for clinical practice.

Fundamentals of Interview

1. **Establish the validity of the informant** – The primary source of information about the patient is called the 'informant'. The informant could be the patient, or someone accompanying the patient, such as a spouse, parent, child, other family, friend, school counselor, colleague, neighbor, etc. The patient might be requesting the initial referral or consultation and may present to the clinic alone. The latter happens when the issue is considered 'sensitive', especially in Asian cultures. In any case, the validity and authenticity of the informant must be established. The patient must explicitly clarify that the informant is authorized to discuss

and disclose information and is the decision maker (often designated as the 'health power of attorney' or 'emergency contact' in Western societies) when the patient is unable to or deemed unable to make decisions.

2. **Be unaffected** - In general, doctors get exposed to the most personal details of people's lives. The psychiatrist gets to hear the strangest, most intimate, most concealed, and unusual of these stories. It is natural to become affected, positively or negatively, or overcome by emotions or judgments upon hearing these stories. Simple news stories, or those seen enacted on screen evoke such strong reactions. The psychiatrist sees and interacts with these stories at arm's length. The mood is infectious, and thoughts are like vines. Yet, to stay unaffected is a necessity to function as a psychiatrist. More importantly, the psychiatrist must continuously and consciously introspect and monitor one's own thinking and language to avoid explicit and implicit bias and judgment. The patient's information, regardless of how deviant it may be, is merely yet another data point in a medical history-taking endeavor. Shut up, hold back comments and remarks, don't air your opinions and views, don't steer the conversation in your preference, but keep listening. Continue your silence even if the patient pauses the conversation or completes talking – you will notice they begin talking again without asking for more information. The patient's talking helps more than history taking alone - it is catharsis at the altar of the psychiatrist, which builds the doctor-patient trust.

3. **Reconstruct the past** - History is taken in two dimensions – cross-sectional, and longitudinal. Cross-sectional history is the elaboration of all aspects of the presenting complaint, and mental status during a given time point, episode, or interval. Longitudinal history is a chronological listing of the evolution of one or more mental health complaints. Cross-sectional history is easier to obtain, more accurate, and easier to corroborate. It is like a 'snapshot', or drawing a portrait of an event, and trying to understand every detail seen on/in a photo. Longitudinal history is more difficult to obtain and corroborate and is less accurate. It is like watching a movie, paying attention usually to the leading actor, while other details sink into the background. Trainees and younger psychiatrists tend to perform well and become more interested in cross-sectional history. Still, longitudinal history is more important to make an accurate diagnosis and draft an effective treat-

ment strategy. My style is to start with longitudinal history first –this is because cross-sectional history is misleading, and the psychiatrist may be led down the wrong path early on and may end up making big blunders. Reconstruct the story, as it might have happened, to fully understand the predicament the patient is in at the current moment. For reconstruction, it helps to know how the patient behaves in his/her surroundings. Corroborating history through multiple sources, or seeing documented information (such as photos, videos, etc. may help). During reconstruction, the psychiatrist's personality may begin to color the reconstruction, which must be consciously resisted. It is better to seek the help of seniors, especially those of a different personality than you are, or are known to be clinically diligent, to ensure that your understanding of history is correct. Also, once you have constructed the history, it may help verify your reconstruction with the patient or informant, but if they disagree, don't argue, or try to prove yourself right.

4. **Talk in simple words, use native language, and be empathetic –** Language is the psychiatrist's Achilles heel. It could be your superpower or your landmine. Be mindful of how you speak. Use simple terms and avoid overly medical terms. Try to use the patient's own words and descriptions as much as possible but avoid feeding into the use of inaccurate terms too. For example, the patient may use the word 'psycho', 'hysterical', or 'narcissistic' to describe others or self, based on what they read on the internet or seen in media – you should avoid endorsing such descriptions unless medically accurate, which rarely they are. You must be familiar with the native language of the people in the region you practice. Language format and syntax must be empathetic and non-judgmental. For example, do not ask 'What is the problem?' when starting the consultation (like during a non-psychiatric medical interview). Also, even if the informant is a reliable source, and the patient is not reliable, do not direct all conversations to the informant, as this would affect rapport building with the patient. In India, this aspect is especially tricky. The family is very involved in the patient's care, volunteers a lot of information, and may take pride in being the caregiver. It is tricky to try and not slight them, while still implying that your duty is primarily towards developing the doctor-patient relationship, not an informant-doctor relationship at the cost of the patient's rapport. Start with simple topics, personal demographics, or lighter topics before discussing psychiatric questions.

5. **Use medical knowledge, not your common sense** – The psychiatrist could take all information presented at face value and may weave a portrait of the patient's history using the data presented. But, if taken at face value, or by the yards used in everyday life, the reconstructions and conclusions arrived are more likely to be inaccurate than if medical knowledge is applied. You have been taught the principles of medicine, logical thinking, the science of probability and statistics, the basics of mind/Ulan, psychoanalysis, and the pathophysiology of diseases. When the information is presented through these lenses, it will make more sense for clinical purposes. And for this, you must know how to 'dissect' information, and probe the patient with tactful questions. Some students are inherently better at these, while others must learn by watching and shadowing experienced and expert psychiatrists.

6. **Organize your thoughts into the Ulan-Mental health concept** – As thought in the Ulan chapter, employ the Ulan concept to organize and consolidate your patient assessment. Ulan is mood, thought, and intellect, working in a harmonious amalgamation. Is the mood appropriate? Is the thought appropriate? Is intellect appropriate? Are they working in harmonious unison? What is the mental health status – is the patient mentally healthy? Mentally non-healthy? Mentally unhealthy? Or mentally ill? Unless you know where the patient is now, you won't know how to lead him/her.

7. **Record for your own sake** – Be elaborate, but not verbose. Document thoroughly, but not redundantly. Document in a way that helps you clarify key aspects even if you had to refer to it years later, and not in a defensive manner to avoid litigation, that it becomes unhelpful or misleading to you. Don't be cryptic – in your absence, another psychiatrist or trainee must be able to use your documentation to pick up the patient where you left.

8. **Stigma is a genuine hurdle, and stigma to mental illness is universal** – In general, even the smartest and brightest, even among doctors, are not immune to stigma. Doctors themselves are more comfortable making a non-psychiatric diagnosis than a psychiatric one. Patients also have prejudices against specific diagnoses and may prefer being diagnosed with one versus the other. Don't fall into this trap, as it is a costly

one. You cannot change public opinion or break the stigma despite the best possible efforts. But you can succeed despite it – but only at the pace of one patient at a time. The only way to break the stigma is by building a rapport. The patient's trust and exalted respect for you will help them move closer to you despite the obstacles placed by the stigma. If you are weak in summoning this respect, no amount of lecturing or showering of data or facts will convince the patient to exit their circle of comfort. And it could be tricky too – I have had female patients ask me my age and marital status so they would be comfortable sharing their personal details.

9. **Be mindful of the applicable laws, those that are relevant to your practice** – Knowing them does not help in clinical outcomes but will save you the troubles of dealing with litigation. Think about what laws are applicable to a case, and think about how they may become relevant, and how you can prevent pitfalls before you start seeing the patient.

The above are the 'Big 9' principles to be considered for successful clinical interaction with the patient. They are summarized in the table next.

Fundamentals of Psychiatric Clinical Interview – the 'Big 9' – Mananalam Clinic Experience

MCE

- **Validate the Informant** - identify the primary informant(s), obtain clarification of decision maker/emergency contact or health power of attorney, verify the validity and reliability of the informant, get corroborative sources, and maintain a good working relationship with the informant.

- **Be unaffected** - all information presented is for medical purposes only, and do not process them at a personal level.

- **Reconstruct the past** - lean more on chronological aspects and reconstruct the history and the evolution of symptoms. Corroborate with information on observed behavior outside the clinic. Verify your assessment but don't broadcast it.

- **Language –** Use simple, accurate language, and communicate succinctly and pleasantly. Be familiar with the native language. Pay attention to sentence grammar, format, and syntax.

- **Medical knowledge –** use the learned knowledge that is learned to perfection. See past face value and interpret information with the psychiatric eye.

- **Consolidate Ulan and Mental health status –**
  organize your assessment in clear and distinct ways
  using the Ulan and mental health concept. If you are uncertain of the status, restart the interview process again.

- **Record –** document diligently, effectively, and thoroughly, for your own clinical benefit.

- **Stigma –** never lose sight of the importance of building rapport and maintaining trust.

- **Laws –** be mindful, proactive, and pre-emptive in abiding by the law.

Fundamentals of History taking

In the field of medicine, 'history' encompasses all details of the patient that have happened up until the point of the current doctor-patient contact. For the initial contact, history includes everything that happened until the patient entered your door. Events and information that occurred after the initial contact would fall under the 'history' during the subsequent contact and documentation. This portion of history that happens between one doctor contact and the next contact is called 'interval history', or 'interim history', with the rest of the history being called 'past history', simply to differentiate it from the most recent aspects of the history. Essentially, history 'grows' during the doctor-patient relationship and accumulates with time. The history of a disease that occurs without medical intervention is called 'natural history'. The history of the disease that occurs after doctor-patient contact becomes treatment or management history. The purpose of therapy is to deflect the illness from its natural history into a better one. During each visit, the doctor must 're-review' the past history with the patient and informant, obtain the interval history, and then reconcile the overall history with the natural history, and the known outcomes with treatment to see if the treatment is making the expected difference. If the treatment is not making the expected difference, then go back to aspects of the history that might have been missed, overlooked, or misunderstood. The latter is the purpose of history taking – if you do not approach history with this objective, it will not be helpful to you.

History-taking serves the following primary purposes – making a diagnosis, strategizing treatment, and assessing outcomes. The bulk of the history goes towards making a diagnosis. The other minor purpose of history taking is for legal documentation. Here, I shall deal with some important fundamental aspects of psychiatric history-taking.

Demographic data

Demographic data is probably the most helpful piece of information in psychiatric history, but its importance is overlooked, because it is not possible to generalize the impact of a demographic data point to all patients worldwide – so it is not discussed much in academic textbooks or probed through research studies. Also, the psychiatrist must be well informed with general knowledge about the local society to be able to deploy demographic information for clinical benefit.

The fundamental principle here, I have learned through experience, is to have the patient write down the demographic information, attest with signature, and save it to the records. Verify the information through the informant, and gather copies of supporting documentation such as driver's license, state-issued ID cards, etc.

Chief complaint

A disease disturbs homeostatic equilibrium and therefore results in disorderly function, leading to one or more noxious experiences. These experiences that 'come together' with the illness are called 'symptoms' (meaning 'together with'). These symptoms, either directly or indirectly bring about suffering to the patient, which the patient brings to the doctor as a 'complaint'. The complaint may or may not be the symptom itself. The complaint may be a result of an underlying symptom too. For example, the complaint may be the inability to work well – which may be due to under-lying symptoms such as fatigue, depression, anxiety, etc. Another complaint could be sleeplessness or anger outbursts, which may be due to other underlying symptoms, each of which could be attributed to a further set of differential diagnoses. Thus, the words 'complaints' and 'symptoms' are not synonymous and must not be used interchangeably. Even if there are multiple complaints, the patient usually puts forth one or two of them as the most important, and bothersome – which is called the 'chief complaint'. In psychiatry, one symptom may produce a variety of complaints – often many of these complaints evolve slowly over time, and most of them get assimilated into the patient's life and become considered 'normal for' the patient's life. For example, depressed mood or irritability is a symptom that could be manifest as 'worry', which the patient might become accustomed to chronically. So, they do not even bring forth these complaints. They become surfaced only through leading questioning by the psychiatrist. Three aspects of the chief complaint must be ascertained –

- **Type** – The complaints may be one or more of three types. They are physical (i.e., somatic), psychological (i.e., non-somatic), or behavioral. Examples of somatic complaints include pain of any sort, weight loss, sensory or motor dysfunction, fatigue, appetite disturbances, and sleep disturbances. Examples of psychological complaints include anxiety, irritability, depression, suicidal thoughts, loss of concentration, memory disturbances, etc. Examples of behavioral complaints include aloofness, self-neglect, risk-taking behavior, abusive acts, deliberate self-harm, attempted suicide, interpersonal conflict, delinquency, disinhibited acts, antisocial acts, etc. The list of examples is exhaustive. In Internal Medicine, there is a tendency to categorize symptoms by organ system, such as respiratory symptoms (cough, dyspnea), cardiac symptoms (palpitations, syncope, chest pain), gastrointestinal symptoms (nausea, emesis, heartburn), neurological symptoms (sensory and motor abnormalities), etc. However, in psychiatry, any of these symptoms may be a manifestation of an underlying psychiatric disorder.

- **Onset and Duration** – this aspect is particularly tricky because the exact time of onset is difficult to ascertain in psychiatry. I like Kraepelin's description of the diseases 'creeping' in. Usually, the duration is derived from when people started noticing the abnormal behavior or found it disturbing enough to bring it to medical attention. It is the psychiatrist's duty to elicit the most probable duration of the symptom causing the complaint. An excellent way to probe it is to ask a reliable informant

– 'When was the last time you found him/her to be perfectly ok? Or without any difficulty?'. Determining onset and duration is especially important in the case of dementia and schizophrenia. After educating the informant and the family about the natural course of these diseases, they may return with more information during the subsequent visits, which have surfaced in their memory. In schizophrenia, the onset is much earlier than believed – being 'aloof' or a 'loner' in adolescence could be the earliest symptom, and when diagnosed this early and treated appropriately, the outcome could be excellent.

- **Periodicity -** Is the complaint persistent and linear in severity progression, or does it occur in episodes? Is there a pattern of acute exacerbations over a chronic baseline? How long do these episodes last? Are they consistent in timing or brought about by identifiable precipitating factors?

History of present illness

After gathering information on the onset and duration of the chief complaint, collect the information from the time of the perceived onset until the time of the first visit with you, and this portion of the history is termed the 'history of presenting illness'. In this section, one must determine three aspects – predisposing factors, precipitating factors, and perpetuating factors. Predisposing factors are those conditions that make the individual more susceptible or vulnerable to the disease but do not result in the eventual manifestation of the disease. Precipitating factors are those that result in the actual expression of the disease. It is usually the 'last straw on the camel's back' – the camel can keep standing as weight is being loaded on its back. The camel does not incrementally slump down, instead, it keeps standing and slumps down completely when the last straw to the load ('the breaking point') is reached. Most younger psychiatrists and trainees spend more time elaborating on the precipitating factors, as it appears to be the cause of the event. The family, informant, and patient tend to 'blow up' the precipitating factor as the cause of the illness. It is essential to resist the temptation, and progress to other aspects of history. Precipitating factors may be physical (medical illnesses such as infection, acute illness, acute trauma, intoxication, medications, etc.) or psychosocial (loss of employment, loss of loved one, separation, divorce, calamities, etc.,). A missed but likely the most impactful aspect of this portion of history is the perpetuating factor – the condition that keeps the disease in an aggravated state. Identify the perpetuating factors and mitigate them.

Next, determine how the complaint and its underlying symptom(s) evolved over time. This requires gathering information on how the disease was influenced or modified by non-personal factors – for example, the family situation, the work situation, interpersonal relationships, living situation, peer group relationships, etc. A history, well-elicited in this regard, does a great deal to clarify the disorderly component of the Ulan – is it the mood, thought, or intellect? Once the latter is established, it is relatively simpler to narrow down the rest of the mental status examination in a time-efficient manner.

Get the treatment history. The latter includes every attempt by the patient to get help –such as seeking counseling, getting self-help books, seeking the guidance of mentors or elders, or even seeking guidance from astrologers, palm readers, or religious godmen.

Do not forget the often-overlooked aspects of the HPI – gender identity-related issues influencing the disorder, sexual orientation, childhood and adolescent history, and social media use.

Do not forget alcohol and substance abuse-related aspects of the HPI – clarifying this aspect is mandatory, as alcohol and substance use will distort the manifestation and evolution of any psychiatric disorder from what has been traditionally taught and written in textbooks.

The living situation ────────────────────

This is a crucial part of psychiatric history, that is often neglected in textbooks, traditional teaching, and clinical practice. In countries like India, the living situation is diverse and complex. The following aspects of the living situation must be ascertained –

- **The 'home'** – 'Home' refers to the people living under the same roof, i.e., in the same house. It could be parents, spouses, children, siblings, relatives, friends, and roommates. The number of people in the home differs and impacts who is in the immediate surroundings of the patient. These people may be perpetuating factors in the disease or may be the source of support in the treatment. It also impacts who has access to the patient's information and affects secrecy and privacy. Determine if the informant is part of the home. If not, inquire how the informant gets firsthand information about the patient.

- **The 'family'** - 'Family' refers to those related by blood or marriage. It may involve common-law partners or long-term living mates. In India, families are distinguished based on the composition of those who live in the same home - as either 'nuclear' (husband, wife, and children only), 'joint' (nuclear + parental in-laws), or 'extended' family (nuclear + non-parental in-laws). Family members may not live in the same home, and all those at home may not be family members.

- **The 'whip'** - 'Whip' is the person who makes decisions. In the USA and other Western societies, the person whom the patient assigns to make decisions on behalf of the patient is considered the legal healthcare power of attorney, and it is often the surviving spouse/partner or the next of kin. In India, Southeast Asia, and the Middle East, I have noticed that the person who makes the decisions in the family may not necessarily be the next of kin or surviving spouse, or even the legal health care power of attorney. It may be the eldest person in the family, the wife's brother, a cousin, or even a close family friend, and that person is the practical 'whip' of the family. The patient, the patient's spouse, and the entire family may need to seek the approval of the whip of the family before doing anything. The presence of a whip may not be readily apparent to the psychiatrist during the first interview. The patient and the family may not consciously realize that there is a third person acting as the whip. This sometimes becomes apparent only during the interview, and sometimes during subsequent visits. (Sometimes it may be a family astrologer, pastor, or religious guru)

Past medical and surgical history

This part of the history is similar to Internal Medical history taking. Give particular importance to those medical factors that influence psychiatric history. History of medication use is especially important. Inquire about surgical history and the indications for the surgeries. History of surgeries with 'soft indications', 'avoidable surgeries', and surgeries that have happened with the persistence of the symptoms for which the surgeries were performed is essential. History of medications or procedures for sleep, weight loss, body image, gynecological complaints, and back pain must be gathered. Do not forget drug allergies. History of alternative therapies, naturopathic remedies, and counseling must also be asked for.

Past psychiatric history

I have dealt with this aspect of history individually in the following chapters. The overriding general principle in this section is to clearly define for yourself what the premorbid status of the patient was like – so that you can use the same yardstick to establish progression or stability of disease, exacerbations, and remissions with reliability. It is especially important in the context of bipolar disorder and schizophrenia. It also helps in understanding if the medications given in the past had any benefit.

Social history

In this aspect, understand what the 'social circle' of the patient is. Who is in the social circle, and how fluid is this circle? Does the patient have long-term friends or mates? Are they of peer age or non-peer age? How involved is the patient with their social connections, and how much are these valued by the patient?

Legal history

This is also an often overlooked aspect of history. Does the patient often interact with the legal system? Does the patient find oneself unwillingly involved by the law? Or is the patient of a litigious nature? Is there a criminal record or any ongoing legal issues in court? Corroborating the information with the informant and documenting it clearly in the medical record is essential.

Family history

The importance of family history in psychiatric history-taking cannot be overemphasized. The impact of family/genetic factors on the development of psychiatric disorders is so strong, that ignoring this aspect of history could lead to misdiagnosis. You must chart the family tree for at least for three generations in the past, and into the future if available. A general question inquiring if there is any psychiatric history in the past is unyielding, or inadequate. Specifically ask if there is any history in the family of suicide, attempted suicide, suicidal gestures, deliberate self-harm, alcohol use, substance use, epilepsy, mental retardation or intellectual disabilities, any family member remaining single until age 40, any family member whose whereabouts are not known, or being separated or living alone for long periods of time, leading extreme lifestyles, frequent displacements, chronic unemployment, homelessness, eloping, being litigious, etc.

In my experience, there is practically no family without some significant family psychiatric history. Also, ask for a family history of medical disorders, which may influence pharmacotherapy strategies.

Personal history

This is a drill down into the personal life of the patient from birth until the time of the first psychiatric interview. Some of the aspects in each portion of this expansive timespan are as follows –

- **Birth –** Was the conception planned or unplanned, pre-, or post-marital? In Asian societies, it is usually post-marital but unplanned. Was it a wanted or unwanted pregnancy? Was it considered a 'precious' pregnancy or an accidental one? Is there consanguinity? Recently, the history of whether the pregnancy was natural or medically assisted, or adoption has become necessary. Birth defects, abnormalities, and medical issues in the early post-natal period must also be asked for.

- **Early development –** milestone developments must be asked for. Any issues during early development such as thumb sucking, bed wetting, sleep problem, etc., are asked for. If necessary, do not hesitate to ask about a history of abuse or neglect.

- **Education –** How was school initiated? Any issues with school performance, delinquencies, frequent school change (and the reason for each change), extracurricular performance, participation in group activities, general level of competitiveness, and peer relationships, are the aspects to be ascertained.

- **Work/employment –** How was the job obtained? Any issues with job performance, repeated changes in employment, history of conflicts in the work environment, history of long-term unemployment, or 'gaps in the CV' must be determined. Trivial reasons for quitting or changing jobs, the value given to the job in the patient's life, and satisfaction in the job are essential aspects to be ascertained.

- **Menstrual history** – history related to age at menarche, regularity, and menopause is gathered (just as taught in gynecological rotations). Important here is ascertaining the emotional reaction or 'value' given to menstrual periods and fertility in general.

- **Sexual history** – age at sexual initiation, method of sexual knowledge acquisition, sexual preferences, orientation, difficulties in sexual functioning, and further workup if the patient wishes more intervention.

- **Marital history** – Age at first marriage, circumstances surrounding the marriage, level of familiarity prior to marriage, the age of the spouse, the reaction or aftermath experience of the marriage, presence of consanguinity, and marital issues such as discord, unhappiness, separation, divorce, etc. The details must be collected for each marriage and the length of each marriage.

- **Progenial history** – I use this term to refer to the history related to the patient's children. Details of the children, their biological parents in relation to the parents, and medical and psychological issues in each child must be gathered.

Premorbid personality and Premorbid functional status——

This section is very important. Personality is different from functional status. Personality is the nature of the person prior to the onset of any disorder or illness. Personality is not an illness. So, if you need to incorporate any aspect of the patient's history into his/her history of illness, it must reconcile with the nature of the patient prior to your deduced time of onset of the patient's disorder. Personality disorders are also not mental illnesses. As per the Ulan concept, some personality disorders fall under the category of 'mentally not healthy' and must not be considered as 'mentally unhealthy' or 'mentally ill'. The nuance here is that patients with stronger personalities or personality disorders may be functioning well, or even better than expected, while patients who do not have any underlying personality issues or disorders may be functioning poorly. Functional status in psychiatric history refers to a 360-degree assessment of the patient's premorbid psychological status, with a special focus on high-yield aspects as follows –

- **Temperament –** refer to the chapter on personality disorders to understand temperament. Temperament affects how a patient reacts to the environment and can be assessed by inquiring about preferences, beliefs, daily routines, habits, and value systems. Explore whether the patient likes and welcomes new responsibilities or significant life changes or shuns or avoids such changes – this could give an idea of the overall temperament.

- **Social role –** does the person assume (or prefer to assume) the role of a leader vs follower, ambitious or 'go with the flow' type, industrious or relaxed, submissive, or dominant, adaptive or intolerant, proactive or reactive, likes or shuns new responsibilities: Probe deeper into interpersonal relationships. These questions could give you an idea of the role the patient plays in his/her social life, so you can work on restoring this baseline, and not a position that you may see as ideal.

- **Habits and routine –** Try to reconstruct 'a day in the life of ... ' the patient prior to your deduced time of onset of the disorder or complaint. Information about habits and routines could give you a pretty good idea in this regard and would inform you of what the patient 'values' in his/her life, and the aspects they try to avoid. Eating habits (including food fads), leisure activities, preferred places to hang out, hygiene/toilet habits, sleep habits, and religious activities provide helpful information.

Examination of a Psychiatry Patient

Examination is an expansive topic, encompassing both physical examination and mental status examination. Physical examination must be focused so that significant clues or organic pathology are not missed. Height, weight, BMI, and vital signs (especially blood pressure, heart rate, and rhythm) must be obtained. Some high-yield physical examination signs include –

- Fundus examination.
- Look for signs of deliberate self-harm (linear scars and bruises on extensor surfaces, especially wrists and thighs, and tattoos, piercings, and marks).
- Surgical scars (abdominal, facial).

- Posturing (voluntary and involuntary).
- Motor activity – tics, weakness, akinesia, akathisia, hyper-
      tonicity, spasticity, rigidity, dystonia, tremor, myoclonus,
      chorea, athetosis, tardive dyskinesia, grunting,
      catatonia, cataplexy, waxy flexibility.

Then comes the core mental status examination, i.e., the 'MSE proper'. The latter consists of two parts, the general appearance, and the Ulan examination.

General appearance

Appearance includes face, dress/attire, and behavior. Facial appearance reflects the mood component of the Ulan, whereas attire and behavior reflect the mood/thought component. Facial appearance faithfully reflects depression, anxiety, and mania quite accurately. The mood is infectious and a mere gaze at the face can transmit the quality of the affect to the examiner effectively. This is why actors can invoke the desired mood in their audiences through facial expressions. Attire/dress reflects self-care, self-hygiene, diligence, and attitude. Behavior includes responses to stimuli, especially those of the psychiatrist interviewing the patient. Suspiciousness, defensiveness, silly smile, inappropriate gaze, unprovoked or needless laughter, restlessness (fidgeting), oppositional behavior, hyperactivity, and echopraxia could be obviously noted. At this point, even prior to the Ulan examination, you should be able to ballpark the level of psychomotor activity status of the patient, which is a broad yet reliable marker for the overall psychiatric functional status of the patient.

Next is the examination of the Ulan. Ulan has three components – mood, thought, and intellect, which all work in seamless amalgamation. First, examine each of these three components individually, and then determine if they are functioning in good coordination.

Examination of the mood component of the Ulan

I have discussed the definition of affect, and what constitutes normal and abnormal mood in the chapter on affective disorders. Please refer to that chapter for a detailed understanding. In MSE, you must be clear about specific terms, and use them accurately while documenting. The relevant terms are – mood, affect, emotions, and feelings.

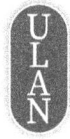

Mood is the general state of quality experienced by the Ulan. Affect is the medical term for 'mood' and is a better term for medical communication. Affect (or mood) is a state of the experience of the Ulan and is typically long-lasting (usually days, weeks, or more). In the ideal state, the affect is not felt in any quality by the person. Affect is readily felt in response to environmental/internal stimuli. In other words, affect is realized as the response (and hence the term 'affect') to stimuli. These stimuli could be environmental or thoughts that Ulan generates. It is the general background state of the Ulan experience. Emotions, on the other hand, are 'specific', and occur in response to a stimulus. They are typically short-lived (usually minutes or hours). A good analogy is the difference between the season (or climate) and weather. Affect/mood is like the season or climate and refers to a broad theme over a more extended period. Emotions are like the weather and change by the hour. Affect is spontaneous and more resistant to simple environmental changes. People wake up from sleep in a certain mood. There may be no reason or object attached to the mood. Emotions occur in the context of ongoing environmental stimuli, against the backdrop of the affective state. Patients (and people in general) focus a lot on their emotions and tend to elaborate on them more, going into more granular detail. However, ***emotions are not a clinical target for therapy*** – it is the mood, which lies further beneath the flurry of emotions that the patient may talk about. The psychiatrist must resist being pulled into extrapolating emotions to the affective state of the Ulan. The mood is broadly reported as a 'good' or 'bad' mood, while emotions are broadly reported as 'positive' or 'negative' feelings. Examples of mood/affect include – depressive state, manic state, hypomanic state, irritable state, agitated state, and anxious state. Emotions include sadness, happiness, excitement, amusement, wonder, anger, hostility, nervousness, shame, surprise, guilt, fear, gratitude, etc.

The affective state, in turn, is understood in two dimensions – the 'subjective mood', and the 'objective mood'. The subjective mood is the mood reported by the patient. Objective mood is inferred by the psychiatrist through deduction using the information collected by his history taking and examination. The subjective mood has certain limitations for use as a clinical target – it could reflect the emotional state (rather than the mood) as the patient may be unable to differentiate between mood and emotion. Second, the subjective mood is subject to the patient's intention, will, and judgment. Sometimes, they conclude this is 'how one should feel in this situation'. In other words, the subjective mood could be the thought about the mood, not the mood itself.   Objective mood is assessed by the examiner, verifiable and more reliable to be used as a clinical target. The objective mood could be assessed again through appearance, dress/attire, behavior, and interrogation.

At this point, determine the following – Is the mood appropriate regarding the quality and intensity of the life situation? If not, it signifies a pathological affective state. Here, go deeper into the examination of the Ulan to determine congruence of the affective state to environmental stimuli, and the thought component of the Ulan. For further clarification on this topic, please refer to the chapter on Mood disorders.

Examination of the thought component of the Ulan ——————

Thought is the product of the Ulan. There is nothing else that the Ulan produces, except thoughts. Mood is the quality of the Ulan, and thought is its content. Thought is autonomous and originates spontaneously. There is no need for any stimulus for thoughts to occur. However, environmental stimuli affect and influence the type of thoughts produced. Thoughts also vary in nature depending on the mood component of the Ulan. For example, if the affect is depressed, the thoughts are congruent to a depressed state. If the affect is elated, the thoughts tend to be of such nature too. Also, the Ulan *can summon thoughts of any nature, at its will*. It does so by the ability of the intellect component of the Ulan. In summary, thought is the product of the Ulan, and is autonomous in production but can be influenced by the other components of the Ulan. Thoughts are formless and dissipate immediately. However, in the physiological state of the Ulan, thought production can be controlled, and thoughts can be dismissed, or retained without dissipation.

Now, let us understand specific other terms and phenomena related to thought. While the affect is 'experienced', thought is 'realized'. Since thoughts are autonomous, they are first produced and are then realized – which is why the word is used in the past tense ('thought') when implied as a noun i.e., We use the word 'thoughts', not 'thinks' for the noun form. Thinking is the conscious summoning of thought production. Even

while thinking, thoughts are realized after they are produced. The quality
and speed of thought production in the normal functioning state
depends on the intellect component of the Ulan. The Ulan can
summon thoughts, can order thought production, but ***cannot
control the type of thought*** that emerges. After the thought has
emerged, it is realized.

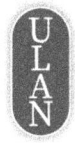

Next, you need to be clear about other aspects of thought such as perception, memory, attention, focus/concentration, and cognition –

Thoughts realized in response to a sensory stimulus are called 'perception'. When an individual receives a sensory stimulus, it produces varied
responses in different people. The type of experience depends on the
Ulan of the individual. Thus, the thoughts produced in response to the
stimulus depend on the person and cannot be generalized. Hence the term
per-ception. Perception does not mean that the patient is unable to recount
the sensory stimulus accurately, in other words, perception is limited
to subjective thought differences in response to sensory experiences. If
the individual reports a variant sensory experience, it is not a perception
problem. It becomes a more profound thought disorder, which is of two
further types – illusion (altered report of sensory stimuli), or hallucination
(report of an absent sensory stimuli).

Memory refers to the recall function of prior thoughts. Once thoughts
are realized, they are 'stored' in the Ulan and may be recalled at will. The
ability to do this is called memory, and this function is enabled primarily
by the intellect component of the Ulan and may be influenced in part by
the affect component too.

Attention is the ability of the Ulan to control the production of thoughts
at will. Since thought production depends on sensory input, the ability to
maintain thought production in an orderly is called attention. The basic
concept here is that thoughts are produced by the Ulan, to enable the
individual to complete a task for one's own benefit. To do so, thoughts
must be produced in an orderly and stable fashion. They must be related to
one another and proceed incrementally in a logical fashion to complete the
task. The ability to maintain thought production in this fashion is called
attention.

Concentration or 'focus' refers to the ability to summon extra force to increase the intensity of attention. In Tamil, 'focus' is translated as 'kuvi', which means 'to heap'. In simpler terms, concentration is nothing but a more intense form of the faculty of attention.

> Just like the Ulan can summon a thought, the Ulan is also capable of dismissing a thought. Unwanted and unpleasant thoughts may arise spontaneously, but the Ulan must be able to dismiss them, with little to no difficulty. If Ulan is unable to dismiss the thought, then it is called an 'obsession'.

Let's recap a bit now – thought production is autonomous, but there is a section of thoughts that occur in response to the sensory stimulus. These thoughts that occur in response to a sensory stimulus are called 'perception'. Innumerable autonomous and perceived thoughts occur every day, but only some are available for recall, which is called 'memory'. The ability to control thought production and flow in relation to a particular sensory stimulus is called 'attention', and the ability to boost attention at will is called 'concentration' or 'focus'. Finally, what is the purpose of this thought process? How does all this benefit the individual? The answer is that all these thoughts are used to construct an understanding of the world around us – i.e., to build a 'system' or 'schema' of all information collected based on these thoughts, for problem-solving purposes. This schema is also used to achieve targets or reach goals, whatever they may be. This constructed 'system' or 'schema' is called 'knowledge', otherwise called 'arivu' in Tamil. I use the word 'arivu' here, instead of simply using the word 'knowledge' or 'knowing', because the word 'know' has two implications – (1) to 'know' means to be aware of data or information, which in Tamil is called 'therivu' and (2) to 'know' means to have a system or framework of information on which problems are approached to get the solution, and this type of knowledge is called 'arivu'. This arivu has now gained the term 'cognition' in English recently. The word 'cognition' is relatively new in the field of psychiatry. It is being used a lot, and many times inaccurately. Cognitive abnormalities in their most severe form have been known to psychiatry as 'delusions'. Cognitive abnormalities, not amounting to delusions are common and are now discovered to be the underlying cause of most life stressors and unpleasant living. Although cognition is composed of thoughts, the construction of cognition depends on various mental faculties, all of which are categorized under the 'intellect' component of the Ulan.

Now that you understand thought, perception, memory, attention, and cognition, examine each individually while conducting the MSE. Remember – you cannot know what the patient thinks. It is impossible to do that. Many lay people also have this misconception, that the psychiatrist knows what others think. It is not so. You, as a psychiatrist, through accumulated evidence and knowledge in medicine in general, and psychiatry in specific, can 'deduce' or conclude through conjecture the underlying processes of the Ulan, thought being one of them. The process of this deduction is solely limited to medical purposes – to relieve the patient's suffering or 'pathos'; and not to solve every unanswered question in the world. In order to begin such deduction, you must examine the patient's Ulan in an organized fashion.

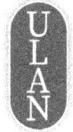

A normal thought process consists of a thought which typically progresses linearly (in one direction), increases incrementally, progresses to a conclusion, and then disappears.

Approach the thought component of the Ulan, in two dimensions – content and flow. The most evident way to examine the thought is to examine the speech. What one says, and how one says it are the two dimensions. Other substitutes for thought delivery include writing, drawing, gestures, facial expressions, or actions. Several abnormalities of speech flow have been described, as follows –

- **Irrelevancy –** is when speech reflects no context of thought with the sensory environment.

- **Coherence –** is when speech reflects no orderly sequencing or continuity of thought

- **Circumstantial –** is when speech reflects the inability of thought to progress to a conclusion. It may be called 'beating around the bush'. The individual's speech is circumlocutory, unnecessarily digressive, has plenty of parenthetical clarification, and goes 'around and around'. This type of speech usually reflects some level of organic brain issues.

- **Tangential –** is when speech reflects a thought process that is not linear. The thought progresses in one direction not for long, before which it branches into another direction, and hence the initial thought never increases incrementally or reaches a conclusion.

- **Flight** – is when speech reflects erratic thought production. The patient talks of one topic and then quickly shifts to another. Thoughts occur in bursts, do not progress, and do not conclude either.

- **Loosening** – Otherwise called 'looseness of association'. It is when speech reflects thought progression that is weak, and hence not able to reach an effective conclusion. Such a person does have a thought process that is 'somewhat normal', but the strength of the process is not reasonable or adequate. Often the link between different thoughts is based on illogical details (which the individual considers as logical). This type of thought move is called the 'knight's move', based on the movement of the knight (horse piece) in chess, where it goes linear for a bit and then could swing either way.

- **Perseveration** – is when speech reflects the inability of thought to progress. The patient typically responds to all questions with the answer to the first question. This condition also may be associated with organic brain problems.

- **Thought block** – is when speech reflects sudden cessation of thought production. It is evidenced as a sudden halt in speech.

- **Fusion** – is when speech reflects fused or combined thoughts. The patient used 'new words' (such as neologisms), representing thought fusion.

- **Muddling** – is when speech reflects an extreme degree of disruption in the thought process. An extreme degree of derailment, or fusion of thoughts.

- **Overinclusive thinking** – is when speech reflects an inability to preserve conceptual boundaries of the topic/subject of the thought. The patient's thoughts 'wander off the reservation' to related topics but not contributory.

- **Pseudologica fantastica** – is when speech reflects fantasy thought production. Fantasy is the mental construction of improbable imagery, often through fusion or extension of real-life thoughts. Fantasy is a function of the Ulan to fulfill a mental need, or express thoughts or concepts that have not become consolidated into words.

- **Approximation** – is when speech reflects a tendency of thoughts to avoid conclusive accuracy to verbal stimuli. When a patient is asked a question, the reply is an approximate answer, even though an apparent accurate answer is readily available.

- **Echolalia** – is when speech auditorily reproduces thoughts generated in response to auditory sounds (like sounds in the environment). The patient takes in the sounds from the environment and reproduces them (i.e., echoes the sounds)

The above are some types of speech that reflect an abnormality in the thought component of the Ulan. Remember that these are ***not speech abnormalities, but speech that reflect pathologies of thought*** that manifested through speech.

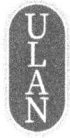

Now let us discuss the other dimension of thought – content. Is it possible to categorize thought as normal or abnormal based on its content? The simple answer is no. As mentioned before, thought production is autonomous, and although thought can be summoned by will, the exact content of thought cannot be controlled. So, a person cannot be held accountable or responsible for the thoughts that occur to oneself. The next question – is it possible to objectively witness the content of another person's thought? The answer is a no again. You cannot witness another person's thoughts, and as a psychiatrist, you can only observe the behavior (including speech) and use reported behavior from other sources to come to a conclusion. The patient can report the content of his/her thoughts, but it cannot be used as the sole source of data to assess the thought component. Evaluation of the thought component could demonstrate one of the following major types of abnormalities, the most conspicuous of which is delusion.

Delusion – As discussed above, thoughts are the building blocks for constructing a system of knowledge about the world, called 'cognition'. When thoughts emerge in such a way that cognition is markedly disrupted, the individual's cognition about the world is so inaccurate and wrong, at which point it is called a 'delusion'. Etymologically, 'de-' implies broken or split, and '-lude' refers to the main play or act (i.e., primary content). 'Delude' implies a broken content of thought. The fundamental delusion is often isolated to a specific aspect of the cognition, but then the rest of the cognition must play catch up to accommodate the primary disordered thought. In other words, the building blocks (thoughts) are abnormal, leading to abnormal cognition. How is a delusion manifested? It is manifested as a system of thoughts that cannot be evidenced (i.e., beliefs) and not agreed upon by the majority of the population causing disruption in the functioning of the individual in the society These are called 'false beliefs'. Delusions (abnormalities of thought) are also generated autonomously (emerging 'out of the blue'). Delusions come in various flavors and forms.

Think of the pathology of cognition as a spectrum, with the least pathological disruption being mild cognitive deficits requiring cognitive therapy, and delusions occupying the other end. Between these two ends is a form of cognitive abnormality that would qualitatively mimic delusions but fall short in intensity to qualify for the definition of delusions, which are called overvaluations, or overvalued ideas.

Based on the scope of the delusion, they are of two types -

- **Encapsulated delusion –** reflects a thought system disrupted in one area of global cognition. For example, the patient may be unable to trust the spouse and have delusions of betrayal.

- **Systematized delusions –** reflect a thought system that has multiple isolated delusions that become interconnected. For example, the patient has an extensive broad cognitive framework that the government or authority is plotting against him/her, their family, neighbors, town or city, etc.

Based on the primary content of the delusion, they are of the following types –

- **Grandoise –** is the term used when the thought content pertains to an unreal elevated sense of the self. The patient thinks they are powerful, supernatural, extraordinarily talented, extraordinarily attractive, influential, resistant to trauma or disease, immortal, etc.

- **Erotomanic –** is the term used when thought content is that another person (usually someone who is much higher in social position than the self) is romantically in love with the patient. It usually occurs in the setting of bipolar disorder, schizophrenia, or schizoaffective disorder, and responds to electroconvulsive therapy. In a sense, erotomanic delusion is the romantic form of a grandiose delusion.

- **Jealous** – is the term used when the thought content pertains to unreasonable suspicion of betrayal by a spouse, intimate partner, or friend.

- **Nihilistic** – is the term used when the thought content pertains to an unreal deflated sense of self. The patient feels powerless or extraordinarily defective. It is the qualitative opposite of the grandiose delusion.

- **Passivity** – is the term used when the thought content pertains to being controlled by another entity (other than one's own self). It is similar in quality to a paranoid delusion.

- **Persecutory** – is the term used when the thought content pertains to being attacked or targeted (spied, surveilled, followed, harassed, etc.,) by another entity. It is also akin to a paranoid delusion.

- **Reference** – is the term used when the thought content pertains to being the point of reference to environmental stimuli. The patient feels that objects present around them, incidents that happen in the environment, or utterances of people all, in a way, refer to them. Another type of paranoid delusion.

- **Somatic** – is the term used when the thought content pertains to being afflicted by a disease. Often by a type of infection, virus, or parasite, or being taken over by a deadly disease. This is also a type of paranoia.

- **Control** – is the term used when the thought content pertains to being controlled or 'operated' by another entity (other than the self).

- **Misidentification** – is the term used when the thought content pertains to the self, or a known other person is being an imposter, or a transformation of another.

The above are some of the flavors of delusion, mainly of the paranoid type. They are not diagnostic but are merely terms used to refer to the content of the thought abnormality.

Now, let us discuss some of the thought abnormalities that are commonly confused or misdiagnosed as delusions.

- **Obsessions** – refer to thoughts that cannot be dismissed. The content and flow of thought, and the speech that reflects the thought are not affected. As mentioned above, in the physiological state of the Ulan, thought production can be dismissed. Once the self dismisses a particular thought, it should stop being produced eventually. If thoughts keep appearing despite dismissal, it is called an obsession. Obsessive thoughts occur in all people, but they rise to the level of being pathological in some people. The affect component of the Ulan senses this abnormal production of thoughts and reacts with anxiety. Behaviors emerge to ward off anxiety, which is called 'compulsions'. When the compulsive behavior becomes consolidated, i.e., becomes well-evolved to the point of what, where, how, how many, and when the compulsive act is to be performed, it is called a 'ritual'.

- **Phobia** – must be differentiated from delusion, in that the thought content is not abnormal in phobias. It is the affective state in response to a thought that is exaggerated. The thought of the target object related to the fear response is not necessarily an abnormal thought – for example, being afraid of heights, spiders, or closed spaces is not abnormal. However, an exaggerated fear disabling the patient's functioning is pathological. However, after phobia sets in, some thought patterns tend to get disrupted to accommodate for the disruption in the affect (because all components of the Ulan function in unison, and a disruption in one component results in a disruption in the others).

- **Illusion** – Etymologically, 'il-' means 'absent', and '-lude' means 'in play' or 'in action'. So, illusion means 'not in play' or 'not in the act'. Illusion reflects an abnormality of thought, in having a perception without a stimulus. There is no abnormality in the content of the thought (as in delusion).

- **Hallucination** – Is a perception (i.e., a thought in response to a sensory stimulus) disorder, wherein the perception occurs without an external sensory stimulus, or more specifically, a brain activity mimicking an external stimulus. The patient is in a clear state of consciousness and perceives a sensation without an external stimulus. Often, hallucination is defined as 'false perception', which is a somewhat inaccurate use of terminology. Perception is the thought of a patient, and hence cannot be categorized as true or false. For the patient, every perception is real. It is the observer (i.e., the doctor) who must determine if the perception is appropriate to the environmental stimulus. Hallucinations, being thoughts, are not verifiable objectively, but can be deduced with accuracy. Any of the five sensory inputs may be involved, and more than one can be involved in the same patient as well. They occur with organic and non-organic etiologies of psychiatric disorders. Some of the commonly discussed descriptions of hallucinations are -

- **Hypnogogic** - occurring prior to sleep, usually visual.

- **Hypnopompic** - occurring at the time of transitioning to wakefulness from sleep.

- **Elementary** - isolated sensory perceptions, such as seeing stars or objects, or hearing whistles, rattles, machinery sounds, etc.

- **Complex** - perception thought complexes, such as fully formed imagery, or a voice talking in complete sentences.

- **Command** - ordering the subject to indulge in a particular action.

- **Autoscopic** - hallucinating of one's own self.

- **Haptic** - involving touch, or tactile-related perceptions.

- **Olfactory** - involving smell or odor.

- **Gustatory** - involving taste.

- **Ictal** - occurring as part of a seizure episode or disorder.

- **Migrainous** - occurring as part of a migraine episode or disorder.

- **First person hallucination** - auditory perception where one's own thought being voiced in words.

- **Second person hallucination** - perception that someone else is talking with or to the patient.

- **Third person hallucination** - perception that people around the patient, or at a distance are talking about, to or with the patient.

There is also a term 'pseudo hallucination', which is a term that I recommend not to be used. The term has been used to refer to those perceptual distortions of which the patient has insight. These are sensory distortions that the patient reports as illusory. For example, the patient may report distortions in visual-spatial schema, such as macropsia, or micropsia, or distortions in color, distance, etc. This term is better avoided as it gives the impression of falsification or feigning and may result in misunderstandings by the patient, and sometimes by other non-psychiatrists. Two other phenomena in the differential diagnosis of thought-related symptoms are depersonalization and derealization. These phenomena are altered perceptual experiences, but there is no evidence of abnormality in the content or flow of thought. They are both 'as if' experiences. Depersonalization refers to a condition where the patient has an experience 'as if' the self is detached from the Ulan. The patient experiences feelings, not as one's own, but of another person, which is the body of the self. Derealization is a much more distressing and disabling condition where the patient has an experience 'as if' all experience of reality (i.e., the outside world) is unreal or vague. Patients find it hard to describe this experience and do recognize it is not imposed on them by outside forces (unlike hallucinations arising from schizophrenia-type illnesses).

In summary, all these types of hallucinations are variations of disturbances of the thought component of the Ulan – the only difference being the subset or dimension of the thought component of the Ulan that is primarily affected. It could be the form, flow, or perception. The individual subtypes are more of academic importance than clinical significance. In the clinic, the most relevant aspects are the content of the hallucination, as hallucinations, in general, may be quietened but not entirely eliminated as they are resistant to standard pharmacological intervention. Non-pharmacological methods and strategies are needed, which must be tailor-made to the content of the hallucination.

Examination of the Intellect component of the Ulan————

Now, let us move on to the examination of the intellect component of the Ulan. Intellect is the faculty of Ulan that builds the framework called 'cognition'. How well cognition is built is based on how effectively thoughts are retained, how well they are recalled, and how they are used in building the cognitive framework that serves the individual for survival benefit, both in the short and long term. Cognition has a broad scope and mental status examination during the initial visit is geared to examine simple thought frameworks – orientation, attention, memory, abstraction, general fund of knowledge, judgment, and insight.

- **Orientation –** refers to the ability of the thought processes to be congruent with the environment. The environment consists of three dimensions - time, space, and context/object. Accordingly, orientation may be tested in three dimensions, namely time, place, and person. The individual must be able to relate to the correct current time (year, month, day, and time of the day), correct current place (country, state or city, and the building), and correct current persons in the surrounding (who he/she is, who are the people surrounding them). In the clinical setting, one of the common questions asked to start with this portion of the examination is 'What is your name?', and 'What is your date of birth?' and to correlate this with the information obtained prior to the examination. These two questions are commonly used in the inpatient setting while examining a patient for altered states of consciousness or delirium. It is possible that the patient could be oriented to time, place, and person, but still not be accurate about the overall orientation. Try these questions – 'Why are you here?', 'What is happening here?', or 'Who is the President?'. These questions can quickly ascertain if there are any abnormalities in orientation. If the orientation is intact, further examination of intellect would be worthy and contributory.

- **Attention –** Attention is the ability to maintain the thought production to one stimulus. It is effortless and involuntary. The ability to summon extra effort to attention is called focus or concentration. Attention is assessed through simple tasks such as counting from 100 backward, reciting the days of the week or months of the year backward, or the alphabet backward. Or you may give them a series of random numbers and ask them to repeat the series after you. Or a simple arithmetic task, such as 'I will give you a number, and you must first multiply that number by 2, give me the answer, and then add 7 to the resultant number and give me the answer again'. Before you conduct these tasks, explain the task and that you are doing so to test their attention. These tests are invalid if the patient is drowsy, or under the influence of drugs or medications that affect cerebral functioning or arousal level.

- **Memory –** After thoughts are experienced by the Ulan, they are then 'encoded' into data. The data is then available for retrieval, or recall. Memory is the ability to recall thoughts. However, deficits in memory may be due to deficits in encoding, or deficits in recall. There is no straightforward way to tease this difference clinically. The best you could do is to first test encoding – ask the patient to see an object, touch an object blindfolded, or hear a sound or audio. Then have them explain what they saw, felt, or heard. If there is an abnormality at this level, then there is a problem with the encoding aspect of the memory. If they can do this adequately, then move on to recall. Recall is tested at three levels –

  - **Immediate recall –** which is testing ultra short-term memory, such as a set of numbers or images of objects seen seconds to minutes ago.

  - **Short-term recall –** which is testing short-term memory, such as the weather that morning, the menu on their morning breakfast, or the news on the radio or TV that morning.

  - **Long-term recall –** which is testing recall of consolidated and notable events in the patient's life, such as events surrounding anniversaries, marriage, retirement, graduation ceremonies, etc.

  Memory can be evident and tested in several dimensions. Declarative memory is the recall of facts, principles, or concepts. Procedural memory is the recall of techniques or skills, often relating to 'doing' something. Biographical memory is the chronological retention of the past events, often associated with mood associated with the events. Confabulatory memory relates to events that are concocted to fill in gaps in memory, and the patient does not realize these are not true memories. Again, deficits in these memories may be due to defects in encoding the thoughts or recall of the adequately encoded thoughts.

- **Abstraction –** Etymologically, 'abstract' is 'ab-' + 'tract', implying 'taking away from the tract'. Essentially, it means 'what you can take away from'... from a larger body of information. It is the concise, or crystallized form of a thought process. The opposite of abstraction would be to hold information in the raw form with details. For example, if there is a room with a table surrounded by chairs, with plates and cups in the table, and fruits, the abstraction is that it is a dinner table.

In the absence of abstraction, the individual would only see the objects, without extrapolating what they mean. This is an example of simple abstraction. Abstraction is the critical force behind cognitive ability. Events, facts, and details are then compounded to come up with simpler expressions, called complex abstraction. A good example is proverbs or wise sayings. Ask the patient to explain a well-known proverb, such as 'all that glitters is not gold'. The patient may have a simple abstraction such as 'all glittering objects are not made of gold', or a more complex abstraction 'external appearances may be deceptive'. Another proverb to ask to explain is 'Don't judge a book by the cover'. A brilliant example of a very complex abstraction, reflecting cognitive process is the Thirukkural. If you have not heard of the Thirukkural, you must look it up. It is an excellent example of a very complex abstraction.

- **General fund of knowledge** – This refers to the 'volume' of knowledge a person has in general. It may be broad-based or relatively weighted towards some regions of relevance or interest to the person. Nevertheless, it is very important. Ask the patient about a wide range of topics and keep it simple and superficial. Then ask more about what relates to them most and see how deep their knowledge is – for example, a farmer may not know a lot about the economy of the country, or world politics, but may have a wealthy repository of agricultural topics, or details of farming methods. The general fund of knowledge is a retrograde method to infer the overall functioning of cognition. Those whose cognition is functioning well will end up with a larger fund of knowledge than those who have a lesser level of cognition.

- **Judgment** – In the clinical context, judgment implies the ability to analyze varying thoughts, and then conclude on how to act appropriately. An example of simple judgment would be 'you are walking on the street when someone asks you for directions to an address. While giving directions, you also observe a child crossing the street unassisted in the middle of traffic. What would you do?'. The answer must not be assessed based on what is right or wrong but on the simple act of being able to conclude what is more appropriate. Crying for help, calling someone else to grab the child, quitting the conversation, and running to help the child are all appropriate answers.

- **Insight** – Insight refers to the cognitive ability of the patient to objectively assess the status of one's own Ulan. Insight has a high prognostic impact, the better the insight, the better the prognosis. Insight also predicts cooperation with the psychiatrist, and compliance with treatment. Insight is measured along as scale, such as 0 - complete denial ('nothing is wrong with me'), 1 - slight awareness ('I am affected, but I need help'), 2 – mediocre awareness ('I am affected, but it is because of others/external factors), 3 – high awareness ('I am affected, the problem is with me, but I don't need help as nothing can be done), 4 - intellectual awareness ('I am affected, it is because of me and my thinking patterns, and I can do something about it), 5 - emotional insight ('I can modify my thinking patterns to avoid problems in future, and I am willing to do so').

Some of the questions that are helpful in exploring insight are – 'What do you think is going on?', 'What do you think is the problem here?', or 'What do you think will solve this problem?'.

In summary, the intellect component of the Ulan is composed of orientation, attention and concentration, memory, abstraction, general fund of knowledge, judgment, and insight. All these together determine the ability of the Ulan to 'survive' in this world (by problem-solving), and the latter is measured as 'intelligence'. Intelligence is measurable by standardized testing and expressed as a relative position of the tested person compared to the rest of the population, i.e., 'intelligence quotient' (IQ). It must be kept in mind that traditional IQ tests weigh heavily on memory, attention, concentration, general fund of knowledge and abstraction, and much less on judgment or insight. However, they are helpful adjuncts.

All the above is only a primer for mental status examination. Each individual diagnosis or presenting problem would require a more detailed examination. The two questions posed to patients that I find very useful, prior to concluding the interview, or if I am unsure if I have gathered all details, or if I am running out of time are (Mananalam Clinic Experience) –

- Is there anything else you would like to tell me?
- Is there anything else you would like me to ask about? (Is there any question that you would like me to answer?)

After these questions, you may have open a whole new Pandora's box, so be prepared!

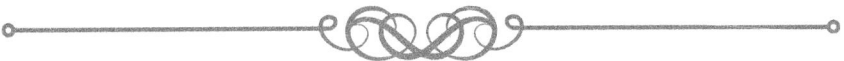

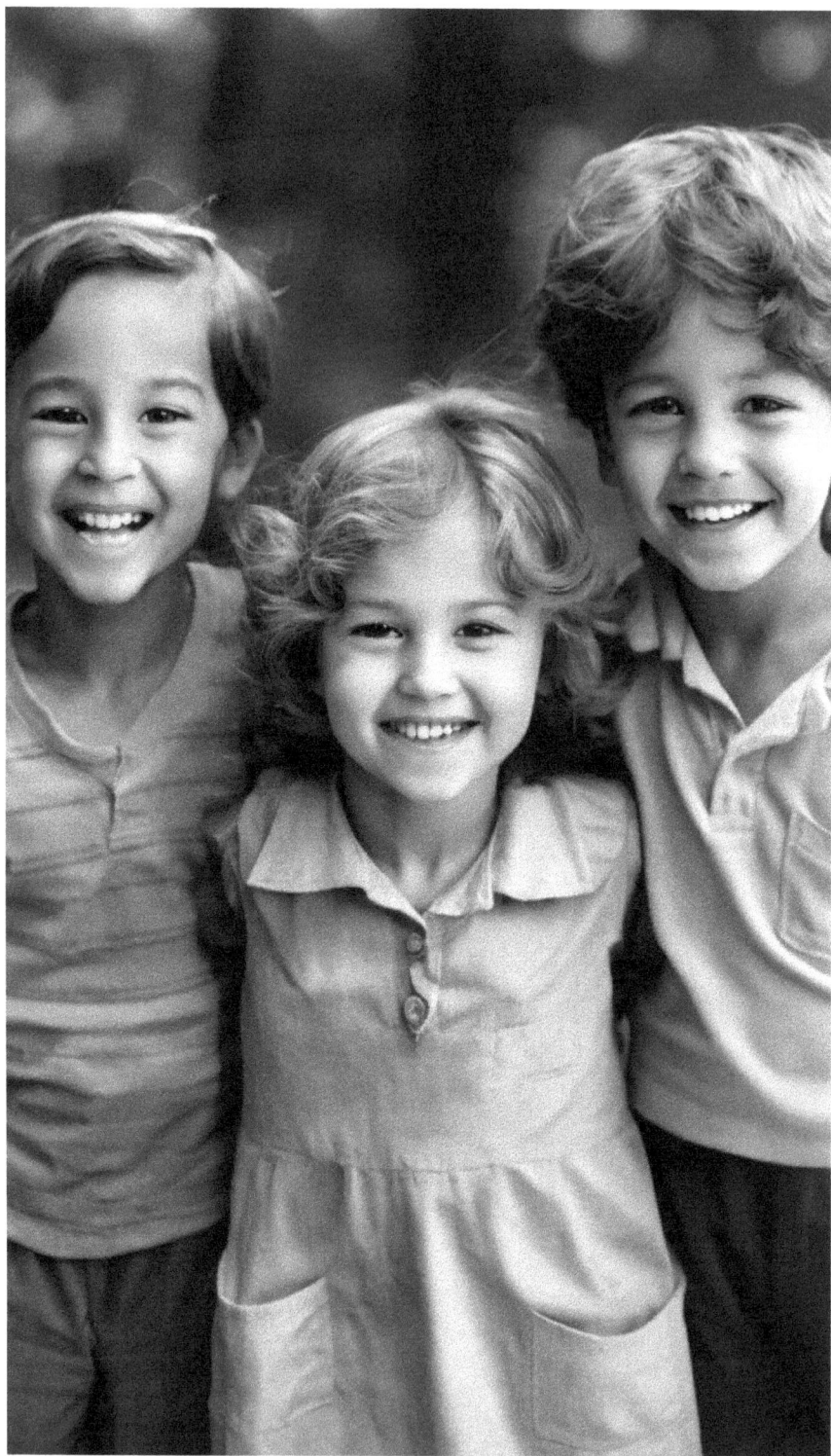

CHAPTER 6

The Child Patient

Other Contributors: Dr. V. Jayanthini, MD, Dr. Thendral

Importance of Child Psychiatry

The acceptance of the concept that mental illnesses are medical disorders in the mainstream medical community is a relatively new phenomenon in the long history of medicine. Accepting the idea that such mental diseases could occur in children is an even newer one. Although the importance of childhood experiences in the development of adult mental disorders has been recognized at least since the time of Sigmund Freud and popularized by him, it did not evolve into a dedicated branch of psychiatry until much later.

One of the medical graduates of the University of Berlin, an Austrian named Leo Kanner (1894-1981), later emigrated to the United States of America, where he founded the first department of Child Psychiatry at the Johns Hopkins Hospital in 1930. Later, in 1934, the first academic journal in child psychiatry in German was published. In 1936, Dr. Kanner also established elective courses in child psychiatry, and eventually, the child and adolescent psychiatry fellows at Johns Hopkins University continued to be called 'Kanner Fellows'.

However, the popular opinion and emphasis on the importance of child psychiatry have seen both extremes. The public has, and still does to a large degree, consider that psychiatric disorders in children are not 'real' but instead a mere sequela of poor education or upbringing. Claims that mental disorders are manifestations of emotional maladjustments that can be addressed through education and counseling alone are still legitimate. On the other hand, the academic community has sometimes gone to the other extreme of suggesting that nearly all adult psychiatric disorders have childhood origins and that dramatic efforts to identify and treat childhood problems could prevent the need for adult mental health care. In my opinion, the latter is just wishful thinking; most mental health disorders can indeed be diagnosed early during childhood, and it is also true that there is a fair proportion of mental health issues that are exclusive to the childhood age, diverse enough not to be boxed into firm diagnostic silos, and likely amenable to successful non-pharmacological intervention alone.

How is Child Psychiatry Different From Adult Psychiatry?

According to the widely used etymology resource etymonline.com, the word 'child' is derived from the proto-germanic word 'kiltham', the old Danish word 'kuld', or the Swedish word 'kulder'. In Tamil, the word, 'kulanda' is used. As per the Merriam-Webster dictionary, the word 'child' refers to a young person between infancy and puberty. Infancy refers to an individual less than 12 months of age. Puberty refers to the milestone of reproductive capability in an individual, which is often considered 12 years of age in females and 14 years of age in males. During childhood, the individual is often incapable of reproductive function, which is still in the stage of maturing until puberty. After puberty, an individual, although capable of reproduction, does not reach mental maturation for another few years until society does not confer civil rights to that individual. Such a young adult between puberty and the legal age of majority is called an 'adolescent'. Hence, this field is often called 'child and adolescent psychiatry' or 'pediatric psychiatry'.

Childhood is a ***fluid state*** of physical and mental growth, which makes it a cherished experience. But such fluidity also makes this period in life vulnerable to injury. Factors such as the helplessness of the newly born infant, the long duration of childhood, and the differential speeds of development between the physical, intellectual, emotional, and sexual aspects of maturation bring forth a unique and diverse set of clinical disorders at each age. Physiological functions such as sleep, eating, excretion, speech, sexual behavior, and emotional sensitivities, which need to be integrated into the growth process, are susceptible to disturbances, thereby becoming the center of symptom formations such as enuresis (bed-wetting) and somnambulism (sleepwalking). Certain other disorders, like truancy and thumb-sucking, almost always disappear without a trace before adulthood. Certain conditions, such as speech stuttering, food fads, and nail-biting, may continue into adulthood. Nevertheless, it is essential to recognize that although all these 'behaviors' are brought to the psychiatrist as the chief complaint, they often manifest an underlying mental health disorder, which may commence in childhood and persist through adulthood. The psychiatrist must be constantly conscious that the underlying mental health disorder is subject to varying influences during childhood and be able to differentiate the temporary and short-term issues from the more long-term ones.

   The role of the family and environment is crucial. Unlike adults, children are passive respondents to their social environment. The child is easily affected by its environment, so the home and family assume central importance. Lack of a nurturing domestic environment results in unhappiness in the child, which may manifest as many behavioral problems. The mother-child relationship must be enjoyable for both the mother and the child. If one of them is unsatisfied with the relationship, it affects the other and generates a back–and–forth cascade of negative interactions and experiences.

   The child not only needs love but ***'dependable' love*** – i.e., predictable, reliable, consistent, and relatively unconditional love. Unpredictable love, randomly dispersed with negative interactions or conditionally expressed, results in anxiety, stress, fear, lack of trust, and unhappiness. Extreme unpredictability and adverse living conditions could also be associated with mental retardation. Terms such as 'maternal deprivation,' 'parental rejection,' 'parental negligence', etc. are often used variably to describe the lack of such dependable love. The study of the dynamics in the social environment in homes lacking such reliable love has led to the academic discussion on the types of homes and their association with childhood disorders.

   In summary, the importance of the family and home environment are critical considerations in the context of behavior problems in child psychiatry.

   Characteristics such as ready submissiveness, weakness of will in the face of temptation, impulsiveness in action guided only by the affective state, lack of foresight, and decision-making under the impact of the present alone are considered 'normal', expected, or acceptable in children, but not deemed acceptable to adults. Hence, ***the presentation or manifestations of disorders in childhood differ from those in adulthood.*** What is considered normal or reasonable behavior in childhood may be unacceptable in adulthood, and what is considered appropriate in adulthood may be regarded as precocious or dangerous if displayed in childhood. It is not unusual to come across mothers who underestimate and find acceptable the abnormalities of their children. Many parents also presume that their children will 'outgrow' their abnormal behaviors with time. However, elderly individuals, such as grandparents and great-grandparents who have been around the family stock across generations, may have an eerily accurate prognostication about the adulthood outcome of these children through observations that may seem relatively insignificant to academic experts.

Child mental health examination is a ***time-consuming process.*** The psychiatrist must depend on the providers of the history, which may be the parents or other caretakers, for accurate and unbiased reporting of information. The history needs to corroborate across different sources of information, and the psychiatrist must be able to reconstruct the flow of events retrospectively and how the narrators of the history might have perceived it. The psychiatrist should be able to see the course of events through their mind illuminated by medical training to objectively determine if the child is 'off course' in the developmental ladder and, if so, the degree to which it is so. Childhood development is a continuous process with substantial variation; the child is always 'in motion' in their life, and the mental health interview happens during that motion. The examiner must get onto the 'conveyor belt' and assess the child during the motion.

Childhood development is not a smooth and linear process. It is irregular and intermittent. Consider the example of a baby's motor development of walking. The baby first tumbles over, then learns to crawl, then exhibits baby-walking steps. However, these stages are not clearly defined. There is a considerable period during which a baby that has demonstrated crawling abilities does not crawl or continues to crawl intermittently, even after demonstrating walking abilities. However, there comes a period when the child irreversibly crosses over to a stage, i.e., after a certain time, a walking child never returns to crawling. Thus, growth is irregular and intermittent progress through certain permanent milestones.

Growth vs Maturity - The increase in height, weight, head circumference, and the development of muscle function and coordination are all objective and measurable and are called 'growth'. But the functional ability to use these bodily structures to crawl, walk, run, etc., is called 'maturity'.

Unlike growth, which is measured as a continuous variable, maturity is measured as a categorical variable by the time of irreversible progress or attainment of a capability (termed a 'milestone'). Children grow and mature at the same time. Furthermore, there are several spheres of such development, such as physical, mental, social, etc., and these all occur simultaneously, irregularly, and intermittently at variable speeds, which all must be considered while determining a child's mental health. Growth without maturity is a waste, and maturity without growth is precocious and dangerous.

Thus, it is necessary to follow the symptoms over a period to understand the context of the problem adequately. These symptoms may be due to a normal variation from the developmental course, a pathological delay in social development, or a manifestation of long-standing anxieties and deficits in social skills.

The influence of parental figures – Parents or other primary caregivers and the family play a critical role in shaping the child's developmental trajectory. The psychiatrist should assess the child's position in the family and try to gather an understanding of the emotional climate at home, including an assessment of the parental agreement and concordance on child-rearing practices. Parents tend to differ from each other about their ideas, attitudes, and expectations toward the child. They tend to have different and sometimes opposing perspectives on the child's upbringing. A child has full realization of its powerlessness and dependency on its parents, as a result of which, it tends to behave in a way that satisfies each parent's expectations and demands. A child's behavior, at least partially, can be explained by the child's attempt to respond to its parents' reaction to environmental stimuli. The psychiatrist must discern the degree of such impact on the child. One or both parents or other family members might be affected or suffering from known or undiagnosed psychiatric disorders, and the child may merely be reacting to such pathological caretakers.

In essence, what might appear as an inappropriate behavior of the child may be an appropriate response of a child to an inappropriate living situation. While handling these nuances, the psychiatrist is vulnerable to appearing as being biased or taking sides within the family disputes and should tactfully avoid being misunderstood.

Manifestations of Psychiatric Illnesses in Children

The stage of the development of the child and the degree to which it may be deviant from the usual course affects the onset, nature, and type of manifestation of the mental disorder. Certain manifestations are specific for the child's age – for example, separation anxiety presents in toddlers and preschool children. In contrast, mood manifestations are more evident in later childhood and adolescence.

Adult psychiatric illness manifests with different symptoms when occurring in the pediatric age group. For example, a depressive disorder often presents as a depressed mood in adults but as an irritable mood in children.

Certain mental disorders are diagnosed nearly exclusively in children. Examples include mental retardation, autism spectrum disorders, pervasive developmental disorder, enuresis, reactive attachment disorder, feeding disorder, separation anxiety disorder, selective mutism, tic, learning disorder, attention deficit hyperactivity disorder (ADHD), conduct disorder and oppositional defiance disorder (ODD).

The presence of one childhood mental health diagnosis often signals the presence or possibility of other diagnoses. For example, a child with ODD may have symptoms of ADHD and conduct disorder. Enuresis coexists with anxiety disorder.

After a diagnosis is assigned, the manifestations of the child's diagnosis may change or evolve in line with the developmental process, leading to diagnostic ambiguities and confusion.

Special attention should be given to any recent significant changes in the child's life, such as a change of school, parental separation, addition or deletion of a member in the family, etc.

Regardless of the diagnosis or the diagnostic category, the psychiatrist must investigate the child's family situation, school environment, and social circle to better understand the full scope of the problems.

Often, the child may not meet the diagnostic criteria for any specific textbook diagnosis; nevertheless, it does not preclude that the child is 'normal' and does not need attention. Also, in such a situation, a more thorough assessment of the child and its environment may reveal other more subtle truths about the psychiatric and social health of other family members, which may have resulted in the referral – in other words, the referral of the child may have been a manifestation or an unintended consequence of other underlying social or psychiatric illness in the child's surrounding – which in turn may need medical or legal assistance.

Child development affects management strategies as well – for example, a child diagnosed with ADHD may have other remarkable medical histories such as premature birth, neonatal ICU care, repeated hospitalizations for severe childhood asthma, parental conflict, parental separation at 4 years, etc., or any combination of the latter. Another child diagnosed with ADHD may have none of those mentioned above issues in the history, but a father with a history of ADHD. The management strategies of each of these two children would be vastly different from each other.

Stages of Child Development

As discussed earlier, child development is a continuous process that spans throughout the entire childhood. However, it is best understood to happen under two broad stages – the preschool age period (0-4 years) and the school-age period (> 4 years until adulthood). This delineation is biologically founded – human brain development develops rapidly from fetal stages until 4-5 years, which is relatively much slower. That is, the basic infrastructural anatomy of the neural networks and the reaction patterns are pretty cemented by age 4-5, after which significant changes are not expected. It is understood that by age 5, the brain has reached about 90% of the usual adult size, and the rest 10% happens over several years from age 5 until adulthood. This is why most societies consider children at 4 years eligible for their first consistent communal interaction with peer-age children in the form of schooling, often referred to as 'kindergarten' (literally meaning 'garden of children' in the German language). Variations exist in the speed at which such development happens across the general population, so kindergarten is mostly a relaxed environment without stringent conditioning. But by age 6, it is safe to consider that most children may not benefit much from waiting any longer to commence organized education, and hence, most societies start the first grade of schooling by age 6.

So, let us explore these two stages in further detail –

Pre-School Age Period (0 - 4 years of age)

The biological substrate of the neural system begins in utero, with the birth of cortical neurons from approximately day 40-125 of intrauterine life. From thereon, neurons connect ('synapse'), migrate, and differentiate. Around the toddler age, thousands of synapses are formed daily, and the total number of synapses could reach 1000 trillion. Not only are synapses formed, but many are 'dropped' or 'discontinued' if not used. This process is called 'synaptic pruning'. In essence, preschool is a vibrant yet vulnerable stage in neurological development, which is why this age group requires a safe and nurturing environment for the children.

Certain core aspects of the preschool age child are essential to clinical practice.

Role of temperament

External (i.e., environmental conditions) and internal factors (i.e., health and disease conditions) could affect the formation, migration, and pruning of synapses. For example, nutrition, alcohol and drug use, stress, etc can affect neurological development and could result in mental retardation, fetal alcohol syndrome, epilepsy, autism, schizophrenia, and other yet unbeknownst conditions. Extremes in such aberrant neurological development are readily recognized as the illnesses mentioned above. But, more important are the subtle, non-extreme variations in such effects that result in different types of human natures. In other words, various characteristics of human nature are mixed in varying proportions among people. Each such mixture is called 'temperament' (from the Latin word 'temperamatum' meaning 'correct mixture').

It is essential to recognize each child's temperament type, as it is pretty stable and not modifiable. Temperament determines the pattern or style of how the child responds to situations or environmental stimuli, especially new or difficult situations. Although there are innumerable types of temperament, certain broad classes of temperament could be identified in clinical practice. Many philosophers and medical professionals have historically classified and elaborated on temperament types.

For practical clinical purposes, a psychiatrist must be able to identify three significant dimensions of temperament –

- **Reactivity –** this temperament pattern is themed on an 'intense' response to stimuli. They tend to express both positive and negative emotions more emphatically, but it's the intensity of the 'negative' response to stimuli that often draws attention. Reactions such as irritability, negative mood, emotionality, distress, anger, etc., are common in this temperament. Often, individuals with this temperament react with fearfulness at novel situations or irritability when faced with obstacles.

- **Self-regulation –** this temperament is themed with a diligent effort to control or moderate one's self to deal with novel or difficult situations. Individuals with this temperament tend to analyze the nature of the task ahead and themselves inwardly and shed more effort and focus on the problem, thereby weathering down the intensity of the difficult situation. They are often persistent, non-distractible, and calm.

- **Approach-withdrawal –** this temperament constitutes a choice of the child to either readily withdraw or proactively withdraw when faced with a new or difficult situation. Children with a 'withdrawal' temperament tend to find it difficult for parents to introduce new learning situations and experiences. Still, these children tend to be more cautious and thoughtful in their decisions, often less risk-taking individuals, and may suit well in their later lives in academia. Children with an 'approach' temperament tend to embrace newer experiences, and hence, often a pleasure for parents. Still, the flip side is that these children may be susceptible to peer thinking, tend to go along with the crowd behavior and engage in risky behavior. They also need to be encouraged to think for themselves.

The critical concept to imbibe here is that a child's temperament is a relatively stable pattern of response to environmental situations. None of these temperaments are necessarily entirely desirable or undesirable, and efforts to change or willfully modify a child's temperament may result in more trouble. Parenting techniques cannot durably modify temperament. However, parenting styles that conflict with the child's temperament may result in an adverse childhood experience, which in turn may impede the synaptic enrichment in the developing neural networks, thereby having lasting effects on the child's future psychology as an adult.

The psychiatrist must be able to identify the temperament of the child and counsel parents to act in such a way to exploit and maximize valuable experiences for the child. It also helps in identifying the source of conflicts in the parent-child interaction. For example, the mother may be an introvert, i.e., with a tendency to function better outside social environments, with relative quiescence and seclusion. Her child, however, may be an extrovert, i.e., with a tendency to be vibrantly involved in social and interpersonal interaction, and often outgoing. An introverted mother would struggle to handle a vibrant, extroverted child. In other words, the relative 'goodness of fit' in the natural temperaments of the parent-child dyad could serve as a facilitator or detriment to the child's secure attachment and hence influence the child's psychological development. Since psychological development co-occurs along with the child's motor functioning, which gives the child more 'physical' independence and access to the environment, the role of temperament in the child's overall development.

Separation and stranger anxiety

A newly born infant does not have the idea of 'permanency' – that is, the infant understands what it sees as that which exists and that which it does not see as non-existent. It is sometime during the latter half of the first year of life that the child begins to grapple with the idea that objects or people that disappear from the field of vision still might and do continue to exist. From this time until its verbal and motor skills are pretty mature (i.e., until 2-3 years of age), the child is at risk of accidents and other significant risks and needs the constant protection of the primary caregiver. The child naturally reacts by protesting any form of separation of the primary caregiver (often the mother) or transfer of care to an unknown person (i.e., a stranger). This protest is manifested as crying or other forms of resistance to separation. These are called 'separation anxiety' or 'stranger anxiety'.

Separation/stranger anxiety is not anxiety but rather an actual protest activity of the child. This is an expected and healthy behavior on the part of the child, as children who are 'universally friendly' to strangers or non-reactant to the separation of the primary caregiver may have severe attachment disorders or psychological derangements. However, working parents living without an extended family of grandparents, aunts, or uncles often find separation anxiety debilitating for their necessary economic income or career development. Stranger anxiety makes it difficult for assigned nannies or maids to care for their children. Parents may engage in extensive parenting techniques to contain separation/stranger anxiety, which may incite or exacerbate childhood psychological problems.

Specific simple methods can help deal with separation or stranger anxiety. Parents are not recommended to expect, instruct, or force their child to show affection or warmth to a new individual. Parents must not 'sneak away' from children when they are asleep or not paying attention, as it breaks the child's essential trust and amplifies the protest behavior.

Usually, children's separation and stranger anxiety issues are resolved by age 2-3. If there is a continuation of these issues beyond this age range, it may qualify as a clinical diagnosis, but the psychiatrist must delve comprehensively into history taking before such a diagnosis.

Children tend to 'cry' in distress or for protest. Crying should be seen as a sign and not as a problem. Excessively crying children may still be less distressed, while less-calling kids may still be more distressed. Crying should not be viewed as problematic behavior, and cessation of crying is not a clinical endpoint or marker for clinical resolution.

Symbolic thought

Symbolic thought refers to the thought process containing abstractions to represent reality. For example, a child may tell a story of a mother dog and a puppy dog, mirroring the relationship between itself and its mother. It may be able to project emotions and thoughts to its favorite doll. It may draw pictures or enact imitations during playtime for such characters. The pivot milestone for the development of symbolic thought is the ability of the child to employ language to consolidate thoughts.

By 3-4 years, children should be able to identify themselves in the mirror, understand the symbolic meaning of language, engage in imitation or fantasy play, draw pictures to demonstrate thought and play cooperatively with other children in games.

By the end of the preschool age period, a child should be able to comfort itself when it does not have its way (such as not getting its favorite candy), limit its aggressive behavior against siblings and friends (such as self-regulate or restrain itself from beating the younger sibling who takes their doll), and call upon figures of authority (such as a parent or elder) to intervene in conflict. These actions are reflections of the development of abstract and symbolic thought. After symbolic thought has been formed, parable stories and nursery rhymes may be exploited to inculcate expected behaviors, value systems, and cultural norms in children.

Awareness of gender identity differences

Between the ages of 2-5 years, the child becomes progressively aware of gender identity and differences in such gender identification. Sexual differences in body image, as well as gender identity roles allied with such bodily appearances, begin to develop. Children become increasingly aware and sensitive to preferences in gender differences in clothing, color choice, characters of toys, selection of games, use of language, etc.

Children preferring to play and clothing choices of their opposite sex may evoke concern among parents during pre-school age.

In summary, the preschool age period is rife with vibrant developmental progress and is susceptible to adverse experiences that may result in long-term effects. Mental disability, mental retardation, learning disorders, communication disorders, and Attention Deficit Hyperactivity Disorder (ADHD) are possible preschool diagnoses.

School-Age Period (5-12 years)

School starting is a significant event in a child's life. Until this point, the child is primarily at home, and its primary caregiver (typically the mother) is everything to the child. Usually, prolonged or regular separation of the child from the primary caregiver has never happened until now, and only a few people have been in the child's environment. After starting school, the child leaves its most comfortable place (home) regularly for progressively extended periods to a place where its primary caregiver is not present and is confronted by many unknown people. The child must negotiate and adjust to new environments, authority figures, rules, social relations, and expectations. For children who have not been in pre-school or daycare, this is quite a dramatic shift in experience. The child's existing cognitive schema of the world gets challenged, and the child will have to accommodate multiple new people and rules of living into its cognitive schema. During this adjustment, experiencing difficulties is expected. Experiencing problems is a sign that adjustment is happening. How each child adjusts is different and depends on the child's temperament (which typically has completed formation before school age). Some children may undergo more than usual difficulties in adjustment and get brought to see a psychiatrist. Not infrequently, the child is adjusting as expected, but it may not be in the way the parents have pre-conceived their child to undergo the expectation. These parents may view expected adjustment difficulties as abnormal and may seek psychiatric attention. Nevertheless, school exposure is an excellent opportunity for the child to learn more, achieve mastery of skills, and face competition.

Learning and criticism

The child is ambushed into a vibrant learning mode due to the rapid flux of environmental changes after school exposure. Children are constantly curious about the world and enthusiastic to acquire new information. They assimilate the constantly incoming new pieces of knowledge by generating assumptions through their reasoning capabilities. Often, they have incomplete information, and their reasoning capabilities are immature; hence, their assumptions, interpretations, and conclusions about the world are inaccurate or erroneous. Adults often find their assumptions and interpretations comical or entertaining. However, children are susceptible to criticism at this age. They build their sense of self, worth, and esteem based on the feedback given to their efforts. Thoughtless criticism of their efforts to know about the world around them can negatively impact their self-esteem, while accomplishment and positive recognition can further a child's motivation to learn and achieve mastery. A child who struggles with school's academic, social, or behavioral demands may feel defeated and develop poor self-esteem. A creative and imaginative child may derive self-esteem in art activities, which in turn may protect self-esteem if they are deficient in academics. Success in sports may also have such a protective effect. Organized physical exertion (such as sports) could be a constructive vent for aggression and energy, especially in children with attention problems. Hence, a school experience must include 360-degree exposure to academics, social, art, and sports.

Sibling relations

During school age, the child may face the birth event of a new sibling, who then takes priority for space at home and attention from mother and other caregivers, and with time, also sees the growing younger sibling as a competition in terms of skill and knowledge.

Play and social relations

Children begin to play games with increasing rules and restrictions during school age. They learn to respect rules and regulations to cooperate with peers. They begin to acquire and master new skills and develop newer and more thoughts and ideas. They learn that peers are competitors while also being playmates and friends. Problems with social relations during this age group can lead to difficulty making or keeping friends and bullying or being bullied.

Sexual and gender awareness

Early school-age children prefer same-gender playmates and gender-specific games. The attention and importance given to sexual differences becomes accentuated as they progress into adolescence. Children also become acutely aware of their physique and appearance. Girls tend to become preoccupied with size and shape, while boys are more concerned about height and strength.

Bodily functions

An early school-age child is expected to have matured in primary motor and autonomic bodily functions. They are expected to be fully mobile, have complete gross and fine motor control, have a reasonable command of language, and express needs and distress with clarity. Most children have obtained daytime bladder and bowel control, even during sleep. However, some children do not; hence, enuresis and encopresis are common clinical complaints in child psychiatry. Such problems may lead to school problems or even school refusal. Conversely, a separate mental health issue may lead to encopresis/enuresis and school refusal. Somatic diseases may lead to school problems, and school-related issues may lead to somatic complaints such as frequent stomachaches, headaches, etc.

Problems with academic performance

Parents and school faculty usually give issues with academic performance a lot of importance. But usually, they are just anxieties from parents and school faculty about underperformance in examinations. Mental retardation, learning disorders, and autism are potential causes too. Usually, complaints about academic underperformance do not arise until educational material becomes more complex and peer competition more demanding.

In summary, the school-age period is a grand and protracted phase encompassing the separation from parents and adaptation to a peer-populated learning environment controlled by non-parental authority figures.

History Taking in Child Psychiatry

Pre-visit preparation

Find out who requested the consultation for the child. In Western countries, it is usually the parents. In India or Asian countries, it is typically the family physician or school authorities. There are also specific cultural variations in who has decision-making influence in the family. In South India, for example, the maternal uncle (the mother's brother) significantly influences family decisions. Also, one parent may have more authority over decision-making than the other. In India, grandparents also have a significant say in the matter. In most cases, these caregivers have differing opinions on the need for the consultation or whether the child is 'abnormal'.

The child itself has less say in the need for consultation. For a child, a doctor visit means pain (such as a needle prick) or something is wrong with them for which an outside authority is approached to assign blame or render punishment. So, parents must be instructed to tell their child that the doctor would understand the child's worries and problems and solve the latter. Parents need to be advised that their child should not be threatened by force or coercion to come to the doctor.

Consulting room milieu

- *Spacing and seating* should be ample and uncrowded. Child-size chairs should be available for the child to sit individually without having to be held by others or seated on the laps of adults.
- *Toys* – Toys in the consulting room serve not only to engage the child while the parents or caregivers are interviewed but also to note any significant deviances in the child's approach to the toys. Toys should be of appropriate selection for age and gender. They should also be safe, unbreakable, and without sharp edges. The toy display must be modest and not extravagant enough to overstimulate or distract the child. The presence of toys makes the child feel at ease and let down its guard to engage socially. The way the child explores the room and the time it spends on each toy should be noted. Does the child stay fixated on one toy for too long? Is it easily distractable by the next new toy and end up not engaging in exploring any toy? Does it engage in fantasy play with dolls? Does it display anger, aversion, or hatred towards a person/family doll while overly cuddly to another? A child's gross and fine motor skills, attention span, ability to cooperate, listen, and obey can also be assessed using toys. While helpful clues could be extracted from such toy interaction patterns, no distinct or clinically impactful conclusion should be drawn based on the interpretations with toys alone.
- *Games* – older children find games more engaging than toys. Games also provide an opportunity to observe the child engaged in mental activity and for conversation. Care must be taken to avoid any competition between the child and the examiner in these games.
- *Pictures and drawing* – The child may be invited to draw pictures or sketches, which may symbolize underlying thoughts, beliefs, and experiences that may be clinically useful. While pictures may be a 'window' into the child's mind about the possibilities of the circumstances of the

child's life experience, they must not be used to make clinical conclusions.

Custody

The word 'custody' means the locus of primary guardianship and responsibility for the child's care. There are legal and practical implications for this word. Legally, it implies the person(s) entrusted with the child's care and the final authority in deciding matters for the child, as sanctioned by the law of the land or the court system. However, the legal custodian may or may not function as the primary caregiver or the day-to-day decision-maker in the child's care or family. In India and other Asian countries, the maternal uncle and grandparents may play a significant role in decision-making and may be influenced by another person. The psychiatrist must understand the nuances in the power structure in which the child's life is embedded. Often, the family paints a different picture during the interview, but details of the actual important person in their lives emerge during the interview or during subsequent visits.

First appointment

Since the widespread use of the internet and social media, it is common for one of the parents, often an internet-savvy and educated person, to contact the doctor over the phone to request an appointment. Usually, such a person also begins to discuss the problems over the phone. The person may also emphasize that they prefer not to discuss these issues in the child's presence or the other parent's presence.

I have observed that the doctor can safely talk in brief sentences to instruct and prepare the family for the first appointment but not listen extensively or discuss details over the phone. In-person conversation is always preferred over telephone communication. Seeing the child in the context of the whole family system is extremely helpful to the treating psychiatrist. Observing the child's position within the family and sibling interaction is beneficial. Information from such observation and clinical examination must be consistent with the interpretations from clinical history obtained from caregivers and the family. It should be probed further if there is inconsistency or discrepancy and reasons clarified. In my experience, the observed family dynamics in the clinical interview are not the same as what happens at home. Parents often try to paint a neat picture during the first interview. Truth emerges with time, and sometimes not at the first appointment.

The 'circle'

Detailed information on the child's social and interpersonal life circle must be obtained. Who are the people that live at home? Who are the visitors –uncles, aunts, stepfamily, maids, nannies, babysitters, chef, driver/chauffeur, employees, etc.? What is the extent of these individuals' relationship or involvement in the child's care? If the child is not living with the biological parents, getting the details of their access and visiting times is necessary. What are the languages spoken at home? Plain, simple, and short, straightforward questions are the best way to extract the most effective method to gather these details.

Does the child go to school, or is it home-schooled? Information about the education system, the syllabus, and the person(s) involved in teaching should be gathered.

Observe who the child prefers to be with or sit with when not instructed. Observe the interaction patterns of the child with the family members and vice versa.

History of the presenting problem

I prefer to use the word 'problem' instead of the term 'illness', as there is no evidence that the child has an illness at this point in the clinical examination. We know that those who have brought the child to medical attention perceive a 'problem', i.e., a 'difficulty' with the child. Hence, use the phrase, 'History of Presenting Problem' (HPP). Comprehensive questioning into the HPP includes the following –

- When did the problem start?
- Did it start without any apparent precipitating factor or event?
- Did it start with any precipitating factor or event?
- Is the problem worsening over time?
- What makes the problem worse?
- What makes the problem better?

- Is it acute or insidious in onset?
- Where does the problem occur? (as in classroom, home, shopping mall, car, etc.)
- Who is around when it happens? (mother, maid, father, etc.),
- Are there problem-free periods?
- Any prior therapy?

During this portion of the interview, the doctor should remember that the parents may often give their conclusions about the child – for example, that the child 'never listens', is 'adamant', is 'lazy', is 'stubborn', etc. The conclusions that the parents or caregivers have drawn based on understanding may be truncated. For example, a caregiver may complain that the child never responds when called by name. However, the child may be focused or engaged with an activity and wishes to respond only after the activity is completed. While these are acceptable adult behaviors, adults complain when a child behaves in such a way. The parents may complain that the child is 'lazy', but the child may be depressed and express decreased psychomotor activity. Another common complaint by parents is that 'the child is difficult to manage at home', but the parents' availability and responsiveness to the child's problems may have contributed to such non-responsiveness.

Furthermore, it is unnecessary to tell the parents or the family your clinical interpretation or opinions, as this might create unintended conflict and mistrust that may disrupt the intended treatment plan.

The expanded scope of the problem, i.e., the extent of the impact of the situation in question and other associated factors, should be gathered during this portion of the interview. For example –

- Has the child's academic performance fallen?
- Is the child withdrawn from friends?
- Does the child frequently have somatic complaints or miss school due to somatic complaints?
- Is the child depressed, tearful, irritable, or angry?
- Impact on the family.

The impact of the child's problems on the family often brings about the consultation, and hence, addressing it directly is crucial to the doctor-patient relationship. How have the child's issues impacted the family? Has it strained or disrupted the relationship between the parents or between parents and the other family members? Often, the family members try to paint a picture of being very tolerant towards the child or coping without any stress. The parents try to display that they are not stressed, when in fact, they might have undergone stressful adjustments for a long time that may have been internalized as 'normal' and not worthy of mention. Parents also do not want to be perceived as selfish and may suffer guilt for contributing to the child's situation.

Chronological developmental history —————————

This is an elaborate component of the initial history taking and is more important in children under 7 years of age. It is also best obtained in the absence of the child. Parents tend to omit certain aspects of the developmental history if the child is in the room or might have considered them minor or unnecessary, which may be useful for the clinician. For example – Was the child slow to talk? Was the child slower than peers to walk or develop other motor skills or delayed in toilet training? The following questions are also needed –

- Was the conception of the child wanted, planned, unexpected, casual, or assisted?
- Was the child delivered full-term or premature?
- Was the child healthy, breastfed, etc.?
- Was the child slow to develop language skills?

What was the nature of the child's temperament (see above for a description of temperament)? Was the child easily settling into a routine of eating, sleeping, toilet habits, etc.? Was the child always fussy and colicky? Was the child adventurous and curious or cautious? Was the child social and extroverted or quiet and introverted? Does the child persist on tasks or quickly lose interest and move on to a newer activity? How does the child respond to being told 'no' to their requests or desires? Any history of temper tantrums? Does the child prefer to be left alone and independent or clingy and dependent? How does the child react to separation?

Have there been any physiological difficulties during development, such as … Any difficulty in toilet training? Any persistent bed-wetting at night? Any feeding or eating difficulties? Any sleep-related disturbances or nightmares?

Does the child experience any issues with peers, like being rejected, bullied, or neglected? Does the child play with only a few specific friends every time? If so, what role in the play does the child assume for itself? These could give certain clues about the possibility of autistic disorders.

Strengths and weaknesses

Identify the strengths and elicit the weaknesses. Identify the goodness and elicit the badness. Strengths may be in academics, sports, arts, or social skills. These strengths provide the scaffold for the psychiatrist to plan interventional or behavioral strategies and offer areas of opportunity to boost confidence and self-esteem. Areas of strength also provide a potential reason for the child to disengage from conflict areas.

Past medical history

This section is like the traditional history taking in routine medical practice. All principles and concepts involved in internal medicine history-taking must be uncompromisingly followed here.

School history

Is the child in a regular school program? Or a specialized curriculum or home-schooling? If enrolled in a modified program, in what way does it deviate from the traditional school model in terms of age, grade, or curriculum?

Are there concerns related to schooling? If so, is the concern put forth by the school or home? If at home, is it the parents or other caregivers? Is it one or both parents who share the concern? Does the child also share the same concern as put forth by others?

Parents often put forth problems with academic performance as a concern. In such cases, comprehensive assessment is required, rather than just relying on the school grades and examination scores. If any prior psychological testing has been performed, it needs to be repeated to confirm its accuracy and validity. Any concern regarding learning disorders should be corroborated with detailed information provided by the child's teachers at school. Learning disorders could be a manifestation of underlying physical and mental disorders, and, behavioral and emotional issues, in turn could affect learning.

How many schools has the child attended? If the child has attended multiple schools, then what is the duration in each school, and the reason for transfer? Change of school could be a stressful or traumatic event and can precipitate emotional and behavioral problems. Adjustment to a new school, teacher, and peer group could be challenging and anxiety-provoking. Is the child having to repeat years, or falling behind or advanced quicker than usual from a grade at school? Any history of delinquency, truancy, suspensions, or detentions? Does the child bully or get bullied at school? If bullied, how does the child cope?

Risky behavior

Fire-setting, vandalism, unsafe sexual activity, and illegal activities are examples of risky behavior, which may indicate the severity of an underlying disorder or a manifestation of the child's attempt to cope with or handle a problem. The history of such behavior is more pertinent in pre-pubescent children. It is not inappropriate to inquire directly about history of legal offenses committed or on record for the child.

Self-harm and suicidality

Like adults, children may also experience thoughts of harming themselves or others autonomously or reacting to acute or chronic stressors. They may express these thoughts by hitting, cutting, smashing, or burning. They may progress to making plans or possess the intention to die. It is important to differentiate between 'thoughts', 'plans', and 'intention' to commit self-harm or suicide. Younger children cannot express the depth of helplessness and hopelessness and instead tend to be quiet and withdrawn. They also tend to be impulsive and act out their urges for self-harm without a clear plan – for example, running into traffic. Older children are more practical and capable of drafting and implementing a clear plan.

The psychiatrist should not hesitate to ask parents about the child's potential for self-harm bluntly. Specific questions on whether their child seems sad, melancholy, or miserable are useful. Ask if the child has discussed topics about death or dying. Some children express their desire to die or self-harm to their parents or others. If the child has done so, then the following questions must be asked –

- What exactly did the child say?

- Do other members of the family or caregivers say such things?
- Under what circumstances did such talk or behavior occur?
- Was it after the child was scolded, rebuked, or punished?
- How did the parents respond to the child's words of death/ self-harm or behavior?
- Is the child aware of anyone who has committed self-harm or suicide?

While straightforward and blunt questioning is more effective for the parents or caregivers, children do not respond to direct questioning about their internal state of mind, intentions, or plans. They must be led slowly into conversation, and then the necessary information must be elicited. Drawing pictures could be a lead point for conversation, too. Also, interviewing the child alone, in the absence of parents/caregivers, could lead to more first-hand information from the child.

Child abuse

Child abuse is often considered to be a sensitive and delicate topic. But, I think it is most effective to deal with it directly without beating around the bush. A few key concepts may help navigate this issue. First, providing a safe and friendly environment may lead to spontaneous disclosure by the child about the information of the abuse. Second, directly questioning the parents about whether they think abuse has happened could be effective. Direct questioning of the child if the abuse had happened is also effective, but the possibility that the child's confession of abuse at home to the doctor could mean negative percussions to the child should be kept in mind by the doctor. Sometimes, physical abuse may arise from severe disciplining methods of the parents, which they may feel is appropriate considering their own childhood experience. There are several models describing how to ask for abuse, but I recommend the doctor construct a model based on knowledge of the local language, culture, and norms. Third, if child abuse is evident during examination, the doctor must comply with the local laws and regulations of the land.

Family psychiatric history

Psychiatric and behavioral history of the parents and members of the family tree of the child may provide helpful information on patterns prevalent in the family, as well as biases held by parents towards the child based on their knowledge of practices of outcomes of individuals in their family. Though most parents are comfortable volunteering information about themselves and their pedigree, some parents may feel that the doctor does not require such information or may feel offended by the doctor for asking about such information. The latter is usually due to the parents' sense of guilt in being responsible for or blamed for the child's problems. Sometimes, parents have had unusual childhood experiences that may have contributed to the current concern about the child. Parents also may have already reached a 'diagnosis', in which case comprehensive assessment is needed before accepting such a diagnosis. Sometimes, the parents are concerned that the child might end up like one of their parents or siblings, who 'never amounted to anything'. Such concerns are common in the Indian population. While such information is not conclusive for a clinical diagnosis, it nevertheless offers a perspective to the doctor about the sources of concern. Eliciting information about their family members' psychiatric history is helpful in these cases.

Clinical Examination/Interview of a Child

The goal of the clinical interview is to understand the child's perspective and mental state, not merely to gather information to see if it satisfies the criteria laid down in textbooks or the DSM for making a diagnosis. The interview must be organized, complete, and not trimmed to confirm or rule out a concern about the presumed diagnosis. I prefer to break down the clinical interview/examination of the child into the following subparts –

Observation

The younger the child, the more important a tool observation becomes in examining the mental state. Observe the following – Does the child always sit with a parent or elder? Does it independently roam across the room? Is it explorative around the room, or withdrawn and quiet? Is it gentle and deliberate? or impulsive and clumsy? Use the information obtained from observation to better draft questions directed to parents and the child.

Physical and cognitive development

Examine and record the child's height, weight, general health, presence of any disabilities or deformities, gait, posture, and nutrition. Observe for fine and gross motor skills – such as sweeping or throwing movements, pencil holding, walking in a straight line, etc. Are there any peculiarities in walking, posture, or mannerisms? Assess the use and comprehension of language and vocabulary.

Look for sensory deficits or hypersensitivities in the child – this is a common area that is overlooked. Some children may have a deficit in their sensations, may be oversensitive in one or more sensory realms, or may be compensating for a sensory deficit – which, when unrecognized, may be perceived as a behavioral problem by adults. For example, a slight auditory malfunction may be the reason for a 'silent child' or a child that does not respond to calling – adults may perceive this child as indifferent or disobedient. Feedback to the child may be based on such erroneous assumptions, which may have evolved into other behavioral or emotional problems over time.

Examination of mood

In my opinion, assessing a child's mood is the most complex task in psychiatric practice. A child's mood is understood by a complex, nuanced, and intelligent conclusion based on multiple components of the history and clinical interview, including but not limited to the child's facial expression, behavior, psychomotor activity, the content of the play, the content of pictures, and the feelings evoked and elicited by the examining psychiatrist.

Scope for human relationability (Mananalam Clinic Experience)

I use the word 'relationability' to refer to the ability of an individual (child or adult) to relate with others and be available to relate with others. Humans cannot survive in isolation. Relationability with other humans is an important survival attribute – the right amount and nature of relationability determine the outcomes of an individual's actions. For the treating psychiatrist, the scope of an individual's relationability with other humans is essential to know. For example, during the first meeting with the child, does the child greet with words or just a smile? Or does it not greet at all? Some children may even hold the psychiatrist's hand and start walking and talking with them. Does the child always cling to one parent? Does it indulge in play with peers? If so, is it parallel play (playing alongside others but by itself) or cooperative play (playing with others)? Does the child respond to verbal or gestural communication? Does it initiate contact proactively? While all these points must be noted factually, it is essential not to draw definitive projections or clinical conclusions based on these observations. Also, the examiner's perception of the ideal level of relationability may affect how they evaluate the child's scope of relationability. Furthermore, the examiner's relationability may affect the expression of the child's relationability, which must also be kept in mind while interpreting the recorded observations.

Anxiety

In general, anxiety and affect are closely related. In children, it is almost fused! Children persist in one affective state for much shorter periods than adults. They could rapidly switch from crying to smiling, happy to sad. Some children have a flat affect by nature, too. A child may display sadness or anger when a topic of difficulty is discussed and pride or pleasure when an issue of its strength is discussed. The latter factors could overshadow or amplify a child's anxiety level.

Is there a theme?

'Theme' means a prominent or recurring entity pervasive in all aspects. The psychiatrist should look if there is a particular idea or message that is present or conveyed in all the child's mental aspects – is there anything that is expressed in the child's speech, activity, mood, facial expression, gestures, drawings, play, behavior, choices, etc., Is the child playing out an inevitable drama? Sometimes, there isn't any theme. Sometimes, there is one, but it may be broken or disjointed.

Examiner's experience

Children tend to evoke strong feelings in all people. The examining doctor is also a human being, like everyone else. Meeting and interacting with the child evoke specific experiences and feelings within the examiner. The examining doctor should look inward and see what emotions the child has produced in themself. How does this experience compare to the reported incidents of others with the child? The psychiatrist should ask oneself – how do I feel in the presence of this child? This aspect of psychiatry involves a superior skill, which is not necessarily required in other specialties.

Talking with children ——————————————————

Talking with children is a skill. For some, it comes naturally. For many, it is a daunting task. The psychiatrist must observe from experts and constantly practice child-interviewing skills. Some broad guidelines are –

- Do not ask direct or close ended questions, especially early in the interview. You will be met with a universal 'I don't know' answer for all questions from thereon.
- Lead the child into a conversation, encourage more talking by the child, and gather information from the information the child brings out naturally in a conversation.
- Start the dialogue with something about pleasure or pride for the child, and then guide the conversation slowly into areas of your interest.
- Invite the child to talk about their wishes, fantasies, and dreams. Some children may express retaliatory fantasies towards their detractors or individuals of dislike.
- Elicit how the child feels or experiences. Sometimes, the parents may perceive the child as destructive, provocative, disruptive, or unpleasant when, in fact, the child may simply be reacting to a negative experience. When parents/caregivers can see what the child is or has been experiencing, their blaming and battling attitude may flip to an empathetic and cooperative one.
- Some children may be difficult to engage in – they would not persist in a conversation and jump from one topic to another, one toy to another, and so on. Do not lose hope. Keep trying by not trying to gather information, but in gaining the child's trust. You may have to spend a few non-productive hours to gain the child's confidence before proceeding with the interview. Use a toy or a game to keep the child engaged with you. You could also invite this type of non-engaging child to discuss their fears and nightmares, as sometimes that may help break their firewall.
- Inform the child that the discussion is private and privileged.

- If the child wishes to be with a specific person at the side or be alone, honor those wishes.
- Do not lecture or dictate advice to the child.
- Talk less.

The 'silent child'

I used to teach my students and residents, 'Silence is the most dangerous weapon'. A silent child is a complex problem to crack. Ask the parents ahead of time if the child is talkative or not. Quiet children may be either universally less spoken and mute or selectively mute. Caregivers may have helpful information about the child's attitude to the interview and topics to open the conversation with. Key points to keep in mind are –

Lack of verbal communication does not mean the assessment cannot progress. Silent children can be adequately assessed through observation of their behavior and activities. In such children, play, and pictures could be pretty revealing.

- The examiner will need patience. The process is often time-consuming
- Do not force, rush, or compel the child into talking
- Do not bribe or coerce the child into talking
- With enough perseverance, the examiner can gain the child's trust, and after gaining the trust, these children could be easy to work with.

The 'angry child'

An angry child is not necessarily a difficult child to assess if the examiner can keep their calm and stay focused. One must approach the angry child with the understanding that angry children typically feel justified in their anger. Often, such children feel victimized or have been victimized or traumatized. Some valuable tips in this situation –

- Do not use the word 'anger' or 'angry' while talking to or in the child's presence. Use other words.
- Allow the child to express their anger freely (while being cautious that it does not physically harm itself or others).
- Use an empathetic approach – presume the child's anger is

justified while exploring the clinical context.
- Allow the child to express or verbalize the reason for anger without arguing, explaining, or critically analyzing it.

The 'hostile family'

Parents and the public in general do not have a good grasp on the nature of a good child psychiatric interview. Even most doctors don't. Parents make the appointment in an anxious attempt to get their assumptions confirmed or to get a 'verdict' on the solution. They would want an instant solution to a complex problem. They tend to think that it might be like a pediatrician's visit. Most of this friction with the family can be prevented by explaining to them before the first consultation, calmly and relaxed, that the process is long and time-consuming and may be boring, annoying, and redundant to the observing family. They should be told that the process may take several visits to make a longitudinal assessment, and recommendations may not be made immediately. They should also be told that hasty or 'instant solutions' could be more counter-productive and may injure the doctor-patient relationship permanently. An ineffective,non-therapeutic, or wasteful first experience with a doctor may taint the child's ability to be amenable to therapy in the future with other doctors too.

The Step-parent family

Being a parent is difficult, and being a step-parent is even more so. Step-parents and children could share a complex relationship as such, as the society's prejudices and opinions about step-parents could bring in a lot of preconceived misunderstandings between the step-parents, caregivers and the children, which must be kept in mind by the examining psychiatrist. The psychiatrist should look past these overshadowing complexities to diagnose the clinical problem.

Hypnogogic hallucinations

Hypnogogic hallucinations refer to vivid hallucinatory perceptions experienced during the transition from awake to sleep. These hallucinations could be auditory, tactile, or visual and may constitute experiences of danger, threat, fear, etc. At times of heightened stress or anxiety, vulnerable children may experience these states. The examiner must be able to differentiate these states from similar experiences arising from an evolving psychotic process.

Clinical experience and expertise are required during these situations.

A 'cry for help'

In certain situations, a child is expressing verbal suggestions of self-harm or suicidal complaints as a 'cry for help' in a distressing situation. The latter needs to be differentiated from actual suicidal ideation. The doctor should refrain from hasty decision-making and, more importantly, misdiagnosing the problem, as it may lead to the child feeling like 'lying' or the parents feeling blamed or perceived as 'bad parents'. Again, clinical experience and expertise are required for these nuanced interventions.

What if you're wrong?

One of the most challenging situations for a psychiatrist, especially in child psychiatry, is when the parents or family of the child contests the psychiatrist's interpretation of symptoms or behavior. They challenge it by providing their interpretation, and the psychiatrist may be dragged into a common-man argument. The family may ask indirectly or directly to the doctor, 'What if you are wrong?'. A trickier question the psychiatrist faces, for his own clinical sake, is, 'Are the child's problems a result of a dysfunctional environment/family, or an independent diagnosable clinical disorder of the child'. Both components are somewhat valid, and an argument could be running along a 'chicken or egg first' logic.

The psychiatrist should explain to the family the following – While innumerable interpretations are possible, only a few are probable. While several theoretical solutions can be imagined, often only one is practical. While the most practical of the few probable solutions may be reached through trial and error, the child and parents could have undergone more damage, and valuable years may be lost in discovering whose interpretation is correct and whose solution was effective. The role of a mental health professional is to learn from the accumulated clinical knowledge and experience gathered over the years, if not centuries, in an organized and scientific fashion to deploy a reduced-risk approach to reach the most practical solution for the most probable explanation, so that the child and family could return to a better life soon, with less damage during the process of treatment.

In summary, child psychiatry requires the pinnacle of the summation of all worldly knowledge, clinical acumen, and interviewing skills in all medical practice. It is a formidable and challenging field but a lot of fun!

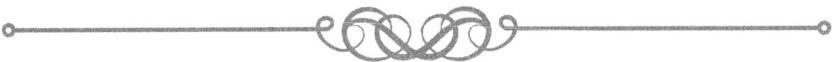

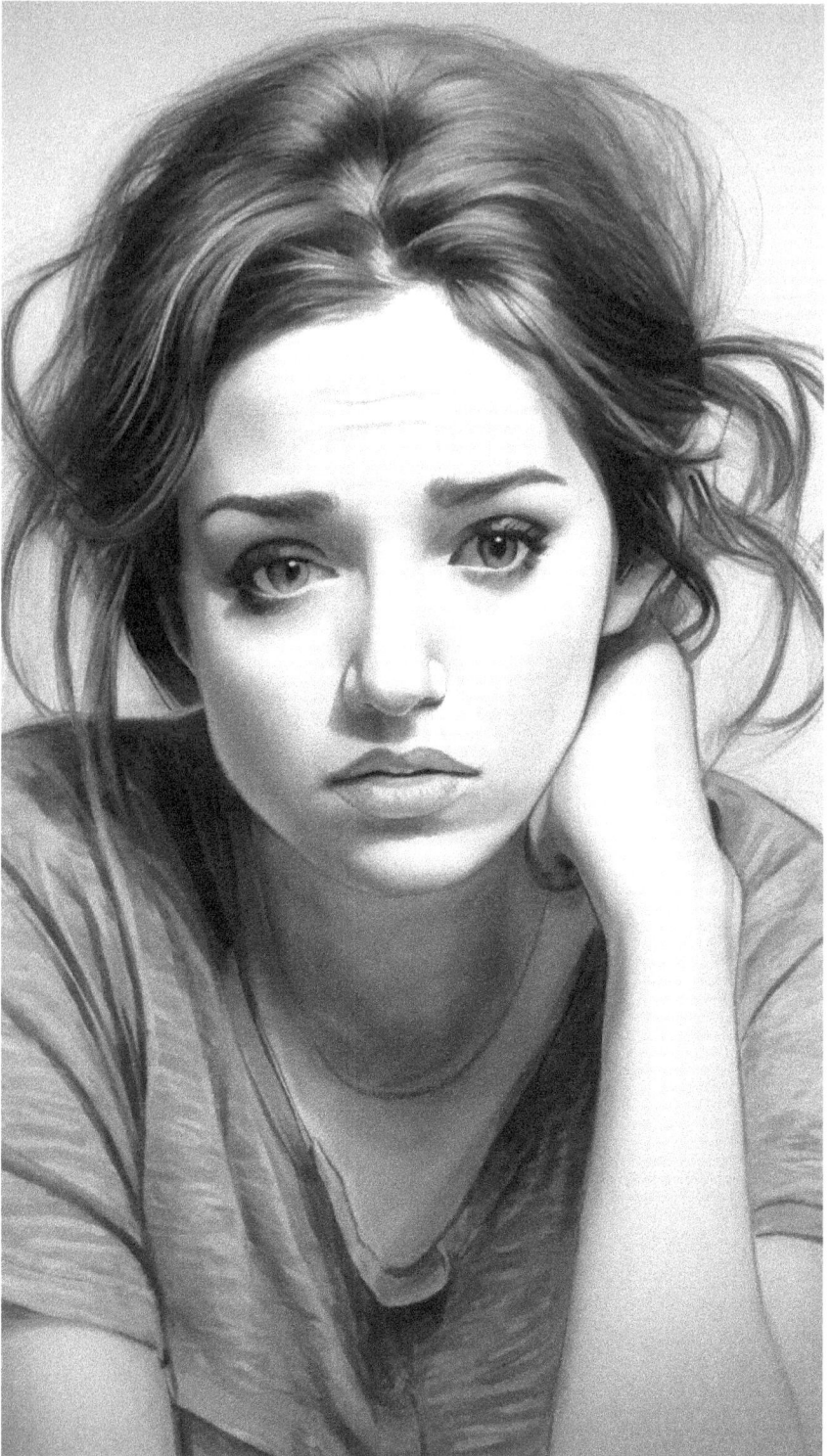

CHAPTER 7

Depression

The Usage of the Word 'Depression'

'Depression' is a term that is used commonly, both in lay language and in medical contexts. The meaning for which the word is intended has many other synonyms such as 'sad', 'unhappy', 'gloomy', 'dejection', 'worry', 'dull', low', 'grief', 'misery', and so on. Each of these words is different but has overlapping implications. Furthermore, the terms used to describe depression differ between languages.

The word 'depression' could convey either a feeling or experience (i.e., temporary, such as an emotion) or a state of being (a constant and pervasive mental theme). Also, depression could be a symptom of an illness or the illness itself. Regardless, depression is used to convey a 'mood'.

What is 'Mood'?

The everyday language use of the mood derives itself from the Proto-Germanic root 'mut', or 'mod', meaning 'angry', 'irritable', or 'wrath'. Essentially, the word mood refers to a negative state of experience. Another etymological association of the word 'mood' is from an alternative derivation of 'mode', i.e., in a specific state of mind to do something, such as 'in a good mood' implying a 'good mode', and an angry mood indicating an 'angry mode' of being. The usage of these words in everyday language reflects another common characteristic of a mood – its temporary nature. A person who is often irritable, sad, or angry is described as 'moody'. We can learn one thing from these linguistic patterns – historically, mood is used to describe a state of depression! For these reasons, using the word 'affect' instead of 'mood' in the medical context is better.

What is 'affect'? Affect refers to how one feels. Since how one feels is presumed to be a reaction to what happens around the person, i.e., how one is 'affected' by the internal or external milieu, the term to describe how one feels, i.e., experiences the present, is called 'affect'. Thus, mood disorders are accurately referred to as 'Affective disorders'.

When is a Mood Considered to be a Disorder?

As described in an earlier chapter, it is better to avoid differentiating between normal and abnormal moods. Instead, it is more accurate to think of mood as 'appropriate' (i.e., clinically unremarkable) or 'clinically significant' (i.e., worthy of further clinical assessment). I delineate affect as appropriate by going through a set of criteria objectively (as shown in the table below) –

Criteria for 'Appropriate affect'
– Mananalam Clinic Experience   **MCE**

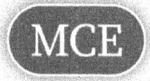

A particular affect is considered 'appropriate' if all the following criteria are met –

- The affect is in reaction to a stimulus.
- The quality of such reaction (i.e., affect) is commensurate with the quality of the stimulus.
- The quantity of such reaction (i.e., affect) is adequate and proportionate* to the intensity* of the stimulus.
- On withdrawal of the stimulus, the mood returns* to pre-stimulus level.
- On frequent exposure to the same/similar stimulus, the individual demonstrates adaptation and conditioning.
- The affect (reaction to a stimulus) must not impair the functioning* of the individual.

An affective state that does not meet all the criteria mentioned above is termed a 'clinically significant' affect.

---

*The intensity of the stimulus, intensity of reaction, and the timing and duration of the affective response are determined as appropriate vs inappropriate, taking into consideration the individual, social, cultural, and societal variations. The clinical acumen of the psychiatrist is essential to the accuracy of these considerations (see within the chapter for further discussion).

When a clinically significant affective state results in 'suffering' of the individual (as reported by the self or others), the affect qualifies as 'pathological'.

In other words, it is crucial to differentiate an appropriate level of sadness from a pathological level of sadness. This area has multiple misconceptions and clinical mistakes, even among doctors and trained mental health professionals. So, let us look at it in further detail –

Patients with a depressed affect often associate it with an adverse event in life, such as death, loss of job, failure in academics, relationship or marital discord, work-related stress, financial losses, etc. It is expected that any individual would feel depressed in reaction to such negative stimuli, which could be an appropriate affect in response to the surroundings. But the mood is an integral part of the Ulan, which has two other components: thought and intellect, functioning in synchrony (Refer to earlier chapters). Thus, when the Ulan works correctly, the other two components (thought and intellect) also get impacted in congruence with the affect. For example, an adverse event (such as the death of a friend) evokes a negative affect (sadness) and negative thoughts (such as worries about one's death or the death of other loved ones, etc.). This is the concept of 'mood-thought' congruence, a functional principle of the Ulan. The intellect also receives this information and begins to work on ways to address the latter concerns. Simultaneously, the thought and intellect restore the Ulan to the pre-stimuli level. The intellect would recognize the impact of the negative stimulus. It must work to restore the negative affect to the pre-stimulus level, i.e., to restore the affect, and hence the Ulan, to homeostasis again. Eventually, the affect is no longer negative, and the individual feels well. However, if the latter restoration does not happen, the individual cannot exit the negative state. The accurate word for such an experience, where an individual feels 'put through', 'made to undergo', 'made to tolerate', 'made to endure' or 'unable to prevent or rectify', is 'suffering'. In summary, 'feeling depressed' differs from 'suffering from depression'. The former is appropriate, and the latter is pathological.

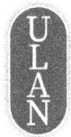

Textbooks and academic societies put forth various diagnostic criteria and symptom checklists to diagnose depression. While these criteria are helpful guides, the most valuable clinical skill is eliciting the presence/

absence of 'suffering'.

'Suffering' from Depression

So, how do we recognize if an individual is feeling depressed or suffering from depression? The answer – pervasiveness. The critical feature that allows the psychiatrist to clinch the diagnosis of depression as an illness (as opposed to just 'feeling sad') is the pervasive nature of the depression – i.e., in depressive illness, the depressed state affects many if not all areas of life – sleep, eating, motivation, cognitive ability, memory, functioning at work, academic functioning, physical activity, negative thought pattern, sexual activity, self-esteem, inability to concentrate, outlook on life, ability to relate or socialize with others, etc., which the patient feels is 'made to endure unpreventably or inescapably' – and that is 'suffering'. As a result, it goes to the extent of thoughts of death/dying and acts of imminent self-harm, including suicide. Essentially, it could turn a patient into a state of practical neuro-vegetativeness.

Key Concepts in Examination

Awareness of certain key concepts and the typical clinical mistakes /misconceptions during the assessment of a patient with depressed affect are –

- **The 'Mood contagion'** – I teach my students and residents that 'mood is infectious'. The mood of one person tends to infect others around. This is why watching a happy movie makes us feel happy, and watching sad scenes makes us feel sad. When one walks into a party, it feels exciting, and on walking into a funeral home with mourning people, sorrow is felt. Similarly, the psychiatrist can quite readily feel the patient's mood. Especially in the case of major depression, the psychiatrist can feel the depression 'in the room' and become more profound while talking to the patient. This feeling is worth more than the multitude of symptom checklists and diagnostic criteria. As an implication of the infective nature of the mood, there is a 'mood contagion' that could get transmitted from the patient to the examining clinician. The mood contagion could draw the examiner to the same mental level as the patient in terms of the tone of the voice, the choice of words, sentence formation, and body language. The mood contagion could also make the examiner concur with the patient's explanation for their symptoms and pessimistic thoughts. The examiner must be aware of this mood contagion and always maintain a neutral tone while empathizing with the patient's viewpoint.

- **Looking for a reason** – Often, the patient or the family puts forth a reason for the depressed mood or associates the onset of the sadness to an adverse event. Examples include the loss of a job, the death of a loved one, monetary loss, job-related stress, etc. They often rationalize the presence of such an adverse event to qualify the affective response as 'normal'. While this is understandable, such a reasonable cause does not rule out a pathological state of depression. In other words, an appropriate stimulus is necessary but not sufficient for considering the affect as appropriate. I have seen even mental health professionals keep interrogating a patient with depression or questioning the family persistently in a manner to fish or look for a reason. A pathological state of depressed affect can and does occur without an adverse event. Due to mood-thought congruence, the thoughts of a pathologically depressed Ulan ruminate with negative thoughts. The intellect also begins to rationalize the negative states of the mood and thought, resulting in coming up with explanations for the negative mood. Any individual's life has adverse events, which the intellect can easily use to rationalize the depression as 'normal'. The psychiatrist should be able to recognize such rationalizations and look beyond the histories given by the patient and the family.

- **Assessing the appropriateness of the affective response to negative stimuli** – While the presence of a negative stimulus is relatively easier to elicit, clinical determination of whether the affect is appropriate in quantity, quality, and duration is not elicited but determined by the examining psychiatrist. A common misconception is that such determinations of whether a particular affective response is 'proportionate' or 'excessive' are subjective and hence unreliable. For example, what is the appropriate duration to be sad about the death of one's mother? People argue that it may vary widely depending on the closeness of their relationship, the local culture, and nationality. While the latter argument is valid, it is reasonable to expect the individual to be able to tolerate the sadness and return to work in roughly two weeks, which is corroborated by the times in most cultures for the funeral/passing away ceremonies or rituals. The psychiatrist must be aware of the local customs and way of living and should be able to decide if the affective response is adequate, excessive, protracted, or unusual.

- **Lack of awareness about depression** – Many people are unaware of a medical condition called depression, and many others do not comprehend that depression can be felt for no apparent reason. Many do not even understand the word 'depression'. Thus, initial direct questioning could be unyielding. Usage of other synonyms such as 'sad', 'gloomy', 'dull', etc. may help.

- **Fatigue** – One of the classic signs of depression is pervasive fatigue. Patients suffering from depression feel 'tired' and 'exhausted'. Often, it is expressed as physical fatigue, lack of motivation, or laziness, and patients may put forth a variety of reasons (such as school start season, marriage, home relocation, travel for work, eating less for weight loss, going to the gym, etc) to explain and justify the fatigue. Inexperienced doctors and psychiatrists may go along in agreement with such justification for fatigue. In situations where women are housewives or stay-at-home mothers, the daily chores and routines that they used to execute efficiently would now seem like a mammoth and enormous task. The psychiatrist must be familiar with the local dialect to describe fatigue. Pervasive fatigue is such a classic expression of depressive illness that in my language, Tamil, depressive illness is translated as 'mana-chorvu', meaning 'mental fatigue'.

- **Atypical symptoms** – As explained earlier in this book, the mind is not outside the realms of natural laws of the universe, such as the law of conservation of energy. So, when a negative stimulus induces a negative affective response, the Ulan 'copes' or 'adjusts' to the stressor by various means. While it may successfully preserve the affect, it may have done so by diverting the impact of the negative stimulus into other areas of Ulan (such as the thought and intellect) or bodily functions. For example, depression may manifest as anxiety (effect on thought), inability to concentrate (impact on the intellect), sleep disturbances, change in eating habits, or somatization (muscle aches, headaches, breathing difficulties, change in bowel habits, etc.). Only through specific questioning will these symptoms become apparent during the interview.

- **Co-existing psychiatric diagnoses** – Depression may exist as a symptom of other illnesses or co-exist with other psychiatric conditions.

- **Poor quality of history obtained** – The effects of depressive illness on cognitive function, communication, memory, and recall abilities, and decreased psychomotor functioning could lead to incomplete, inadequate, and inaccurate history. Patient's slowed responses may make it difficult to extract all necessary information within the allotted clinic time.

- **Perceptual disturbances** – As described earlier in the Ulan chapter in this book, the affect, thought, and intellect work in unison, and hence affective disorders could alter the perception of reality. The psychiatrist must keep the latter in mind while interpreting the information provided by the patient with depressed affect.

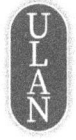

Care should be taken to consciously address the above concepts during the examination of a patient with a depressed mood.

Impairment in functioning

As explained in the chapter on Ulan, every psychiatric condition should be assessed for its impact on the self (i.e., patient) and others. I explained earlier that the clinching feature of depression as an illness is the presence of suffering. However, suffering is an internal experience, and it alters the other components of the Ulan, such as thought and intellect, which results in significant changes in a person's functioning ability or behavior, which in turn need to be elicited during the examination. The latter allows for determining the burden of the illness in day-to-day life and is essential for strategizing treatment to enable the return to pre-morbid functioning.

I find it easier to broadly classify impairment in functioning into three broad categories – achievement-related, interpersonal, and intrapersonal.

- Achievement-related impairments include decreased academic performance, decreased work productivity, and job underperformance.
- Interpersonal impairments include changes in interactions with the family, social life, leisure time activities, and reli-

gious activities.
- Intrapersonal impairments include hopelessness, self-blame, guilt, self-depreciation, and low self-esteem.

One of the implications of intrapersonal impairments such as guilt, low self -esteem and blame is excessive involvement in religious or charitable contributions and donations. Donating large sums of money to charity, indulging in remedial activities such as rituals for sins committed in the past, and excessive religious involvement to 'surrender to the Almighty', all the latter, unlike the pre-morbid level of functioning, could be manifestations of intrapersonal impairments of depressive affect.

Classification of Depression

There are multiple classifications and categorizations for depression, but none is entirely comprehensive. There is general agreement that the severity of the change in mood, acuity/chronicity of the mood state, and relationship of the mood to external life events are valuable elements. Certain clinically applicable descriptive classifications are -

- **Endogenous vs Reactive** - Endogenous depression is depression that occurs with no recent stressors or precipitating events. Here, symptoms such as sleep and appetite disturbances are prominent. Diurnal variation is noticeable in endogenous depression. Reactive depression refers to the onset associated with a recent stressor or precipitating event, such as the death of a loved one, and symptoms, such as sleep and appetite disturbances, are less prominent.

- **Psychotic vs Neurotic** - Psychotic depression refers to depression that presents with severe psychotic features and marked changes from baseline functioning. Neurotic depression, on the other hand, presents with more of the traditional symptoms of depression and is milder, tends to be more chronic, and occurs without psychotic features.

- **Primary vs Secondary** - Primary depression is idiopathic and is not caused by another systemic illness. Secondary depression refers to depressive diseases caused by organic causes such as traumatic brain injury, stroke, etc., or systemic diseases such as hypothyroidism and other endocrine disorders.

- **Unipolar vs Bipolar** - Unipolar depression refers to patients who only
  display depressed affect, termed as Major Depressive Disorder (MDD).
  Bipolar depression refers to patients who exhibit both depressed and
  manic affective states alternatingly.

Specific clinically-relevant descriptive subcategories of depression include –

- 'Agitated' – associated with irritability, anger, and agitation.
- 'Anxious' – associated with anxiety as a predominant feature.
- 'Atypical' – absence of typical features like increased appetite,
  weight gain, increased sleep.
- 'Bipolar' –depression and mania are present, but depressive
  symptoms tend to be atypical.
- 'Chronic' – refers to a duration greater than two years.
- 'Endogenous' – refers to idiopathic etiology, with no
  apparent reason, biochemical in origin.
- 'Major' – refers to a severe form of depression.
- 'Minor' – refers to a milder form of depression with fewer
  symptoms.
- 'Melancholic' – refers to a severe form of depression.
- 'Premenstrual' – refers to the timing of depression associated
  with menstruation.
- 'Postpartum' – refers to the timing of depression within four
  weeks of childbirth.
- 'Psychotic' – refers to depression associated with psychotic
  states, used exclusively in MDD.
- 'Reactive' – refers to depression precipitated by a recent
  stressful event.
- 'Substance-induced' – refers to depression associated with or
  caused by the use/abuse of drugs.
- 'Seasonal' – refers to onset and remission at specific times
  during the calendar year.
- 'Unipolar' – refers to depressive state in MDD.

Although such varied descriptions and subcategories of depression exist,
the symptoms often overlap, and such classifications have severe limitations. Endogenous and reactive elements seem to co-exist in most cases
of depression, both in MDD and bipolar disorder. A purist, dichotomous
differentiation of psychotic vs neurotic depression is oversimplistic. Most

epidemiological studies in the field of depression make no distinction between depression and mania. Thus, the utility of most categorizations is limited to identifying the 'flavor' of depression and understanding the patterns in clinical manifestations and outcomes.

In my opinion, the most useful clinical distinction in depression is to identify if depression occurs as a persistent state or alternates with distinctive manic episodes because it has crucial implications in strategizing pharmacological and psychological interventions.

Constitutionally Depressive Temperament

As mentioned in a prior chapter on child psychiatry, each human being has an innate temperament – i.e., a particular mixture of specific characteristics of human nature in a certain proportion. Temperament determines the pattern or style in which one reacts to situations or environmental stimuli. The temperament of an individual is relatively stable and not modifiable. One such temperament that could overlap with a diagnosis of depressive illness is constitutionally depressive temperament.

This temperament is often overlooked, passes unrecognized, and is misdiagnosed as depression. Individuals with this temperament are quiet, reserved, and like to be in the background rather than 'standing out'. They may perceive everything as a heavy burden and are inclined to see the sad side of any event. They may come across as pessimistic or lacking in self-confidence. They may quickly move to tears or exhibit prolonged brooding over minor adverse events. They respond readily to depressing events and may be profoundly religious or pious. They are genuinely emotional creatures without bigotry or fanaticism. They do function as lacking in energy and drive but are efficient within specific controlled environments. They prefer to live a secluded life with few friends but are not unsociable. They may be perceived as the 'nervous' type and develop minor obsessions and hypochondriacal preoccupations.

I have delineated this temperament with a specific focus on educating readers about the risk of misdiagnosing this temperament (which is not a disorder requiring pharmacological intervention) as depressive illness (a psychiatric condition amenable to pharmacological intervention). Again, you could stay away from misdiagnosis if you follow the criteria from the

Manannalam clinic experience for determining appropriate affect, and identifying the presence of 'suffering', as mentioned above

Clinical Presentation

The textbooks and academic society guidelines provide checklists and criteria for diagnosing depression based on the presence of a certain number of symptoms. They qualify specific symptoms as more important than others and specify a duration for these symptoms to be considered diagnostic. Furthermore, they guide the categorization of depression as mild, moderate, or severe.

While it is essential to know and appreciate the information in these well-intentioned guidelines, it is not practical to adhere to them strictly in daily clinical practice, especially in the non-academic outpatient clinic. Furthermore, patients rarely present with the textbook symptoms. Instead, they present the consequences of depressed mood, subject to individual, loco-regional, and cultural variations.

Specific examples of common presenting complaints of depressive illnesses, as I have learned over several decades of experience in my clinical practice, are enumerated in the below table.

Presenting complaints in Depressive illnesses MCE
– Mananalam Clinic Experience
(This is a list of common presenting complaints and not a checklist.)
• Multiple somatic complaints (such as headache, body aches, unexplained pain)   • Heaviness over the shoulder, posterior scalp, neck   • Feeling weak   • Feeling lethargic or lazy   • Feeling 'run down' or exhausted   • Gastrointestinal complaints (dyspepsia, nausea, abdominal pain, bloating, constipation, diarrhea, flatulence, loss of appetite)   • Sleep disturbances   • Unable to relish food (unlike pre-morbid state)

- Unable to concentrate
- Procrastination
- Shunning or avoiding responsibility (obligations as a mother, wife, parent, family head, etc, are not fulfilled) Not keeping or fulfilling promises
- Subjective memory loss
- 'Every task seems enormous' (unlike premorbid state)
- 'The day is very long or 'awfully long'
- 'Life is miserable'
- Easily irritable or impatient
- Restlessness
- Working to the minimum possible level (unlike premorbid state)
- Ambivalent attitude towards God
- Feel like crying but unable to cry
- Feeling emotionally numb
- Avoiding social activities and obligations
- 'Life is not colorful
- 'Not feeling cheerful'
- Excessive preoccupation with health issues
- Neglecting self-care
- Unintentional weight loss
- Self-destructive tendencies and acts

Symptoms of Depression

In general, some mnemonics could help with easy recall of the symptoms of depression (which are already available in many books).

SAD FACIES – **S**leep, **A**ppetite, **D**epressed mood, **F**atigue, **A**gitation, **C**oncentration difficulties, **I**nterest loss, **E**steem decrease/**E**xcessive guilt, **S**uicidal ideation.

SIGE CAPS – **S**leep, **I**nterest loss, **G**uilt, **E**nergy loss, **C**oncentration difficulties, **A**ppetite changes, **P**sychomotor changes, Suicide.

DEPRESSION – **D**epressed mood, **E**nergy loss, **P**sychomotor changes, **R**educed concentration, **E**steem decrease/**E**xcessive guilt, **S**leep changes, **S**uicidal ideation, **I**nterest loss, **O**ther **N**utritional changes.

However, it is better to think of symptoms of depression in 3 baskets – physical, affective, and cognitive; below are the classic symptoms in each basket.

- Physical – Loss of energy (i.e., Fatigue), Weight changes (loss/gain), Sleep changes (Insomnia/hypersomnia), Psycho-motor changes (agitation/retardation).
- Affective – Depressive mood, Anhedonia.
- Cognitive – Guilt, Worthlessness, Disturbances in attention/concentration, thoughts of death/dying.

In total, there are nine typical symptoms in these three baskets. As per the DSM, depression is diagnosed when there are 5 out of 9 symptoms. The severity of depression is decided based on the number of symptoms and the degree of functional disability resulting from these symptoms. However, in daily clinical practice, such a rote inventory checklist-based approach is neither simple nor practical. The clinician must use their judgment and must decide on outpatient vs inpatient treatment based on the extent of impact of the patient's functional impairment and the timeliness/urgency of intervention to prevent significant damage to the patient's life. Although the cut-off of 2 weeks is a reasonable yardstick, it is within the discretion of the psychiatrist to choose to apply it rigidly. For example, guilt, feelings of worthlessness, or hopelessness do not need to be reported for more than two weeks, especially in the presence of mood contagion, pervasive fatigue, and suffering to be considered worthy of intervention.

Furthermore, the clinician should inquire about each symptom's duration, frequency, and intensity rather than simply enumerating the patient's symptoms. For example, if a patient reports 'feeling like crying', inquire if it persists throughout the day, how many days a week, or if it is intense enough that the patient feels like having failed as a responsible parent. The clinician should explore the extent to which each symptom has affected daily functioning rather than just enumerating the total number of symptoms or the duration of each symptom.

Let us now discuss how to explore the depth of each symptom in detail. These have been summarized in the next table –

Exploring Depressive Symptoms
- Mananalam Clinic Experience   **MCE**

(The patient reports some of these, while others are evident on diligent observation or elicited through questioning.)

Depressed Affect

- Patient uses or relates to words such as 'sad', 'depressed', 'low', 'blue', 'gloomy', 'down', 'in the dump', 'miserable', 'awful', and 'intolerable'.
- Patient or family reports that the patient is easily irritable, losing tolerance, and angry.
- Ask for diurnal variation in moods.
- Easy tendency to cry or be tearful.
- Unable to control emotions or crying.
- Prefers to cry alone.
- Unable to cry.

Decreased Energy

- Routine activities seem unsurmountable (unlike pre-morbid state).
- Unable to complete a task/project/assignment.
- Procrastination.
- Avoiding work.
- Shunning responsibilities.

Concentration disturbances

- Is the patient able to follow a conversation?
- Is the patient able to read the newspaper or finish reading an article in a journal?
- Can the patient sit through an entire movie?
- Indecisiveness implies the inability to concentrate.
    - Indecisive about what to wear.
    - Indecisive about what to cook/eat.
    - Indecisive about what to do with spare time.
    - Indecisive about what to do on the weekend.

Guilt

- Guilt of 'letting down' family/friends/colleagues.
- Guilt of unkept promises.
- Guilt of not completing tasks or missing deadlines.
- Guilt of adding or being a burden to others.
- Blaming oneself for unfortunate events to others.
- Self-loathing over trivial events.
- Belief in that they are 'bad to the core.'
- Feeling of being punished by God/some higher power for their sins ('karma').

Please note that although guilt is a state of mind, it may be a trait in some individuals. I have seen many people with persistent feelings of guilt as part of their character. In such cases, the guilt is inappropriate, making it difficult to differentiate from the inappropriate guilt seen in depressive illness. Patients with chronic medical diseases or psychiatric conditions also develop guilt over time. Thus, the pre-morbid level of guilt must be established, and then its evolution must be correlated through the time of onset and progression of the depressive illness.

Sleep disturbances

- Feeling unrefreshed on awakening.
- Feeling of needing more or better sleep.
- Early morning awakening.
- Difficulty falling asleep.
- Awakening in the middle of the night and unable to go back to sleep.
- Sleeping more than usual.
- Feeling sleepy all the time.
- Ask if the insomnia is initial (while falling asleep), middle (in the middle of sleep) or terminal (early morning).
- Ask what the patient does or thinks of while not able to sleep.

Please note – Some form of sleep disturbance is present in most patients with depressive illnesses, and patients would greatly appreciate and trust the treatment when sleep improves. So, do not fail to understand this symptom fully.

Suicidal ideation/Thoughts of death or dying.

- Do not ask for it directly, at least in the initial stages of the interview. Ask like this –
    - 'Do you wonder if life is worth living?'
    - 'Are you brooding about death or dying?'
    - 'Why should one live?'
    - 'Do you ever think about what the point of life is?'
    - 'Have you ever thought it might be better to end life?'
- Once suicidal thought is established, explore in more detail –
    - How often does the thought occur?
    - What time of the day is it more profound?
    - Is the thought compelling or forceful?
    - Has the patient tried to enact according to the thoughts?
    - Has the patient done any preparation for it?
    - Is the patient afraid that they might execute the thought?
    - Has the patient tried to express these thoughts to anyone? Or try to discuss it with someone?
    - Does the patient find these thoughts autonomous, meaningless, and unwarranted? Or reasonable and meaningful?
    - Does the patient try to ward off these thoughts? Or try to justify them?

Please note – This is a complex area to explore through interviews, especially with the patient's family around. Many family members (usually in orthodox cultures) are sensitive to discussion of suicide. Suicidal ideation is frowned upon and considered a taboo topic for discussion. In some societies, the family does not prefer the psychiatrist to discuss suicidal ideation. They feel that the patient's suicidal ideation or eventual suicide was initiated by the examiner who 'put the thoughts' into the patient's mind or legitimized it through casual talk. So, it befits the psychiatrist to enter the topic from the flank and discuss the 'worth of life' or 'meaning of living' rather than confronting 'dying'.

Anhedonia

- Is there a loss of interest in activities that occur frequently? (e.g., work)
- Is there a loss of interest in activities that occur infrequently? (e.g., vacations)
- Is there a loss of interest in routine unexciting activities? (e.g., watching TV, listening to music)
- Is there a loss of interest in exciting activities (e.g., sex, dating)
- Is there a loss of interest in readily available activities? (e.g., going to movies)
- Is there a loss of interest in activities that require planning?

Sex/Libido

- Desire – Is there a need, desire, or passion to want sex?
- Initiating – Is there effort and interest to initiate sexual activity?
- Maintaining/Completing – Can they continue sexual activity to completion?
- Satisfaction – Are they enjoying the act while indulging in it, and attaining satisfaction on completion?
- Anticipating – After completion of the sexual act, do they anticipate renewed interest?

Please note – Sexual medicine must be practiced methodically. It helps to categorize the components of sexual activity into the components mentioned above for an objective understanding of the details.

Appetite and weight

- 'I am not feeling hungry at all'
- 'I don't feel like eating'
- Have your eating habits changed?
- Do you eat more or less than usual?
- Has there been weight gain or weight loss?
- Do you enjoy food?

Please note – It is essential to differentiate between hunger, appetite, eating, and weight. Each of these entities is different and should not be confused with each other. Hunger is a compelling physiological urge to consume food. It is a physical drive. Hunger disappears after eating. Appetite is a desire to eat food in the absence of hunger. It is a psychological drive. Appetite may persist after hunger has disappeared. Eating is a behavior, a physical activity of consuming food. Weight is an objective and measurable vital statistic that depends on eating (not appetite or hunger).

In depression, appetite is affected, but hunger is not. Eating may or may be affected, depending on the pre-morbid eating habits of the patient. Also, certain medications can cause weight gain and need to be enquired about.

Cardinal signs

As mentioned before, the presence of suffering differentiates a genuine depressive illness from an appropriate reactive response to a negative. However, suffering may occur due to other psychiatric diseases (such as thought disorders). I find the following three clinical signs uniquely characteristic of depressive illness and help diagnose the depressed affect as the etiology for the suffering, as opposed to other psychiatric disorders. These symptoms, which I call the 'cardinal signs' of depression' are –

1. Anhedonia
2. Angst
3. Depressive rumination

Let us explore each of these in detail.

- **Anhedonia –** 'Hedon' in Greek means 'pleasure'. The word 'anhedonia' means 'without pleasure'. As I have explained in the first chapter of this book, the strict medical definition for the word 'pleasure' is the experience resulting from the satisfaction of the id (basic/innate urges), i.e., hunger, temperature correction, and sex. In depression, hunger and the need to seek ambient temperature are preserved, and patients with depression appreciate the satisfaction (i.e., pleasure) of these drives. Thus, 'anhedonia', in the word's strict etymological sense, is a misnomer in the context of depressive illnesses. What happens in depression is a 'loss of interest', 'loss of motivation', or 'loss of drive to function'. The psychopathology here is as follows – Affect refers to the state of mind responding to the environmental stimuli. When the affect is so severely depressed or paralyzed, the individual's mind cannot respond to environmental stimuli – which is realized as a feeling of 'numbness'. Thus, the individual cannot enjoy the activities they once enjoyed. So, they no longer feel motivated to expend their already low energy on such activities. Essentially, they are 'not in the mood' to do anything. This state of being 'unable to enjoy' has been labeled 'anhedonia' in mainstream medical vocabulary. So, what is 'interest' then? Interest refers to the sense of curiosity or concern. Interest begets more interest – i.e., interest leads to the pursuit of the object of curiosity or concern, leading to more activities to keep the interest alive. For example, one is curious about what happened, reflected in the interest in listening to story-telling, manifested as an interest in reading novels, watching movies, listening to narrations, etc. The latter activities then lead to actions that keep such an interest alive, such as visiting a bookstore, subscribing to a movie channel, etc. In depression, this 'interest' is lost – there is pervasive loss of such interest, i.e., loss of interest affecting many aspects of life. This is labeled as anhedonia and is a classic sign of depressive illness.

- **Depressive rumination –** Animals such as cows and goats have the habit of constantly chewing already chewed food. Their physiology is such that their previously chewed food that has been swallowed is regurgitated from the gastric lumen back into their mouths, and they keep chewing the chewed food redundantly. This process of chewing chewed cud is called 'rumination'. Patients with severe depressive illness tend to 'regurgitate' processed thoughts and keep processing the

thoughts again and again persistently. This is called 'depressive rumination'. Rumination is much more critical than other symptoms, as it
has far-reaching implications. Going back to the Ulan being an
amalgamation of the mood, thought, and intellect operating like
the wheels in a clock, any disturbance to one of the wheels leads
to the malfunctioning of the others. Rumination implies a stage
when the disruption of the affect (i.e., depression) has evolved to
significant thought disturbances, wherein thoughts are regurgitated and
re-processed endlessly. Due to the mood-thought congruence principle,
these thoughts are 'negative', leading to a pessimistic outlook on life.
This could further result in perception disturbances about life events
and may progress enough to affect intellect and cognitive function. The
latter leads to the construction of pervasive negative cognitive schema
about the self, future, and the world in general. Such thought and
cognition disturbances then lead to decisions resulting in interpersonal/
relationship struggles, impaired coping behaviors, hopelessness, and
eventually a cognitive structure in which there is 'no escape' or 'no
chance of improvement' of the miserable condition. The latter evokes
suicidal thoughts and may lead to suicide. Thus, depressive rumination
must be considered a cardinal sign of depression and should not be
missed during mental status examinations.

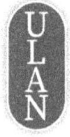

- **Angst –** The dictionary describes angst as anxiety, apprehension, or
  insecurity. Angst is also often confused with anxiety. Angst is a tran-
  scendent emotion of unbearable desperation for hopes of overcoming
  a seemingly impossible situation without the element of hope! It
  manifests as a feeling of constant struggle with the burdens of life,
  where salvation from the battle seems impossible. This sense may lead
  to disturbances in thoughts – believing they are unloved, unlovable,
  and incapable of loving. Then, it leads to low self-esteem and a sense
  of loneliness. Such attitudes then lead to disruption of essential and
  worthy relationships. The signs of angst are

  - **Emotional lability –** being easily moved to tears, incessant crying.

  - **Emotional incontinence –** unable to control crying, crying in
    front of others.

  - **Emotional phantomness –** a feeling of 'losing control' of one's emotion and expression of emotion. It's a feeling of 'losing their mind', 'fear going mad'. Patient may fear becoming insane, is often ashamed of having a 'weak mind'.

In summary, anhedonia (unable to enjoy), depressive rumination (unable to discard processed thoughts), and angst (unbearable anguish and desperation) are cardinal signs of depression and of great practical importance to a psychiatrist for clinching the diagnosis of depression. The latter cardinal signs may override the duration and number of textbook-described symptoms in importance.

Another unique manifestation of depression is the sense of 'being alone in this world' or 'lonely in this world'. Depressed patients may feel that there is no one in this world 'for them', despite having a whole army of family and friends to support them. This is also found in patients with psychosis, or a psychotic type of depression, where they feel that no one is helping them or that everyone is against them. This type of cognition is particularly damaging to the patient, as it makes them become aloof and not nurture a supportive environment for themselves. They end up kicking out supportive individuals from their life – the pathophysiology of this type of depression is that it concocts a cognition that allows the disease to thrive by dismantling all anti-disease mechanisms that may emerge to subdue the illness.

Special Situations

- **Child harm –** Depression in adults makes them feel restless and irritable, resulting in child physical abuse, maltreatment, or neglect. The latter must be diligently noted and documented. Amateur or beginner psychiatrists and trainees must seek the guidance of experienced psychiatrists while dealing with these situations.

- **Agitated patients –** These patients may feel that the psychiatrist's questions are unnecessary or unnecessarily time-consuming. Focus on high-yield areas and keep the interview brief.

- **Shut-down patients –** These patients are expressionless and withdrawn. They look 'blank'. They respond to questions with evasive answers such as 'not sure', 'don't remember', 'may be', 'don't know', etc., and communicate in single words. These are manifestations of social indifference and lack of interest in placing an effort to convince. It is difficult to establish rapport with these patients, and if not approached with empathy, the patient may turn passive-aggressive toward the examiner. A wise approach would be to start the conversation on a broad note, ping a topic of interest to the patient, and develop rapport through such issues first.

- **Defensive patients** – These patients are pleasant, cooperative, and forthcoming but answer questions in a way that pre-emptively minimizes the negative effect of their symptoms or problems. They come up with their own explanations, rationalizations, and theories to explain their symptoms, portraying their symptoms as reasonable reactions to environmental situations. They expect the psychiatrist to concur with their views; if they are not concurred with affirmation, they get disappointed. Some of this defensiveness is due to the anxiety associated with being labeled with a psychiatric diagnosis and the stigma attached to the latter. In these situations, the examiner must not appear dismissive of the patient's explanations, listen to them, and try to explain the mental health viewpoint and that you are there to help them. Usually, they are cooperative and understanding once they feel safe at the hands of the psychiatrist.

- **Tearful patients** – These patients are in despair and overflowing with sadness. They are easily moved to tears and unable to stop crying, but not in a dramatic way. The psychiatrist must empathize with their crying but find a nuanced way to move the interview forward. The examiner must avoid becoming pulled into the patient's depressed tone and pessimistic thoughts. The examiner must be neutral in tone, language, and expression, and should refrain from agreeing to patient's negative assertions as it may confirm the patient's worst fears. Examiners must remember that the patient is depressed and not the situation or interview itself!

- **Suicidal patients** – When a patient dies of suicide, it is excruciating and hurtful for the psychiatrist. I have experienced such pain, and it is more than losing the patient. I found it challenging to overcome such pain. I shall discuss this topic further in the forthcoming chapters. The critical concept to remember here is to be vigilant while assessing suicidal risk. Be empathetic and non-judgmental of the patient.

Discussing About Depression

Discussing the patient's illness with their family is both a crucial skill and an art. Some tips in daily practice are –

- Find out what bothers the family the most and elicit their expectations.
- Unassign blame – Some family members or relatives may be eager to assign responsibility for the patient's depression to themselves or others. Educate them that it is a medical illness, and no one is to be blamed for it.
- Do not make promises – While it is accurate to state that depression is a treatable illness, do not make promises of the time frame for resolution of the patient's symptoms.
- Brief and focused psycho-education – In simple and short sentences, educate that depression is a medical condition. You can briefly touch upon the neurochemical aspects to elucidate that chemical imbalances are related to the symptoms experienced by the patient. I tell them this: 'The patient is *suffering due to an illness called depression. Like other illnesses, depression is also treatable, and the right medication treatment can provide faster and more durable relief. Once the patient experiences relief of the symptoms of the illness, other methods such as non-pharmacological intervention may be tried to prevent further episodes, but to reach that point, treatment now is mandatory'.*
- Educate about self-harm and suicide in a non-judgmental way.

Depression scales

These scales are tools to measure and objectify the presence and severity of depression. Numerous scales have been validated and published. Some are clinician-administered, while others are self-reported by the patient. A few key concepts about these scales -

- **Beck Depression Inventory -** Developed by Dr. Aaron T. Beck (1921-2021), Professor of Psychiatry at the University of Pennsylvania. The advantage of this scale is that it has a meaningful cut-off and is self-reported, incorporating atypical features in the later version. The limitation of this scale includes under-emphasis on neuro-vegetative symptoms and the inability to use it for the depressive episode itself.

- **Montgomery-Asberg Depression Rating Scale (MADRS)** – is a clinician-rated scale that is easy to administer. However, not all symptoms are represented on this scale.

- **Hamilton Depression Rating Scale** – Often considered the gold standard, used ubiquitously and clinician-administered. Limitations include lack of focus on concentration, overemphasis on vegetative symptoms, and underemphasis on cognitive and emotional symptoms.

Take home points

In summary, affective disorders, especially depression, are biological in origin, often transmitted genetically, and characterized predominantly by a condition of the affect/mood, usually acute in onset, cyclical, and episodic in occurrence. Inter-episode recovery may be complete but not guaranteed. It is often self-limiting, but irreparable severe damage and complications (including suicide) may occur. Traditionally considered to be a relatively good prognostic illness (considering other more severe psychiatric diagnoses), but it may cause enough loss and damage, too. Hence, prolonged management (pharmacological and non-pharmacological) is required.

The examining and treating psychiatrist must be fluent and familiar with the local language and the lay slang/vernacular to deploy more than one word to express depressed affect. Be non-judgmental and non-professorial, and avoid lecturing or giving advice. Examine the pervasive effect of depressed mood across all domains of life and determine the presence of 'suffering'. Look for the cardinal signs of depression (as mentioned above) and be vigilant while assessing suicide risk. Develop your own personal and effective method of screening questions for self-harm and suicide, tailor-made for the geographical and cultural region of practice.

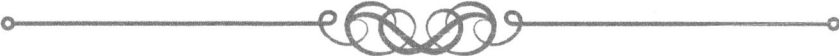

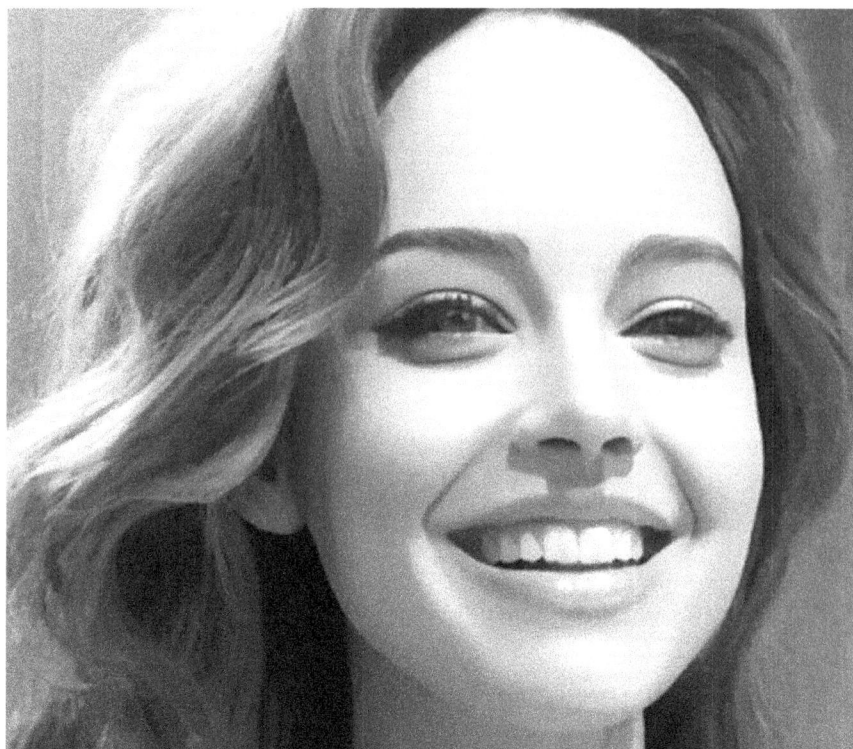

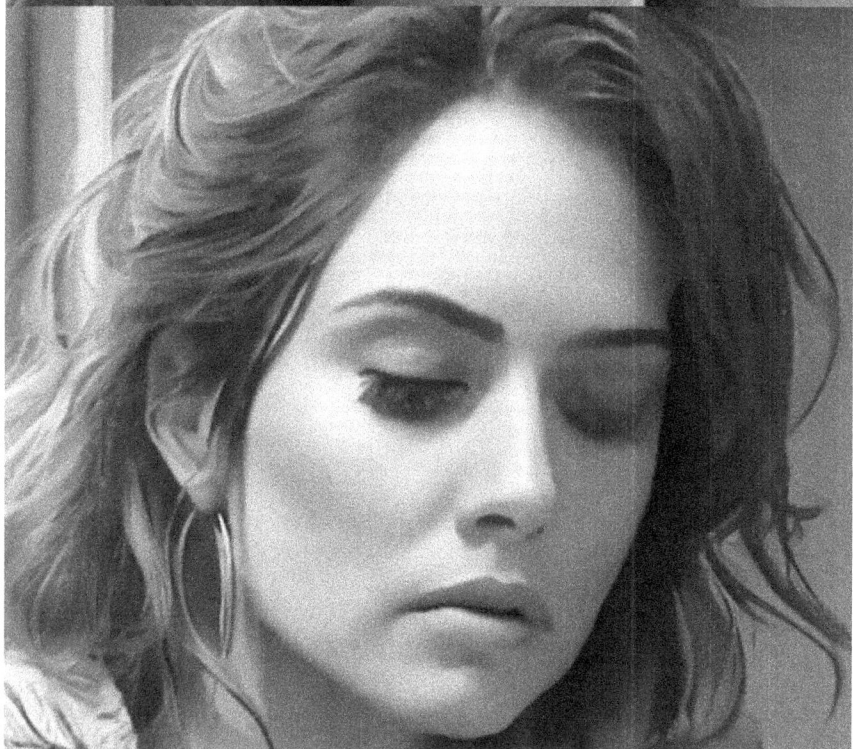

CHAPTER 8

Bipolar Disorder

What is bipolar disorder?

As the name indicates, this disorder is characterized by two extremes, i.e., 'poles' of affect – a depressed affect and an elated affect. Simply put, the mood dips below baseline and then returns to a steady state in depressive disorder. The mood alternatingly oscillates between dropping below baseline and then spiking above baseline in bipolar illness. Bipolar mood disorder was first discussed academically in Germany in the 1850s as 'madness in double form' or 'double insanity'. Because the patient's mood cycles between depression and elation, it was also called 'cyclical insanity'.

Depression in bipolar disorders is clinically similar to the depression that occurs in depressive illnesses. What sets bipolar illness apart (from depressive illness) is the presence of a clinically distinct state characterized by an elated mood, often referred to as 'mania'. Nevertheless, depression predominates the scope of the illness in bipolar disorder too. Depression lies at the root of misery and suffering in bipolar disorders and is typically more severe than depression in run-of-the-mill depressive disorder. Self-harm and successfully executed suicide are more common with bipolar depression than unipolar depression.

One might wonder why we must differentiate between unipolar depression and bipolar depression. A more challenging question is - if the presence of elated mood is the differentiating factor between bipolar depression and unipolar depression, how can one differentiate elated mood from the relative feeling of happiness that is felt during the remission of depressed affect to baseline in unipolar depression? More importantly, how can one differentiate between an elated mood and the constitutional nature of an individual displaying a higher level of cheerfulness and optimism?

These are crucial conceptual questions, and lack of clarity on these concepts has led to unwarranted academic arguments, clinical confusion, and misdiagnoses. So let us explore the above questions.

Elated affect vs appropriate happiness

How do you differentiate between an appropriately happy or usually cheerful affect from an inappropriately elevated one, i.e., elation? The answer to this question lies in returning to the basics - the criteria to identify an appropriate mood as described in the previous chapter. It is reproduced again in the following table –

Criteria for 'Appropriate affect'   – Mananalam Clinic Experience   **MCE**
An affect is considered 'appropriate' if all the following criteria are met –   • The affect is in reaction to a stimulus.   • The quality of such reaction (i.e., affect) should be commensurate with the quality of the stimulus.   • The quantity of such reaction (i.e., affect) should be adequate and proportionate* to the intensity* of the stimulus.   • On withdrawal of the stimulus, the mood must return* to pre-stimulus level.   • On frequent exposure to the same/similar stimulus, the individual must demonstrate adaptation and conditioning.   • The affect (reaction to a stimulus) must not impair the functioning* of the individual.   An affective state that does not meet all the criteria mentioned above is 'clinically significant'.
*The specific details to demarcate the intensity of the stimulus and the reaction, and the time to the presence of the affective response are determined through clinical acumen, in consideration of the individual's personal life, cultural and traditional variations (see within the chapter for further discussion)

Thus, if the affect is either elevated without a stimulus, or despite the presence of a negative stimulus, or disproportionately elevated to the intensity of the positive stimulus, does not return to baseline even after withdrawal of the stimulus, or impairs the functioning of the individual, then the elevated affect is clinically significant to be considered possibly pathological.

So, the next question is - when does a clinically significant elated affect qualify as a 'manic state'? The answer is irritability. People who are constitutionally (i.e., by nature) more happy, cheerful, and optimistic than others in the face of adversity are typically not irritable. A manic state, on the other hand, is typically characterized by irritability. *'Irritability'* is a state of intolerance to environmental stimuli. Irritable individuals are often perceived as impatient or angry. The word 'mania' derives from the Greek word *'menos'*, meaning 'angry' or 'mad'. Another manifestation of irritability is impulsive behavior. *'Impulsivity'* refers to a lower self-restraint from indulging in an act.

Diagnosis of manic state

While the presence of irritability along with elated mood (as defined by MCE criteria in the above table) is typical of manic states, the latter two are not sufficient for the clinical diagnosis of a manic state because there are individuals who are constitutionally irritable, too (i.e., temperament of irritability). Such constitutionally irritable individuals could also have elated mood, in which case further diagnostic clarity is needed.

Thus, I use the following criteria to identify a manic state (see below table)

Criteria for Manic state
– Mananalam Clinic Experience

MCE

A manic state is considered to exist if the individual demonstrates all the following –

- Clinically significant elation of mood (as defined above).
- Irritability (i.e., impatient and impulsive).
- Elated thought pattern.
- Eventual remission.

In other words, a manic state is characterized by a spike in the mood level, irritability, associated changes in thoughts, and the impermanence (i.e., remission) of elation of mood, irritability, and elated thought patterns with time. In other words, a manic state is a temporary state, i.e., an episodic state. No one remains in a constantly manic state, which I consider impossible.

Types of Manic states

All manic states are not the same. There are several shades and flavors of manic states. However, for practical purposes, they can be understood as three major types -

- Mania
- Hypomania
- Pre-mania

All three manic states satisfy the MCE criteria of a manic state, as mentioned in the above table. Mania and hypomania are similar in terms of symptoms and signs. The DSM says that the manic state must exist for at least four days to be qualifiable as hypomania and for at least seven days to be qualifiable as mania. I think this criterion is impractical for use in the clinical setting because these time limits refer to the 'minimum' time for diagnosing the type of manic state. For example, if a manic state has existed for 10 days, it could still be hypomania or mania.

In clinical practice, what differentiates mania from hypomania lies in the third criterion of the utilitarian model of mental health (Refer to previous chapter on Ulan and criteria for mental health). In hypomania, the patient's mental state affects only the self; in mania, the patient's mental state affects the self and others. To use accurate terminology, ***hypomania is a mentally unhealthy state, mania is a mentally ill state*** (please refer to prior chapters for the definition of 'mentally unhealthy' vs 'mentally ill').

Here are some examples from my clinical experience – I have treated a patient with bipolar disorder, who, during his manic state, would have elated thought patterns leading to marrying someone without considering the consequences; and eventually ended up with multiple marriages during his illness. The latter would not happen in hypomania. In mania, patients are uncontrollable, indulge in significantly high-risk behavior, and may need to be physically restrained or hospitalized. In hypomania, patients display higher-than-usual risk behavior but do not behave in a way that requires hospitalization. Nevertheless, the acceptable level of risk requiring hospitalization is subject to national and cultural variations. Hence, the differentiation between mania and hypomania through the need for hospitalization is not applicable universally. The only possible universally applicable criterion that is clinically applicable is the extent of the effect on self and others (mentally unhealthy -hypomania, mentally ill-mania).

What I find more clinically useful is a prodromal state that precedes mania, called 'pre-mania'. Pre-mania refers to a transient and rather clinically subtle manic state that often precedes overt manic outbursts. Patients with pre-mania begin to entertain thoughts or indulge in preparatory behaviors to set the stage for overtly deranged activity that characterizes mania. Identifying pre-mania allows the psychiatrist to take prompt preventative measures through pharmacological and non-pharmacological means to diffuse the eruption of mania or mitigate deleterious behaviors during the manic state. These measures dramatically impact the patient outcome and allow the psychiatrist to manage bipolar illnesses successfully. However, identifying pre-mania requires an experienced and astute psychiatrist with plentiful knowledge of general worldly matters.

Purpose of Identifying Mania

So, let us go back to the larger conceptual question posed earlier in the chapter. What is the clinical utility of identifying the presence of a manic state? In other words, what is the purpose of differentiating unipolar depression from bipolar depression? Here are the following reasons –

- The treatment of unipolar depression and bipolar depression are vastly different; thus, misdiagnosis could lead to wrong treatment.
- Use of antidepressant drugs traditionally used for unipolar depression, in bipolar depression, could lead to a lack of improvement of depression which then could lead to severe depressive states or self-harm/suicide.

- Use of antidepressant drugs traditionally used for unipolar depression, in bipolar depression could lead to abrupt eruptions of mania, which in turn could be severely damaging to the patient's life, and may require hospitalization
- Use of drugs traditionally used in bipolar depression, in unipolar depression, could lead to non-improvement of the depressive state and unwarranted adverse effects.

In summary, although depression predominates the scope of bipolar disorder, accurate diagnosis of bipolar disorders rests in the unique clinical skill to identify manic states, especially subtle, early, and mild versions of manic states. Overt mania is easy to identify and does not require special skills or knowledge. It is the elicitation of the milder and camouflaged symptoms and signs that require extraordinary skill and significantly impact treatment success rate. Thus, I have devoted the rest of the chapter to identifying and comprehensively examining manic states.

Symptoms of Manic States

The pathophysiology of a manic state can be best understood through the 'mood-thought congruence' principle of the Ulan (Please refer to the Ulan chapter). The elated mood is felt by the self as 'heightened confidence', which leads to overly positive thoughts, and such thoughts lead to impulsive behavior. They think fast, lose shyness, and behave uninhibitedly. In its milder form, such a demeanor could be attractive, captivating, and charming. They are more sensual, which is pervasive in all aspects of life. They feel invincible, financially omnipotent, and euphoric. They think fast and have a flurry of ideas. Memory is sharp. But all the latter are a transient honeymoon phase before it quickly becomes excessive where they cannot keep up with the multitude of ideas (leading to confusion), heightened irritability, anger, fear, and sometimes uncontrollability.

In addition to the elated state and depressed state, there may be periods of baseline functioning, which must be differentiated from the prior two states. For example, an elated state may be mistaken for relative betterment of affect while emerging from depression, and vice versa. Sometimes, the onset of depression after a hypomanic state may be misunderstood to be a return to baseline from mania, and vice versa. Sometimes, symptoms of depression and elation may coexist simultaneously, and this is called a 'mixed state', a difficult-to-diagnose clinical state. Hence, identification of pre-morbid and baseline functioning is essential.

Unlike depression, manic state symptoms (except those of overt flagrant mania) are difficult to identify. In Mananalam clinic, the manic state is explored in a very systematic fashion, as shown in the following table -

---

Manic state symptoms
– Mananalam Clinic Experience

MCE

Mood symptoms

- Infectious jollity, hilariousness, and charm – they make a great first impression!
- Tendency to domineer and order things around
- Responds to conflicts or disagreements with temper and rage, but this temper and rage would soon dissipate, without leaving any remorse and stain about the incident in the patient's mind, and then instantly returns to the sunny side, i.e., 'volatile irritability'

Mischievousness

- Takes sides instantly and vehemently.
- Passes judgments, comments, or jokes on others without the least tact, not with ill-intent, but the nature of these comments is such that they are likely to wound or hurt others' feelings
- Expresses one's feelings with a childish-like lack of restraint
- Lacks insightfulness into others' minds as one's own

Please note - Mood symptoms in manic states are not identifiable directly as elated mood but through behavior. Generally speaking, manic states bring out the underlying fundamental characteristics more clearly and hence may be overlooked or dismissed as being similar to the pre-morbid state. Characteristics such as jollity, hilariousness, charm, and excitement are differentiated from otherwise benign cheerfulness by its propensity to lead to conflict. Applies also to the tendency to domineer.

Thought symptoms

- Stream of thought is more rapid than usual
- Flight of ideas – ideas are not connected by sequence of meaning but by casual associations
- Thoughts associating objects in the environment
- Thoughts of word associations, rhyming words, word puns, wordplay, and sound similarities
- Distractibility of thought and attention, and leads to confusion in severe manic states
- Ideas of inflated confidence and achievability, i.e., (delusional), but fixed delusions are rare
- Decision-making impaired in severe states
- Increase in interest in sex
- Writing letters or contacting distant and less known family, friends, and acquaintances 'out-of-the-blue'
- Writing letters or contacting people in positions of power, or higher walks of life about matters outside their circle of knowledge/competence
- Lack of insight – on direct questioning about delusions of grandeur, the patient's response is typically negative; they feel more self-confident and an expansive feeling of the self. Patients with mania also reassure the doctor that 'everything is normal and under control

Please note - At face value, the patient comes across as one with a 'great mind' or 'impressive range of ideas', but comprehensive examination reveals a limited range of ideas with rather illogical flow. Also, this type of idea stream in manic states can be differentiated from the otherwise constitutional ability to multi-task from the inability to sustain attention to a thought or discuss it through to completion.

Speech symptoms

- More talking, sometimes incessantly
- Flow of speech could break down in severe manic states
- Does not finish sentences or elaborate on a topic

Sexual symptoms

- Less shy and disinhibited
- Sexually provocative and advancing
- Comes across as more 'sensual'

Please note - Sexual symptoms are not evident readily to the examiner. However, behavior related to sex during a manic state may lead to serious life problems and interpersonal conflicts, which may be the presenting complaint.

Psychotic symptoms

- Heightened experience of colors, smells, and sounds (bordering on hallucinations of the respective type)
- Propensity to end up in conflicts (due to delusional or paranoid assumptions of others)

Please note – Apart from manic states, psychotic symptoms may exist due to a psychotic state/disorder (please refer to the earlier chapter) or as a part of schizoaffective/schizoid personality disorders. Comprehensive history/MSE is essential for accurate diagnosis.

Anxiety symptoms

Traditional symptoms of anxiety may coexist in patients displaying manic states. Coexisting anxiety makes overall management more challenging and may be associated with higher severity of manic state, increased relapse frequency, and higher suicide rates.

Other symptoms

- Physically exhausted (despite a feeling of limitless energy)
- Sleep deprived (despite a feeling of not needing sleep or not feeling sleepy)
- Changes in eating behavior

Clinical examination

A detailed history and mental status examination should precede bipolar disorder management. In addition to the principles of mental status examination (refer to the earlier chapter on MSE), the following concepts must be adhered to –

- **Appropriate ambiance** – The examination room must be safe and not accessible to objects that might aid accidental violence of a manic state patient. Being accompanied by family is helpful. Acutely manic patients may be impatient and non-cooperative, but the examiner must progress tactfully while not appearing dismissive of the patient.

- **General information** – As mentioned before, the examiner must have broad knowledge about worldly matters to pick up on subtle signs of mania. Residential details, work/employment information, marital status, income, socioeconomic status, living situation, etc., are vital to understanding the changes in the patient's life.

- **Referral source** – Much can be gleaned from the referral source or the person who has encouraged or activated the need for psychiatric help for the patient's sake. It could be a family member, physician, police/law enforcement, employer, or a non-profit/NGO-type organization.

- **Presenting problem** – As mentioned in an earlier chapter, it is best to avoid the term 'chief complaint', as in psychiatric cases in general, and in manic states in specific, the patient usually does not complain of anything. It is often a life problem that the patient's behavior has brought about that becomes the 'presenting problem'. Plunge in detail about the presenting problem – establish the pre-morbid level of functioning and carve the onset of the presenting problem. Corroborate the information with multiple lines of history from friends, colleagues, family members, etc. Elaborate on the current episode and establish the longitudinal history by looking for subtle/subsyndromal past episodes to understand the chronicity better and identify the precipitating factors (if any) for the manic episodes. The key pitfall here is that inexperienced psychiatrists tend to underestimate the duration of these episodes or the chronicity of the disorder.

- **Mood contagion –** As mentioned in the earlier chapter, the mood is infectious, and there is a mood contagion dispersed by the patient that could infect the examiner's mind. The examiner should plan conscious self-evaluations during the interview to ensure they are not swayed in the conversation path advanced by the patient. Sometimes, the patient's heightened sense of humor may incite laughter, and instead of laughing with the patient, use it to engage a distracted patient.

- **Seductive distractions –** Seduction refers to persuading or swaying a person from their duty, loyalty, or allegiance. The power of seduction lies in the infectious and positive affect of the manic state patient. The patient's transient charm could distract the examiner subtly or overtly in going along with the patient. Manic state patients indulge in uninhibited gestures or expressions and may cross interpersonal boundaries during conversation. The examiner should refrain from engaging the patient personally or answering any personal questions and redirect the interview along the clinical path. Some of the seductive gestures may incite smirks or laughter from the examiner, who should refrain from laughing at the patient.

- **Construct a narrative –** While and after gathering the history and mental status examination information, try constructing a narrative or a visualization within yourself of how the events might have unfolded to appreciate the richness of the experience undergone by the patient and the family. Then, constantly corroborate by getting more details and clarifying doubts or gaps in your narrative to increase the accuracy of your understanding. Then, keep focusing on the progress of the narrative rather than asking for or eliciting a symptom, sign, or diagnostic criteria to fulfill a presumptive checklist for diagnosis.

- **Establish the chronological course –** Go back in time, as far back as possible, to inquire about early signs of the disorder. Enumerate the number of depression/manic episodes, frequency per year, length of each episode, and association with major life events such as marriage, childbirth, moving of residence, new job, etc. Explore for change in the nature of the episodes, any need for hospitalization, and response to treatments. Identify any precipitating factors, if any. This portion of the history-taking is time-consuming and best done without a hurry.

- **Look for subsyndromal states** – It is generally believed that patients are symptom-free and euthymic during the inter-episode intervals in bipolar disorder. In my opinion formed through decades of clinical experience, these patients are almost never symptom-free, even during the inter-episode intervals. They are relatively less symptomatic during these intervals, but in-depth interviews and examination could often reveal a mild state of symptoms. These subclinical or subtle states of disturbed affect that do not qualify to be characterized as depression or mania are referred to as 'subsyndromal states'. These patients could also have a higher rate of comorbid psychiatric diagnoses, such as anxiety, OCD, etc. which may reveal more prominently during these intervals. Whether the disturbed affect in subsyndromal states is a part of the bipolar disorder or due to the comorbid conditions remains to be answered and could be partly clarified through thorough mental status examination. Seeking the opinion and guidance of experienced psychiatrists in these situations is wise.

- **Functional history** – Explore how the illness has affected the patient's routine, daily activities, goals, and ambitions. Self-reported mood status or observer opinions on the patient's mood status may not indicate an affective disorder. For example, when a patient who endorses a depressed mood continues daily exercise, work appointments, and attending social events/parties, it raises doubt about the presence of a depressive illness. As I have mentioned before, affective disorders have a 'pervasive' way of affecting a patient's life and activities. Explore how the illnesses have affected interpersonal relationships and sexual interest/activity in general. Sexual information is better elicited during subsequent interviews after establishing patient-doctor trust and confidentiality.

- **Substance use** – Substance use is increasingly common in the current era of expanding acceptance of recreational drug use. Associated drug-related psychiatric comorbidities may exist. Drug use may also precipitate episodes of bipolar disorder. Sometimes, even widely accepted psycho-affective substances such as coffee may be associated with the precipitation of symptoms, especially anxiety. Although patients report amelioration of symptoms with substance use, substance use is associated with poor compliance and overall poor outcomes in affective disorders.

- **Spending –** Often overlooked symptom of manic states is increased spending, especially on luxury items, or buying items in surplus of need. The patient overwhelmingly feels the impulse to spend, so the psychiatrist should not be judgmental or condescending to the patient in this regard. Patients may spend more on self-care, make-up, or beauty salons, reflecting increased sensuality during the manic states.

- **Suicide/self-harm –** The importance of this region of history taking in bipolar disorder cannot be overemphasized. Be thorough, comprehensive, and vigilant in this regard.

- **Past medical history –** General medical history is important; any hospitalizations for apparently non-psychiatric reasons should also be obtained.

- **Medication history –** Organize the medications in your mind into groups such as antidepressants, mood stabilizers, anxiolytics, antipsychotics, ECT, and other drugs. Obtain the dosage, route of administration, duration, response to therapy, adverse effects, and reason for discontinuation in each medication category. Non-pharmacological measures such as counseling and marital therapies are often overlooked.

- **Family history –** Bipolar disorders, psychotic disorders, and certain behaviors (such as elopement and self-harm) may have a positive family history. History of psychiatric medication intake can also give clues in this regard.

- **History of legal issues –** History related to being on the wrong side of the law or being a litigious personality of suing others frequently is important. Examiners may be hesitant to inquire about these issues, but it is essential. This may provide insight into the patient's thought processes, cognition and perception.

Typical clinical narratives in Bipolar disorder

As I have mentioned above, constructing a narrative or a visual screenplay of the patient's life helps the clinician diagnose and plan a management strategy for the patient. Here are some of the relatively 'typical' narratives of bipolar disorder, depending on the patient profile, that I have come across in my experience (see the next table)

Common clinical narratives in Bipolar Disorders MCE
-Mananalam Clinic Experience

Please note – the descriptions below are not necessarily gender-specific, and overlapping features may occur.

'The Housewife'

- After a short sleep, she rises early to a day of continuous and enthusiastic activity.
- Completes most of the routine work much earlier, even before breakfast time, and spends the rest of the day over-cleaning, over-organizing, re-organizing, or unnecessary work.
- Running around making unsolicited or unplanned visits to family and friends, even distant acquaintances (regardless of whether they wanted to see her).
- Dresses up in brighter colors.
- Plentiful and inartistic use of cosmetics and make-up.
- Spending more than usual on beauty salons
- Increased indulgence in religious and community events (increased praying, rituals, etc.).
- Excessive use of cell phones and social media.
- Forwarding unnecessary messages and texts to multiple people or groups of people.
- Increased shopping and impulsive spending, including online purchases.

'The Businessman'

- Multiple entrepreneurial ideas and endeavors – he is 'full of ideas' and 'full of plans.'
- Discusses these ideas and plans with uncritical optimism.
- Indulges in considerable and unjustifiable risks in carrying out these endeavors (which are poorly planned).
- Boastful, overly assertive, and irritated at others who do not endorse his optimism – 'no one understands me.'

'*The Businessman*' - *continued*

- Impatient about plans coming through – 'nothing is done quickly', 'nothing happens fast enough.'
- Over estimation of abilities – 'no one matches my speed and efficiency.'
- Often views the past and present with satisfaction and the future with radiant self-confidence.
- Easily tickled – even simple trifles could incite loud laughter and brash comments.
- Excellent sense of humor.

'*The youthful man*'

- Tendency to pick up quarrels and brawls.
- Passes unwarranted comments on peer group.
- Criticizes teachers, professors in schools/colleges.
- Comments on others' gestures, mannerisms, and appearances without inhibitions.
- Questions authorities, meaningless rebellion.
- Organizes groups or events for flimsy reasons.
- Behaves in an attention-seeking or popularity-seeking manner.
- Makes promises but does not follow through to keep them
- Ventures on projects that appear promising without pursuing or seeing them to completion.

Constitutional temperament – An important differential diagnosis

As mentioned before, temperament refers to a person's innate nature, in medical terms, a certain mixture of traits and personality features that the person possesses by nature, i.e., constitutionally. Many temperaments have been historically described. Although they are not clinically relevant, there are a few temperaments that the psychiatrist must be familiar with to avoid misdiagnosis. In the context of affective disorders, I approach temperaments in the following categories, along the lines of Emil Kraeplin's approach to temperament types, but with some modifications.

- Constitutionally depressive temperament
- Constitutionally elated temperament
- Constitutionally cyclical temperament
- Constitutionally irritable temperament

Please note that these temperaments are not pathological or disease states. These states refer to variations of the appropriate affect (please refer to criteria for appropriate affect/mood above). Temperaments may be a reason for being a misfit in a relationship, employment, or social situation, resulting in complaints that bring the individual for psychiatric consultation. However, ***an individual's temperament cannot be incomplete.*** Misdiagnosis of temperament as an affective disorder could lead to unwarranted pharmacological interventions, with the attended risks of the medications. On the other hand, there is a risk of missing the diagnosis of a certain affective disorder under the presumption that it might be a constitutional temperament type. Temperament types must be recognized because certain temperaments are considered high risk or a 'fertile ground' for certain affective disorders – for example, constitutional cyclothymia or Kraeplin's description of constitutional hypomania may be associated with a higher risk of bipolar disorder. So, the psychiatrist must be vigilant for the eruption of disease states in certain temperament types. Let us understand these temperament types in further detail -

- **Constitutionally depressive temperament -** I have written about this temperament in detail in the chapter on depression (please refer to the prior chapter). It is a temperament characterized by a 'gloomy' affect and a thought pattern predominated by looking at the downside of every event or circumstance. The differential diagnosis is a depressive illness, and the correct diagnosis can be clinched by using the MCE criteria for appropriate mood, described above.

- **Constitutionally elated temperament -** This temperament is essentially the opposite of the constitutionally depressive temperament. The affect is generally positive but still within the boundaries of appropriate affect (as defined by the MCE criteria mentioned above). This temperament is like Emil Kraeplin's description of 'constitutional hypomania'. However, the latter name is misleading, as this temperament is not a manic state or hypomania. Constitutionally elated temperament displays more energy (they seem resistant to fatigue), enthusiasm, and liveliness and appear more sociable. They express versatile interests, are quick to grasp opportunities (but may also quickly let them go), and tend to show interest in mastering a skill or technique. They usually have more friends and acquaintances and are well-networked. This type of temperament is more commonly seen in people occupying positions of power or leadership, such as CEOs, company directors, politicians, journalists, commercial travelers, etc. When faced with a physical illness, they could display more preoccupation with the disease (a tendency for hypochondriacal behavior). They also tend to have a higher-than-usual tendency to be litigious (fighting people through legal battles, etc.). Nevertheless, this temperament does not include antisocial or asocial tendencies.

- **Constitutionally cyclical temperament -** As the name indicates, this temperament is characterized by alternating periods of constitutionally depressive temperament and constitutional elated temperament. The periods of each temperament are typically much longer, lasting for months, seasons, or years. The affect is within appropriate limits. This temperament is similar to what was previously described as constitutional cyclothymia and is more commonly evident in artists such as musicians and authors, where their timing of productive work coincides with periods of elation, alternating with periods of constitutional depression when they are dormant and struggling with lack of creativity. Often, these individuals tend to learn to live through these episodes. There is a belief that this temperament is associated with a higher risk of bipolar disorder – but to confirm if this association is true, more stringent studies are needed, as there is a possibility that subsyndromal states are misdiagnosed as this temperament. I suggest using the MCE criteria for appropriate mood and applying MCE criteria for a manic state (as mentioned earlier in this chapter) to differentiate between constitutional elated temperament and the constitutional elated period in constitutional cyclical temperament to clinch the diagnosis accurately.

- **Constitutionally irritable temperament -** As mentioned above, irritability is a crucial feature of diseased affect. Both depressive illnesses and manic states are characterized by irritability. The latter irritability must be differentiated from a temperament of constitutional irritability – i.e., people generally described by others as being more irritable. Constitutional irritability is differentiated from irritability of affective disorders in two ways

- Affect is appropriate (defined by MCE criteria) in constitutional irritability temperament.
- Constitutional irritability temperament is not associated with periodic impulsive behavior that is typical of irritability with manic states.

However, manic states or affective disorders in general, may happen in individuals with constitutional irritable temperament, and the onset of such illness can be differentiated by the features characteristic of depressive illness and manic states described in this and the preceding chapter – i.e., presence of suffering, depressive rumination, impulsive behavior, angst, etc.

Summary - Take Home Points.

Bipolar disorder is an affective disorder, which is more common than previously believed. It could be significantly damaging to the patient's life. The necessary clinical skill is diagnosing subtle manic states, such as hypomania and pre-mania. In contrast to depressed states which are more evident through depressed affect, manic states are more evident through elated thought pattern, irritability, impulsive behavior and a pervasive change in how the individual conducts through life. Differential diagnoses include constitutional variations of temperament, and unipolar depression – and misdiagnosis could be severely damaging and detrimental to overall outcome. Clinicians also tend to shy away from diagnosing bipolar disorder, which could also lead to irreversible damages and poor outcomes. Clinicians must not underestimate their skill to detect and manage bipolar disorder, and must not hesitate to seek help and guidance from more experienced psychiatrists.

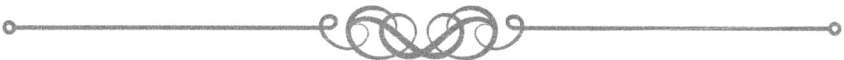

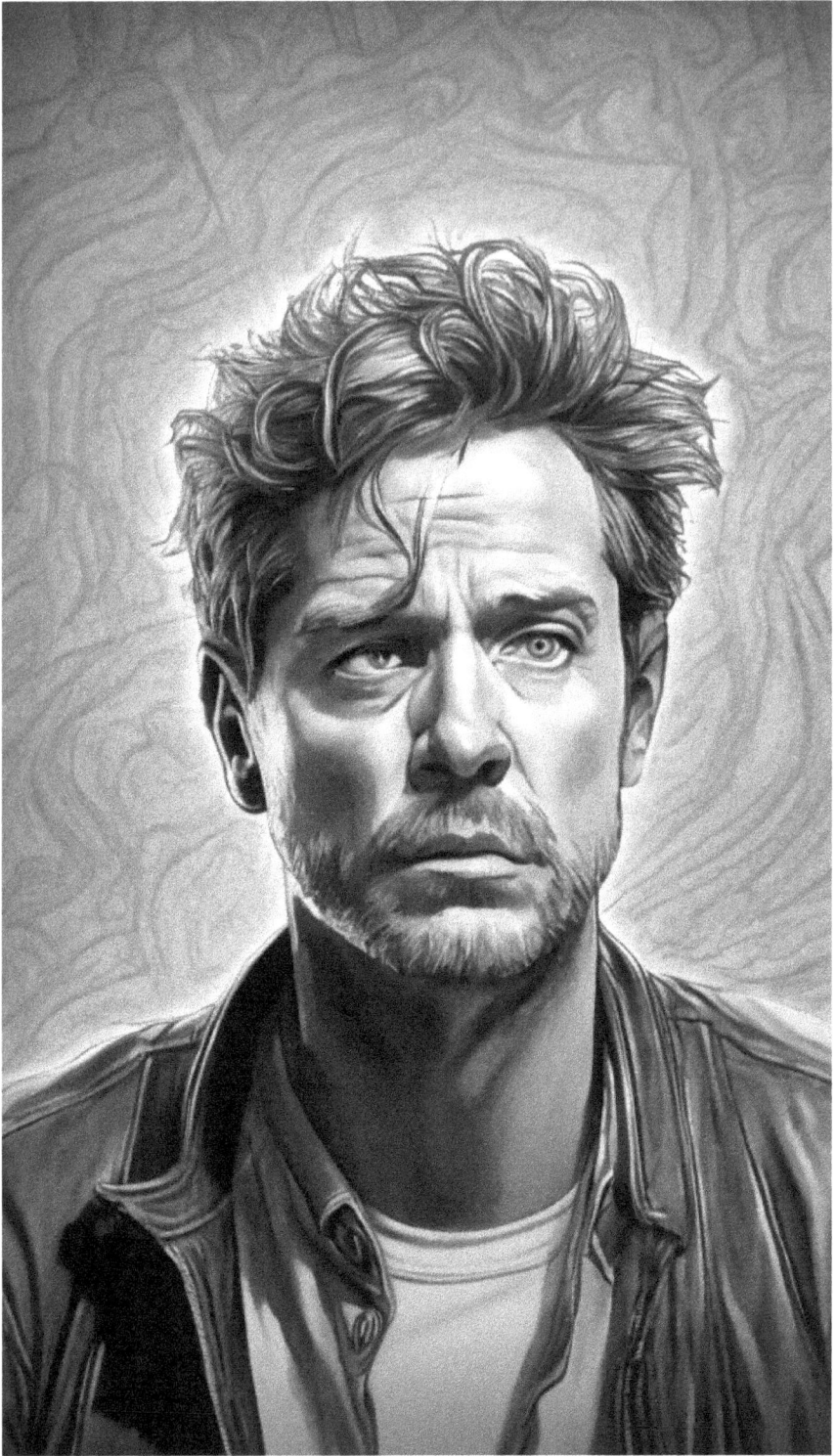

CHAPTER 9

Psychosis

One of psychiatry's most challenging tasks is managing a patient with psychosis. Before we dive into this topic, it is essential to know the importance of psychosis in psychiatry.

Psychosis has predominated in the mental health field since the inception of medical care. The root word of 'psychosis' is 'psyche', which refers to the 'mind'. Anyone who behaves like having 'lost his or her mind' was considered 'psychotic' or 'mental'. The small fraction of patients with mental health conditions that behave irrationally, have extreme or eccentric beliefs, have illogical thoughts, and display violent or aggressive behavior were considered 'psychotic' or 'mental'. It is these patients that society readily agrees with without any need for convincing that their mind or mental health is affected. Hence, for centuries if not millennia, psychotic individuals were the only ones brought to the psychiatrist. Since such patients are disruptive in domestic and public settings, they were rejected from their homes, work, and public areas. Sometimes, they were even abused or traumatized. Hence, they sought 'refuge' in mental health hospitals, and thus the term *'asylum'*, which means 'refuge' in the Greek language is used to refer to housing psychiatric patients. Psychosis is also the reason for the stigma attached to mental health patients as those who have 'lost their mind' and hence of inferior abilities, and for the stigma attached to the psychiatrist as one who is sought only for those who are 'psychotic' or 'mental'.

Since the word 'psyche' is the root of the term 'psychiatry', the common public tends to incorrectly use these words interchangeably. *A 'psychiatric patient' is not the same as a 'psychotic patient'.* This is another reason for avoiding the term 'psyche' to refer to the issues related to the entity that is affected by mental illnesses and use the word 'Ulan' instead. Please refer to this book's initial chapter (if you have not done so already) to understand the term 'Ulan'.

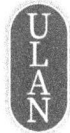

ULAN

Psychosis vs Schizophrenia

Another common misconception even among physicians, is that psychosis and schizophrenia are the same. The symptoms of schizophrenia (a thought disorder), often referred to as Schneider's first-rank symptoms, are not the features of psychosis. While it is true that patients with schizophrenia have features of psychosis, patients with psychosis are not all afflicted with schizophrenia. Pharmacological agents, called 'anti-psychotics' used in treating schizophrenia, are effective in controlling the psychotic features of schizophrenia but do not remove the underlying disorders of thought. If so, what is psychosis?

What is Psychosis?

Psychosis is not a disease but a state – a state of mind. A pathological state of mind. Psychosis may be a component of other known psychiatric disorders. There are certain psychiatric disorders with a 'psychotic' subtype as well. Furthermore, there are different types of psychosis too. Given such overlap in the presentation or manifestation of psychosis, the symptoms of psychosis vastly differ between patients and associated conditions. The conventional understanding is that psychosis is a state of mind characterized by an inability to differentiate reality from what is not. However, except in extreme situations, such an inability cannot be easily recognized, especially in the clinical setting.

I conceptualize psychosis as a pathological state of mind that is clinically recognizable through a sequential pattern such as follows –

- First, the individual is not able to recognize events that happen within the context of reality from those without it.
- Second, the individual misunderstands events happening within and around one's self.
- Lastly, the individual blames or accuses others of misunderstanding them.

In the clinical setting, if it becomes possible to elicit the presence of this 'triad' in a patient, then it is safe to consider that it is a 'psychosis'. Patients with various disorders, such as mood disorders, thought disorders, and personality disorders, may exhibit psychosis.

Schizophrenia represents one such disorder with a particular type of psychosis that is biological in origin, familial in occurrence, insidious in onset, runs a protracted course with remissions and relapses, characterized by thought and perceptual disturbances, manifested by either negative or positive symptoms. While schizophrenia often responds well to treatment, there are situations where patients may never return to complete normalcy despite active treatment. They may return to near normalcy, but near normalcy is very much an acceptable outcome, as no one is truly completely normal! (Please refer to the earlier chapter on 'normal').

Stigma of Psychosis

Historically, to the common public, the image attached to mental illness is a person who is aggressive, violent, uncontrollable, irrational, illogical, and dangerous. Essentially, it is the image of a psychotic state. Most people believe that mental illness implies one condition, and one condition only –psychosis. Furthermore, they also think that psychotic individuals are always in such an extreme state, incapable of rational decision-making in all aspects of life, unable to care for themselves, and are eligible to be denied the usual respect and privileges others enjoy. For this reason, mentally affected individuals are ignored and not brought to medical attention until violence or unmanageable behavior occurs. The extremely bizarre nature of certain psychotic states is also why mental health was associated with magico-religious beliefs and explanations and why mentally affected patients were escorted to religious godmen with hopes of getting relief from their misery.

Positive and Negative Symptoms

A psychotic state, especially in the case of schizophrenia, could manifest through a wide variety of symptoms. They are generally classified into 'positive' and 'negative' symptoms. Positive symptom refers to the excess of a previously present behavior, while negative symptom refers to the loss of a prior behavior. For example, excess talking, an overly excited state, unsolicited overzealous interaction, or 'creating a scene' is a positive symptom. In contrast, withdrawal from social situations, aloofness, and quietness is a negative symptom. To the commoner, positive symptoms are more concerning than negative ones, which are dismissed or overlooked. Positive symptoms respond well to treatment by pharmacological methods or institutionalization, and the public often sees such reduction of positive symptoms as signs of significant clinical progress. However, trained mental health professionals know that positive symptoms are more sensitive to treatment than negative symptoms, often resistant to conventional treatment. We also know that while the disappearance of positive symptoms is encouraging, the real challenge in returning the patient to pre-morbid level functioning depends on the success in managing the negative symptoms.

In the yester era, the examination of a patient with psychosis involved specifically querying for the presence of positive symptoms and Schneiderian symptoms. Pharmacological response in the form of the disappearance of positive symptoms, i.e., 'quietening' of the patient, was considered a clinical improvement and enough to tolerate their presence at home or public places. Electroconvulsive therapy (ECT) played a vital role in achieving this goal. Even today, ECT and the older class of antipsychotic medications form the mainstay of the management of psychotic states. However, in the current era, we understand that quietening positive symptoms alone is not enough. Negative symptoms need to be reversed, so rehabilitation can result in functional re-integration of such patients as productive citizens.

Impact of Psychosis on Prognosis

It was presumed that psychosis would only be associated with increased morbidity and decreased quality of life. But more recent evidence has demonstrated that the longevity of individuals with psychosis is also reduced, and quite alarmingly so. Some argue that it might be due to newer antipsychotic drugs which could cause chronic metabolic derangements, but this is debatable. A more plausible explanation could be the negligence of the medical fraternity to the complaints of psychosis, which could be picked up earlier, and subject to more effective treatment. Furthermore, the legal rights and social privileges of individuals affected with psychosis are also at stake and must be duly protected by the psychiatrist.

Differential Diagnoses

Prodrome of schizophrenia, schizotypal personality, brief psychotic disorder, schizophreniform disorder, acute psychosis, toxic psychosis, first episode psychosis, borderline personality disorder, delusional disorder, schizophrenia, schizoaffective disorder, major depressive disorder with psychotic features, bipolar disorder with psychotic features, Substance-induced psychotic disorder, and early dementia are the important differential diagnoses for a patient with a psychotic state.

Clinical Interview

It is truly an art that must be mastered. It requires diligence, clinical acumen, general knowledge about worldly affairs, and nuanced communication skills. I teach my trainees that while dealing with psychosis, it is not about how to ask a question but about when to ask a question and what questions to ask when. A few critical principles for a successful interview of a psychotic patient are –

Avoid the question, 'What is your problem?', or similar questions that convey to the patient that you are convinced that the patient indeed has a 'problem'. Such questions make suspicious patients defensive, and they might stop answering the examiner's questions or provide evasive answers for the rest of the interview.

- Sacrifice ease of questioning to build trust with the patient. Although it is more time-effective to stick to the traditional and comprehensive format for psychiatric and medical history taking, such simple, direct, and closed-ended questioning may make the patient feel prejudiced and alienated. New trainees and inexperienced psychiatrists may prefer to elicit the symptom checklist to arrive at a DSM diagnosis. In contrast, more experienced psychiatrists may expend time framing the right question and waiting for the right time to ask such a question to build a rapport and therapy-facilitating trust with the patient. Given the thought disturbances of a patient with psychosis, simple talk with the patient might seem absurd and weird, but it paves the way for smooth eliciting of the psychopathy. Simply put, talk with the patient – but remember that the purpose of talking is an examination, and so talk with shrewd observation!

- For a successful interview, the patient must feel safe and comfortable; for the latter, the examiner must first feel safe and comfortable. So, arrange the seating so that there is ancillary staff or a reliable caregiver by the patient's side until the examiner feels the patient is not a danger. Once the examiner feels safe, the ancillary staff/caregiver may be dismissed so that the patient may feel safe to trust the psychiatrist with information. Also, it is essential that seating is not arranged so that the patient feels that they are being observed or monitored.
- The patient must know or be able to understand to some extent why they are there for the interview and be aware of the expectations and the probable outcome of the interview.
- The patient must be made to understand that the details of the interview are confidential.
- Be knowledgeable and talk in the native language and if possible, in the local dialect.
- Discuss at a level that is congruent to the level of intelligence, literacy, education, and culture of the patient.
- Keep in mind that patients with psychosis have features of disorganization and disturbances in attention and concentration, and conduct the interview accordingly to accommodate for their disorganization.
- Be aware of the time duration of the interview and formulate the style and module of the interview accordingly.
- Questions must be brief and straightforward but not confrontational or judgmental.
- Avoid leading questions.
- Avoid questions, gestures, attitudes, or statements that may appear critical or judgmental of the patient.
- Introduce yourself as the therapist or psychiatrist – families, especially in Asian societies, may request the psychiatrist to be introduced as the family's friend or relative. However, this is unprofessional and would be counter-productive to the doctor-patient relationship in the long run.
- The initial phase of the interview should be broad-based

rather than specific, which is a tension-easing approach to examining psychosis in general.

- All questions may not yield answers from the patient. The patient not answering a question is also an answer. It might mean 'I don't know the answer', 'I do not want to answer', 'There is no need to answer', 'The question is not warranted', or simply a sign of protest.

The chief complaint

By virtue of their predominantly textbook knowledge, beginning trainees in psychiatry think that the complaints or presenting symptoms of psychosis are hallucinations, delusions, ideas of reference, etc. These are not the typical presenting complaints. The usual presenting complaints of psychosis at the time of initial presentation may not overtly reveal the diagnosis of psychosis, as they often pertain to problems in daily living or behavior, such as - hostility, irritability, avoidance, abusive behavior or speech, assaultive behavior, aggression, suspiciousness, wandering behavior, refusal of food, preoccupation, withdrawn or aloof behavior, not going to work, sleeplessness, deliberate self-harm.

During the initial encounter, after the psychiatrist has diagnosed psychosis as having been the underlying etiology for the manifestation or any of the above chief complaints, they could educate the patient and the family on the psychopathology, after which the patient or the family could better recognize and describe the symptoms of hallucinations or delusions as complaints in subsequent encounters.

History of presenting illness

It is difficult to follow the traditional order and flow of a psychiatric history taking in a patient with psychosis. The psychiatrist must be able to tactfully rearrange the order of the elements of the MSE to fit the patient's condition. But it helps to preserve the essence of the orderliness and thoroughness of MSE. Some practically useful concepts during this portion of the interview with a psychotic state patient are -

- Signs and symptoms in psychiatry overlap. So, what is presented to the psychiatrist as a complaint and what the psychiatrist needs to elicit may overlap. Asking clarifying questions and pursuing in detail the information provided to the psychiatrist may help unearthing the truth.

- Direct and confrontational questioning may be unyielding. Start with broad conceptual questions in an agreeable tone, then gradually hone in to chisel out the unwanted information from the delusional content of the patient's thoughts.

- Inquire more about the nature of the psychotic episode and ask for the triggering and precipitating factors of such episodes, and then trace the events in both antegrade and retrograde fashion, keeping these psychotic episodes as a reference point.

- Some daily life examples that may be manifestations of psychosis include – a fall in academic performance, picking up brawls and quarrels with friends and family unlike before, shifting homes or residence without a firm or valid reason, striking changes in lifestyle or religious conviction.

- ***When was the first time help was sought?*** – This is an essential piece of information often occult in the eastern half of the world. Let me explain – the symptoms of psychosis, manifest as problems of living or behavior (as mentioned above), may have been recognized as 'problems' by the patient or the family, but misconstrued as a one-off occurrence, bad luck or personal deviance. Care might have been sought through non-medical platforms such as going to temples, pursuing astrologers, undertaking pilgrimages, performing rituals/sacrifices to ward off evil forces, native redressal methods, etc. This information allows assessment of the chronicity of the problem.

- Apart from the presenting chief complaint, the manifestations of a psychotic state may be evident in a diverse set of circumstances, which need to be asked for, as they may not be recognized or volunteered by the patient and family. In my 40 years of clinical practice in psychiatry, I have learned the 'early signs of psychosis', which are compiled in the following table –

Early signs of Psychosis
– Mananalam Clinic Experience

MCE

Physiological

- Excessive sleeping
- Inability to fall asleep

Social functioning

- Social withdrawal
- Isolation
- Reclusiveness
- Deterioration of social relationships
- Shift in basic nature/personality

Affective changes

- Depressed mood
- Bizarre behavior
- Inability to cry
- Excessive crying
- Inappropriate laughter
- Indifference
- Inability to cope with minor problems
- Extreme reactions to criticism
- Inability to express joy

Changes in occupational performance

- 'Dropping out' of activities in life in general
- Decline in academic performance
- Decline in athletic interest
- Absenteeism from work
- Sudden resignation or quitting from work

Cognitive changes

- Unusual forgetfulness
- Inability to concentrate
- Preoccupation of mind
- Remembering and blaming childhood activities and memories
- Blaming parents for academic failures

Behavioral changes

- Unusual sensitivity to stimuli
- Strange posturing
- Hyperactivity
- Inactivity
- Extreme preoccupation with religion or occult philosophies
- Excessive writing without any meaning
- Peculiar use of words
- Odd language structures or sentence formations
- Shaving one's head hair or body hair for no valid reason
- Cutting one's body/ Self-mutilation
- Staring without blinking
- Blinking incessantly
- Flat 'reptile-like' gaze
- Rigid stubbornness
- Refusal to touch others or objects
- Sudden change in food preferences, such as vegetarianism
- Cooking for oneself (unlike before)
- Avoid eating with family or others
- Not leaving the home
- Not leaving one's room
- Prefers to be inside a room without any lights
- Sealing the entry of light into the room
- Increased religiosity
- Long prayer sessions.
- Increased interest in magical and religious activities (unlike before)

> ### *Behavioral changes - continued*
> - Unprecedented aggression
> - Unwarranted hostility

Premorbid level of functioning

After the history of the presenting complaint is interrogated in detail, inquire into details of the level of functioning prior to the illness's morbidity. During the pre-morbid period, preoccupation with self, extreme sensitivity to criticism, difficulty initiating relationships, pseudo-scientific and pseudo-philosophical beliefs may have sporadically erupted, and patients might have acted upon those thoughts too. But such behavior might not have been mainstream, and no morbidity might have set in. Interpersonal relationship disruptions, behavioral disturbances, and odd behaviors must be inquired and ruled out. During this time, it may become apparent that the patient may have schizoid or schizotypal traits – these traits are also associated with thought and perception irregularities, with the difference being whether such traits are pervasive and consistent throughout a person's behavior over time (i.e., 'schizoid'), or episodic and erupting in bouts (i.e., 'schizotypal').

Since psychotic states start insidiously, and progress very slowly during the initial stages, patients in continuous long-term contact may either fail to notice irregularities in the patient's behavior, rationalizing them to not be of concern, or as a unique response to a stressor. However, those who interact with the patient intermittently or for a short term, such as colleagues, friends, and neighbors, may have noticed their abnormalities readily but did not undertake reporting them. This is a proximity paradox – and understanding the latter could help the psychiatrist elicit a more comprehensive history of the illness.

The prodrome

Certain illnesses may be characterized by a period of subtle and simmering symptoms before the manifestation of overt symptoms – that early period of simmering symptoms is called 'prodrome'. While the family and friends of a patient are generally more concerned with clearly psychotic behavior, there might have been milder symptoms during the prodrome that might have been ignored or overlooked. Mild symptoms may be transient too. During this time, the patient may develop new interests, alterations in thinking, perceptual changes, and bizarre ideas based on their pseudo-philosophical and pseudoscientific thoughts. Due to judgment influenced by disordered thoughts, they entertain risky propositions such as change of residence, work, affiliation, faith, or investments. I have seen patients make terrible decisions and suffer significant losses, including indispensable relationships. During the interrogation about the prodromal phase, also look for cognitive difficulties. In this stage, cognitive irregularities such as impaired executive functioning may exist without overt cognitive deficits.

Mental status examination

The principles of mental status examination described in an earlier chapter must be followed. However, certain fundamental principles must be considered during the mental status examination of a patient with psychosis or if psychosis is suspected.

- Irregularities or oddities in thinking alone do not qualify as psychosis. Diagnosis of psychosis through the presence of a delusion requires ***conviction.*** Using words such as 'I think...', 'I feel...', 'I hope...', 'I say...', and 'I believe...' is insufficient to establish a diagnosis.
- Pursue and establish in detail the content of the thought, as it is essential for managing the psychosis. Remember – the nature of the content of the thought or belief in question does not matter much to diagnosis but to management. That is, the diagnosis of delusion is not decided by the content of the thought or belief but by how that thought occurs or the belief is held. Nevertheless, the thought content helps draft nuanced and patient-specific treatment strategies.
- Give due importance to both positive and negative symptoms. Look for Schneiderian symptoms (i.e., the first-rank symptoms of schizophrenia), as they are necessary for diagnostic reasons. However, Schneiderian symptoms pertain only to the positive symptoms, which are easy to treat and respond well to pharmacological interventions but are not enough for the patient's recovery to a pre-morbid

level of functioning. Specifically, interrogate and examine for negative symptoms (such as social withdrawal, quietness, etc.), as these symptoms need to be resolved for a meaningful recovery.

- Thoughts of grandeur or nihilism do not necessarily imply the presence of delusions. Grandeur or nihilism may be a manifestation of affective disorders or thought disorders. The best way to differentiate between them is to look for *'mood-thought congruence'.* This concept has been explained in detail in the publication on Ulan (refer to Chapter 2).

- *Indulgent inquiry* – Perception is not reality, but no individual can tell them apart for oneself! A third person, i.e., the examiner, may be able to tell them apart from the individual in question. Still, the examiner inevitably becomes a part of the perception, and hence the reality, of the individual being examined. Therefore, the examiner must walk into the patient's mental sphere and get a taste of their experience by walking in their shoes. This is why perceptual disturbances are hard to elicit – the examiner may want to slide past or avoid much effort in this area of examination, as it requires the examiner to move out of their comfort zone. For the patient, their perception, including delusion, hallucinations, etc., are real – so direct questioning, such as 'Do you feel that other people are harming you?' may not bring forth helpful answers. The examiner should avoid terms such as 'thinking', 'feeling', etc.; instead, it is better to ask, *at the right stage of the interview,* 'Is there anyone plotting against you?' 'Is there anyone harming you?', 'Are you under surveillance?', 'Is there a force watching you?' etc. This style of examination, which I call *indulgent inquiry,* makes the patient feel that the examiner is part of his perception/reality. As the individual lacks insight, it is better to ask about the perceptual and thought disorders as if they are happening. Examples include, 'Do people plot against you? Is anybody planning that you do not achieve your targets? Are people deliberately preventing you from achieving your goals? Are you perplexed or worried that you cannot trust

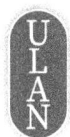

your family members? Wherever you go, people follow you, so is your privacy at stake? See the associated table on sample questions and statements for this interviewing style.

- Imagination, fantasy, illusion, delusion, and hallucination are all different phenomena but may manifest with overlapping symptoms, resulting in diagnostic mistakes. Delusions, thought disorders, and perceptual disorders are ***not imaginary*** thought content. Suppose the individual is conscious and aware that a subset of their thoughts are not real and can exercise control over such thoughts and contain them within the will of the individual. In that case, such thoughts qualify as 'imagination'. On the other hand, if thoughts occur 'out of the blue' and are not within the will and control of the individual, then they qualify to be within the diagnostic bucket that includes thought and perception disorders.
- Cognition must be examined. Insight is a part of this area of the mental status examination. Insight is best established through an informal style of inquiry. The presence or absence of insight is one of the most clinically valuable elements in a patient with psychosis. Grading of insight, however, is merely an academic exercise. Also, as mentioned before, in psychosis, cognitive disturbances range from simple or focal impairment in functioning to pervasive or noticeable cognitive deficits – a patient may progress from the former to the latter during the progression of the condition associated with the psychotic state.
- If the psychotic state is due to schizophrenia, the examiner should broadly approach the examination to fulfill 5 clinical symptom domains – positive, negative, affective, cognitive, and aggressive. All these domains need to be explored – it helps to start the discussion broadly, then narrow down to more specific details using particulars from the individual's life given by the individual itself. Finally, explore in the most detailed way the different elements of the delusions and hallucinations at a stage when the patient and examiner are both within a relaxed and mutually trusting state.
- Concurrent psychiatric comorbidities may exist alongside psychosis. All symptoms do not need to fit within a single

diagnosis. One of my professors used to say, 'Every patient has the right to have more than one illness!'. This is a rule of thumb, not just in psychosis but for psychiatry in general, that screening for depression, anxiety, obsession, phobia, suicidality, and other such diagnosis must be performed. The skill of comprehensive analysis, but not wasting much time, is the most difficult to attain in psychiatry and requires experience, constant learning from experience, and collegial learning.

- *Diagnostic mistakes related to psychotic states could be costly and damaging.* Mistakes in diagnosing the presence/absence of psychosis and the clinical disorder associated with the psychotic state could lead the examiner down the wrong path and the patient along with it, resulting in irreversible loss of time, polypharmacy, and poor clinical outcome. Seeking the help of experienced colleagues and taking time to double-check or even triple-check one's diagnostic algorithm can help prevent such mistakes.

In summary, mental status examination is not about going through the diagnostic and symptom checklist in a rote manner. The latter style is a recipe for making diagnostic mistakes! It is not about eliciting or making the patient commit to the information required for diagnosis. Instead, the examiner should examine the whole patient in a wholesome manner. It starts from the time the examiner sets eyes on the patient – hygiene, self-care, dress/attire, comfort level, signs of intoxication, level of consciousness, adverse drug reactions such as dystonia, akathisia, affect, energy, catatonic symptoms, formal thought disturbances, etc all form part of the mental status examination. Active questioning is only a minor part of the examination, it is more of 'observing during questioning'. The examiner must be able to observe the patient, then walk into the patient's mental bubble, get a glimpse of what the patient perceives as reality, and then walk out of it and continue the examination.

Indulgent inquiry style interviewing
- Mananalam Clinic Experience

MCE

(These are sample statements or questions uttered by the psychiatrist during the mental status examination, and their affirmation by the patient elicits delusions. Hallucinations are better elicited through questions rather than by statements)

Delusions of persecution

- 'Somebody is trying to harm you.'
- 'Someone is planning/plotting against you.'
- 'Some is preventing your success and achievements.'
- 'Your life is in danger.'
- 'Your own people are against you.'
- 'You are not able to get things done for yourself.'
- 'People are taking photos of your activity without your knowledge and sending it to everyone.'
- 'You are under surveillance.'

Delusions of control

- 'Some outside force is watching your activities and controlling your actions.'
- 'What you do is not per your will, but by the will of someone else.'
- 'It is not you who is responsible for the actions happening.'

Delusions of grandiosity

- 'You have some special power, talent, or skill suddenly gifted to you.'
- 'You have been suddenly assigned a major task that nobody can do or execute.'
- 'You can perform or achieve anything, and how it can be done is a secret.'
- 'You are the heir or waiting for a position to be assigned to you.'
- 'The Almighty /God has selected you for a special mission.'

Delusions of mind-reading

- 'Someone knows what is in your mind, and you are thinking within yourself even if you do not disclose it.'
- 'People read your thoughts and act accordingly.'
- 'There is no secrecy for you as everybody knows what you are thinking.'

Thought insertion

- 'Someone else is putting the thoughts in your mind; it's not yours.'
- 'You are not responsible for your thoughts as they are not yours.'

Thought broadcasting

- 'Your thoughts are known to everybody because they are being broadcast by evil forces or utilizing some technology.'

Thought withdrawal

- 'There are no thoughts in your mind because they are being stolen or removed by some force.'

Passivity phenomenon

- 'You are not doing anything; you are being made to do everything.'
- 'Nothing is in your will or choice.'

Delusions of reference

- 'Whatever happens around you has a special meaning for you.'
- 'Wherever you go, people are talking about you.'
- 'People are discussing you and making gestures referring to you in unknown places which disturbs you.'
- Somatization.
- 'Something is grossly not right in your body.'

Thought block

- 'Suddenly, there is nothing to say.'

Auditory hallucinations

- 'Do you hear people talking to you even when they are not physically present before you?'
- 'Do you hear known or unknown voices talking to you even when they are absent?'
- 'Do you get perplexed hearing voices without persons?'
- 'Can those voices be heard by others near you?'
- 'Do the voices come from within you or from an outside source?'
- 'Is it one voice or many voices?'
- 'Are they talking to you? Or amongst themselves?'
- 'Are they passing a running commentary of your actions?'
- 'Are they commanding you?'
- 'Are they compelling you to do something?'
- 'Do you talk to, or converse with them?'
- 'Do you reply to them in your mind, or by voice?'

Interview pertaining to differential diagnosis

There are certain common pitfalls during the examination of psychotic states, which the psychiatrist needs to be acutely aware of –

- Substance abuse history must be thoroughly established. Cannabis, weed, and vaping are now ubiquitous, especially in youth. Alcohol use history must be obtained in detail. Recreational and 'party drugs', stimulants, sedatives, and hypnotics should also be specifically asked for. The patient's family may be sensitive, stigmatized, or in denial of this examination area; hence, this interrogation may need to be done privately. In these cases, it is wise to perform urine or blood analysis for a drug panel. The use of intoxicants with prescription medications is not uncommon and must be explored.

- History of head injury must not be forgotten.
- Inquire for symptoms of organic brain conditions, especially when the illness is acute in onset, bizarre/atypical in description, or associated with cognitive impairment. In these cases, obtaining a thorough neurological and neuro-physiological assessment and imaging studies is wise.
- Explore the presence of sexual disorders and gender identity disorders, which may present with odd or atypical symptoms that may overlap with manifestations of psychosis.

Certain Special Situations

Each patient is different, and every patient is different when they are alone compared to being around others and may behave differently depending on who is around. Sensitive issues such as ongoing substance abuse, details on interpersonal relationships, sexual functioning, conflicts with family members, and adverse effects of medications may need to be addressed in private and sometimes inquired from family/caregivers in the absence of the patient.

Adolescents with psychotic issues need a more comprehensive examination, incorporating principles of child/adolescent psychiatry (as explained in an earlier chapter) and the principles described in this chapter.

Aged people with psychosis must be investigated for organic pathologies, which are more common with advancing age.

Uncooperative patients with psychosis pose challenging obstacles to examination. In these situations, avoid asking about symptoms – questioning must be broad and general, focusing on what is distressing to the patient until cooperation develops. Avoid confrontational questions, disagreement, and judgmental approaches. Remember what I had said earlier in this chapter - While dealing with psychosis, it is not about how to ask a question, but about when to ask a question and what questions to ask when.

If a patient is violent, agitated, and poses a risk to self, environment, or others, pharmacological interventions to sedate the patient are an option. Do not hesitate to call for assistance.

Documentation

Drafting a case sheet does not entail writing everything the client tells verbatim. Documenting everything said by the patient and family could require extensive writing and essential details may be lost in such verbosity.

Concluding the Examination

Examination concludes after diagnosis is arrived. However, the examination may not conclude at the end of the interview session or patient encounter. In general, trainees and rookie psychiatrists tend to make the diagnosis at the first encounter and may appear proud and confident of the diagnosis. Experienced psychiatrists are more cautious and hesitant to make the diagnosis as they are more aware of the differential diagnoses.

Concluding the Interview Session

Concluding the interview session is a crucial event in the interview process. It must address the patient's concerns and the family/caregivers' concerns. Counseling the family is a critical component of the concluding method.

It is natural that the family and caregivers 'want an answer right away'. The family may be divided on their opinions and anxious to settle their dispute on who is correct or to establish the other party is at fault. In this era of internet information, the family and caregivers walk in with a pre-existing bias that psychosis or schizophrenia means bad news or a terrible prognosis. With pre-existing bias or internet knowledge, they may bombard the psychiatrist with loaded and preposterous questions, the answers to which are either not warranted or not available to the psychiatrist readily after the first encounter.

The psychiatrist must educate the patient and the family on the complexities of diagnosis and management. Education on what psychosis means and dispelling serious myths and misconceptions of psychosis must be undertaken regardless of whether the patient has psychosis. Informing patients that psychosis and mental states, in general, are associated with the chemical functioning of the brain, just like diabetes or thyroid disease, could help in understanding the biological nature of the condition, which in turn may undo the anxiety and stigma associated with the diagnosis. The psychiatrist must be able to employ various techniques, without misrepresenting facts or presenting half-truths, to break the news of psychosis or schizophrenia or any bad news associated with the disorder and its prognosis.

It helps to tell the patient and family that psychosis is a 'provisional diagnosis'. When sufficient information is available, the diagnosis can be confirmed with confidence. Emphasize and re-emphasize that disease is a continuously changing phenomenon; hence, periodic re-evaluation and re-assertion of the diagnosis is necessary. Once the diagnosis is given, the next question faced by the examiner is the prognosis. In the case of psychosis associated with schizophrenia, I have found it beneficial to say, *'In present times, people with schizophrenia are fortunate compared to earlier times because if recognized early and treated appropriately with a multimodal approach right from the beginning along with the help of the family and caregivers to ensure compliance, recovery could be impressive'.* I have seen that such a statement reassures the worries of the patient and the family.

In my personal experience, I have seen remarkable recoveries from psychosis and schizophrenia, with patients living their lives and performing professionally even better than before their illness. Like with any illness in medicine in general, some patients will get well, some will improve but not recover completely, some will stay as they are, and some may get worse despite treatment – but everyone is better under the appropriate medical care than without it. After the advent of long-acting drugs, multimodal therapy, and rehabilitation, the prognosis in this condition is much better than what was believed to be.

Often, the family, or the immediate caregiver, such as the parent or spouse, is significantly stressed psychologically by the patient's symptoms, which are often directed mainly at the closest and dearest person. For example, a spouse may be distraught about persecutory delusions directed at them or delusions of infidelity. In these situations, I counsel the imme-diate caregiver in this way – *'the amount of suffering the patient would be undergoing in believing that somebody that he/she loves so much (i.e., the caregiver) is acting against them would be far more than anybody else's suffering.* The latter statement allows the caregiver to empathize with the patient's suffering and alleviate the caregiver's suffering. Emphasize that psychosis could make the patient not realize the extent of their suffering and that the nature of the condition prevents them from seeking a remedy. Remember - Infusing such rationality and pragmatism facilitates nurturing qualities of the people around the patient to the patient's benefit! Make it clear to the family that patients with psychosis may not seek treatment independently when the disease is active. Hence, it is not just a legal obligation but a binding moral duty to facilitate the process of the patient seeking psychiatric care and ensuring compliance.

In summary, the psychiatrist must infuse hope within the realm of truth and be optimistic while being realistic. Do not conclude the interview session with counter arguments to patient's statements, or with disagreement. The goal of the concluding moment in the interview is to leave the patient and family intending to continue pursuing treatment. Let the have the patient have the last word!

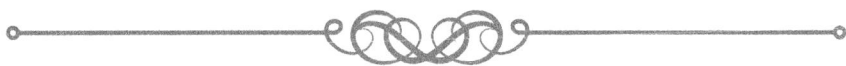

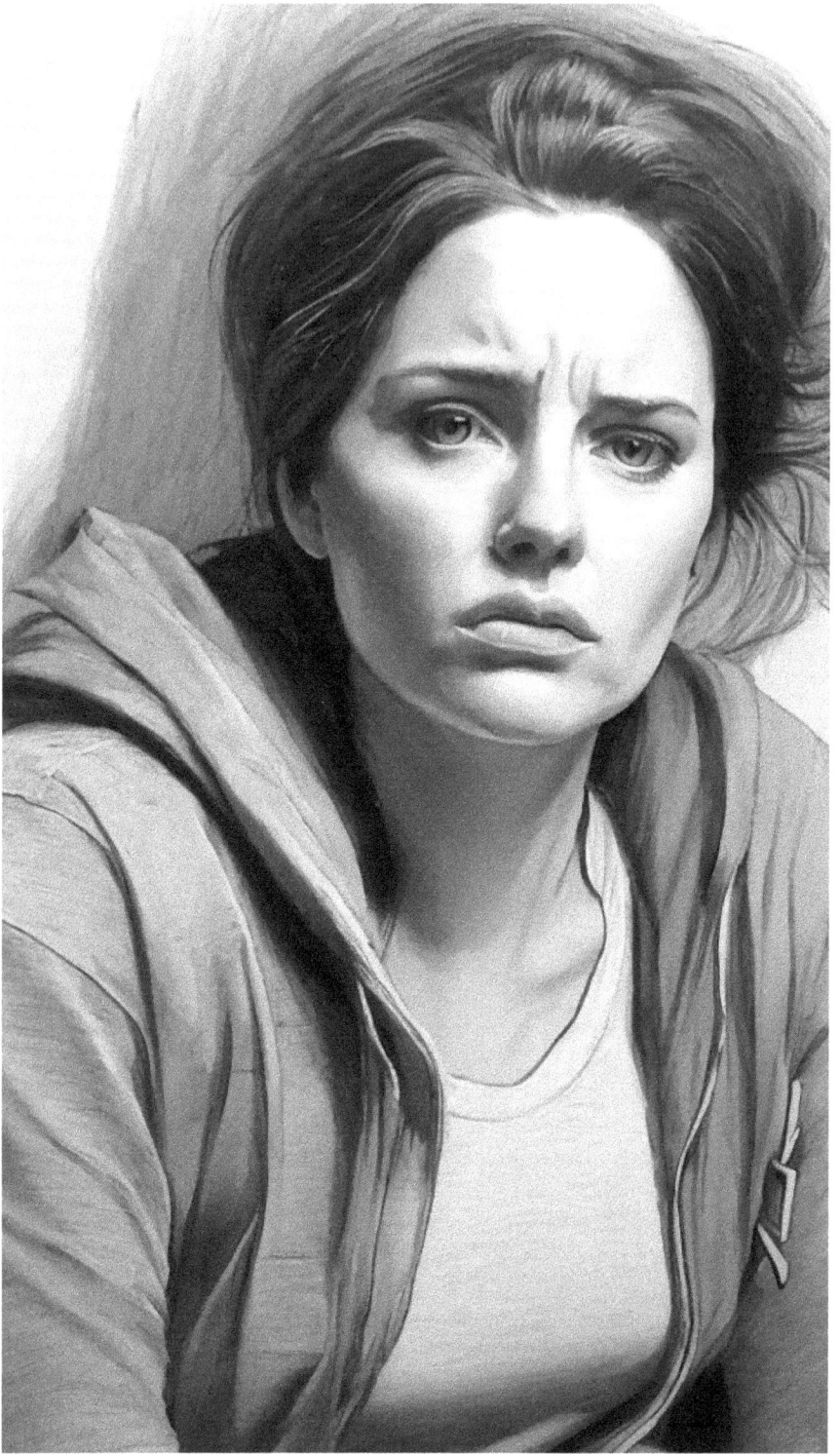

CHAPTER 10

Anxiety Disorder

What is Anxiety?

Anxiety comes from the Latin root 'ango', meaning distressed, troubled, or fearful. In clinical practice, anxiety is defined as the ***affective state of increased arousal***. It is an unpleasant state associated with increased autonomic activity. For practical purposes, it is nothing but fear – a heightened fear state, a sense of impending danger. In an everyday conversation, people use words such as 'stress', 'nervousness', 'tension', or 'nervous breakdown' to describe anxiety.

Anxiety is universal and is the most frequently experienced negative affect. Anxiety could be a physiological response to certain stimuli or a pathological state. Anxiety as a physiological response is a valuable and necessary survival mechanism. Anxiety is an *'alarm signal for danger'*. It occurs physiologically as a response to unusual, out-of-the-ordinary, highly stressful, or dangerous situations and is intended to enhance chances of success or survival. This type of anxiety makes the individual act in a way that escapes or neutralizes danger and is beneficial. However, such physiological anxiety is typically brief and dissipates quickly. Even if the stressful stimuli persist, adaptive mechanisms kick in, and anxiety dissipates.

On the other hand, anxiety that is frequent, brought about by relatively trivial or non-extreme conditions, persistent for more extended periods, non-dissipating, or severe in intensity enough to disrupt performance are pathological forms of anxiety. Though not life-threatening, anxiety is the cause of tremendous loss in personal life, social situations, and employment-related opportunities. It may result in severe disability and poor quality of life. It limits the individual's potential to perform optimally or excel in social and occupational situations and may hamper personal interactions. Essentially, it results in many 'lost opportunities', the loss of which is unmeasurable.

As per the DSM, anxiety is approached through six different clinical categories – Phobias, Panic disorder with or without Agoraphobia, Generalized Anxiety Disorder (GAD), Obsessive Compulsive Disorder (OCD), Acute Stress Disorder, and Post Traumatic Stress Disorder (PTSD). Traditionally, anxiety is approached as a 'minor' mental health issue. However, per the Ulan concept of mental health (refer to earlier chapters), anxiety is classified as a 'mentally not healthy' condition, as the individual suffers significantly, with little to no suffering to others. In my experience, ***anxiety is probably the most damaging mental health disorder*** and is difficult to treat. It is curable, but tough to do so and requires exceptional clinical acumen, psychoanalytic skills, and expertise in cognitive therapy.

Anxiety vs Fear

Fear is a commonly used term to describe the affective state of anxiety. It is indeed an accurate description. However, there is a crucial difference – anxiety is a ***de novo*** response, while fear is a ***learned*** response. Anxiety occurs in newborns and infants and may happen without an apparent reason. Fear, on the other hand, is not innately present in children. They learn fear as life progresses. The anxiety response, however, is manifested through the autonomic nervous system, through various symptoms depending on the organ system that displays it. Examples include respiratory symptoms like dyspnea, cough, gastrointestinal symptoms like nausea, heartburn, diarrhea, constipation, cardiac symptoms like palpitations or chest pain, etc. The response type and pattern are idiosyncratic. On the other hand, fear response is typically manifest through behavior patterns that are also learned and are specific to the individual, social, and cultural factors. This differentiation is crucial because fear is not pathological and is not a clinical diagnosis, even if it occurs in atypical situations or with atypical severity. Being fearful is a trait and does not by itself cause mental distress. Anxiety is not a trait, but a physiological response or a pathological condition.

Anxiety as a Standalone Diagnosis

Anxiety, an 'alarm signal' erupted by the brain, is probably the trickiest clinical situation to analyze. Anxiety could be due to various underlying medical or psychiatric diagnoses, some of which may remain undiscovered in contemporary medicine. Anxiety, in the clinical scenario, may be encountered in any of the following contexts –

- Anxiety co-existing as a physiological response to medical or psychiatric diagnosis.
- Anxiety as a co-morbid diagnosis in the presence of other medical or psychiatric diagnoses, with both of these diagnoses being unrelated to one another.
- Anxiety as a presenting complaint or symptoms (i.e., manifestation) of another medical or psychiatric diagnosis.
- Anxiety as a standalone clinical diagnosis and being the predominant causative factor for other diagnoses that may emerge due to unresolved anxiety.

Let us discuss each of these contexts in further detail –

Anxiety as a physiological response to other medical or psychiatric conditions could be differentiated by onset after the emergence of the other diagnosis, brief periodicity, presence of insight, and emergence of adaptive mechanisms to temper the anxiety. Anxiety from separation from a caregiver is quite common and more common in children, termed separation anxiety. The latter may persist into late childhood and adolescence, at which point, its understanding as a normal physiological phenomenon becomes questionable and must be investigated further.

Anxiety as a co-morbid condition (as a pre-existing diagnosis established by another physician) usually requires repeat comprehensive mental status evaluation to ascertain if it is related to other medical or psychiatric diagnoses. This is important because anxiety is often a presenting complaint of multiple other diagnoses, especially medical disorders, including endocrine (such as hyperthyroidism and hypercortisolemia), cardiac (arrhythmias, cardiomyopathy, mitral valve prolapse), neurological (such as traumatic brain injury, epilepsy), and substance abuse disorders (in both intoxications and withdrawals). Pharmacotherapies (especially stimulants and atypical antipsychotics) can also result in anxiety. The most common co-morbid condition for one type of anxiety disorder is another anxiety-related condition.

Anxiety co-exists with other psychiatric diagnoses. For example, anxiety could occur during hypomania, manic episodes, or major depressive episodes. Anxiety is not necessarily a symptom in these cases and may cease after the associated psychiatric diagnosis is treated. In these cases, anxiety as a separate diagnosis is not needed or warranted. Patients with anxiety and depressive disorder as co-diagnoses are associated with increased suicide risk.

Anxiety could be a presenting symptom in certain psychiatric diagnoses. For example, anxiety is one of the earliest symptoms of psychosis and may present even before overt symptoms of psychosis happen. Here, anxiety presents in heightened frequency. If anxiety occurs only at the time of delusions or hallucinations, then a separate diagnosis of anxiety disorder is not needed or warranted. Anxiety is also an early symptom of dementia.

Anxiety as a standalone clinical diagnosis is warranted whenever the fear as an affective state is inappropriate. For criteria defining 'appropriate affect', please refer to the earlier chapter in this book on depression. Essentially, an affect is appropriate if it occurs in response to a stimulus, is proportionate in quality and severity to the stimulus's nature, disappears after the stimulus's removal, elicits adaptive mechanisms on the persistence of the stimulus, and does not result in functional impairment. Anxiety that is, ***de novo***, disproportionate to the stimulus, persists despite removal of the stimulus, does not wane down with time in the long run, results in functional impairment, and occurs temporally exclusive of other psychiatric diagnoses, is indeed pathological and warrants consideration for being an independent diagnosis.

Due to the high prevalence of anxiety disorders in the general population, it is a common clinical problem for internists and general practitioners, who, when trained well to identify anxiety, become a significant referral source for the psychiatrist. Disregarding anxiety as a trivial problem, dismissing the need for a psychiatric referral, or kneejerk treatment of anxiety with anxiolytics are major clinical mistakes.

Understanding Anxiety

Anxiety is a universal phenomenon, and all individuals might have felt it at some point. It is so widely experienced that it is overlooked as a pathological state, even in its most abnormal form. For this reason, patients and some clinicians prefer not to label anxiety as a 'disorder' or 'diagnosis'. In academic circles, anxiety is approached from varied perspectives.

The most common perspective is the life history or event perspective, where anxiety is viewed as a response to a particular stimulus in the environment, often a consequence of a significant life experience or event. The separation of the caretaker of a child, causing separation anxiety, becomes the model to explain this perspective. Stressful life events, such as severe physical or mental trauma, are used to explain various anxiety disorders in adolescence or childhood. Anxiety is thus rationalized as the adaptation to stressful events during developmental phases- loss of a parent, abandonment, parental alcoholism or substance abuse history, emotional and personal insecurities, etc.

Another perspective is the ***behavioral perspective***, wherein anxiety is viewed through the lens of the type of response mounted to a life event rather than looking at the life event as a causative event. The same event provokes anxiety in one person, while another remains unaffected. Thresholds for anxiety and propensity for heightened anxiety are traits related to the individual's personality type and can explain the development of anxiety disorders from the behavioral response pattern determined by their personality.

Next is the ***medical perspective*** – Here, we consider anxiety disorder as a medical illness, where abnormal levels of anxiety (with the presumption that there are normal physiological responses of anxiety in all individuals) as a biological phenomenon qualifying for a diagnosis of anxiety disorder, with the presence of life events or specific personality traits as mere risk or predictive factors, and not as causative factors. For example, average blood glucose elevates after ingestion of sugar. However, we still identify a cut-off for this elevation as a criterion for abnormality and call it a disease condition when it remains elevated above the cut-off level (i.e., diabetes). We merely identify sugary foods or body habitus as precipitating factors, not causative ones. This perspective is more practical and valuable in the clinical setting. Studies in brain neurochemical pathways have supported this perspective as well. In general, emotional memories of stressful situations are stored in the amygdala, and those of pleasurable experiences in the nucleus accumbens and other related structures, while declarative memories diffusely in the cerebral cortex. A stress 'thermostat' modulates all these neurobiological systems that regulate emotions such as anxiety, pleasure, and sadness, which are linked to other systems that control memory, planning, and judgment. This encompasses a complex interconnected network involving a variety of chemical mediators and a variety of excitatory and inhibitive neurotransmitters. The brain's responses to potentially harmful or pleasurable circumstances, while adaptive under most circumstances, could become maladaptive and thereby a source of pathology. This is possible when individuals are subject to events such as bereavement, acute trauma, excessive chronic stress, serious illness that affects bodily levels of glucocorticoids, monoamines, and other neurotransmitters, direct injury to relevant brain regions, or ingestions of substances that directly stimulate brain reward centers, bypassing the indirect linkage between environment and brain physiology, or factors that make the brain more susceptible to neurochemical abnormalities during developmental phases brought about by genetic factors.

The developmental period of childhood, adolescence, and young adulthood Is a crucial time of high risk for the onset of anxiety disorders. Separation anxiety disorder and specific phobias are the earliest forms of anxiety disorders, with 50% of all onsets occurring before the age of eight, with nearly all affected cases emerging by age twelve. Social anxiety disorder begins later in childhood, showing a steep increase in incidence in early adolescence. Although agoraphobia, panic disorder, and generalized anxiety disorder may emerge in childhood, the most high-risk period is later adolescence and early adulthood.

Typically, anxiety disorders are widely prevalent in the community, but they do not exist at a constantly elevated level above the diagnostic threshold and hence escape clinical attention. Instead, they wax and wane around the diagnostic threshold so frequently that it is overlooked as a persistent problem requiring clinical attention. Spontaneous complete remissions or 'cures' are extremely rare.

As discussed earlier, anxiety is an affective state, but traditionally, it is not included under affective disorders along with depression and mania. This is because mental illnesses were classified as either psychosis or neuroses, and anxiety was approached as a type of neuroses. With time, the more serious mental illnesses (such as major depression and schizophrenia) came to be studied separately and removed from the neuroses category. At the same time, anxiety was still viewed as a 'minor' mental disorder. This misconception still exists.

Clinical Interview

In general, patients with anxiety have difficulty scheduling and showing up for appointments with psychiatrists. This problem is usually more prevalent in patients from other countries making appointments to see me, as they usually live alone, or deal with their anxiety alone. Patients in India, especially women, are often accompanied by someone (family or friend) and tend to be more compliant with their appointments. Sometimes, patients may have acute exacerbations of anxiety, panic attacks, or ritualistic behaviors before upcoming appointments, which may lead to no-shows and non-compliance. For many patients, the mere act of making it to the meeting involves a significant encounter with their fears. Also, patients who fear heights or closed spaces may avoid appointments if the clinic appears closed or on a high floor level. Some patients may indulge in some preparatory safety behaviors to attend the treatment interviews (as a ritual to ward off their anxiety) or make special requests, and it is acceptable for the psychiatrist to make changes to accommodate these requests if it is reasonable. Identify any barriers to successful appointment compliance and address them beforehand.

The psychiatrist must endeavor to examine the adult anxiety patient alone, as the patient may be hesitant to discuss their fears in front of others, especially family or close friends. If an accompanying person is present, start the conversation in their presence, but maneuver a strategy to eventually send them outside the room before diving deep into dissecting their fears. However, keep the accompanying person outside the room at easy call so they can be summoned into the room in no time.

Your gestures and body language are essential. You must act in a way that eases, comforts, and calms the patient. As a general principle, looking at the person is necessary for a person to relate with another. Face the patient and look at them empathetically. The next step is to smile. You will notice that both these gestures – looking at the face while talking and smiling are challenging tasks for the anxious person, especially those with social phobia. Another hallmark feature of anxiety is avoidance. They may try to avoid questions or find excuses to conclude the interview and leave the clinic. They may keep checking their time. In Western societies, shaking hands, holding hands in consolation, or assisting in disrobing winter jackets on entry are hospitable gestures available to the clinic staff or the psychiatrist to ease the patient's anxiety. In India, these are not possible. Facial expression and words are the only tools available for the psychiatrist in India. Also, anxiety is associated with a short attention span, making these patients easily distracted. So, use simple and direct questions to converse or redirect the patient to attention. Don't lecture, be verbose, or give advice.

The patient may suffer a panic attack during the interview session. If this happens, you must not get panicky. Remember, it is a non-life-threatening, short-lived spike in the autonomic arousal level of the patient, a heightened bodily response to fear. Assure the patient and accommodate their demands to comply with any rituals that they believe might provide relief. Assure the patient that they will be safe and that it is okay and normal to feel this way. Complying with their demands, even if it doesn't seem 'medical', is OK, as it helps cement the trust in the doctor-patient relationship.

The symptom profile of anxiety is vast, arguably the widest of any medical diagnosis. It spares no part of the body or faculty of mental functioning. These symptoms are categorized as somatic, cognitive, and behavioral for ease of understanding.

- **Somatic –** Symptoms range from head to foot! Heaviness of the head, hollowness of the head, reeling sensation, blurring of vision, brightness of vision, diplopia, tinnitus-like sounds, buzzing sound, giddiness, dryness of the mouth, dryness of the throat, increased blinking, shortness of breath, difficulty in breathing, hyperventilation, heaviness of the chest, hollowness of the chest, epigastric sensations, burning in the chest, nausea, sweating, trembling, shaking, tremor, increased appetite, loss of appetite, palpitation, muscle tension, increased gastric motility, increased frequency of micturition, butterflies in the stomach, heaviness of the limbs, weakness of the limbs, fainting and so on.

- **Cognitive –** Essentially a thought pattern of 'losing control' and is described by patients as 'I am going to fumble', 'I am going to mess it up', 'I am losing control', and 'Something bad is going to happen'. These thoughts bring about a subjective sense of weakness and may have beliefs like, 'only weak people are anxious'. The thoughts are disorganized and may manifest as confusion. Easily distracted and have difficulty concentrating. The patient may report subjective memory disturbances.

- **Behavioral –** The hallmark feature of anxiety is avoidance. Anxious people tend to avoid pervasively. Slowly, the avoidance behavior expands from a few specific situations to all situations, from facing certain people to avoiding people contact and particular activities to all activities generally. Procrastination, missing deadlines, and shunning responsibilities are common manifestations of the avoidance behavioral pattern.

The key lesson here is that all these symptoms are interconnected, and there are usually multiple symptoms. The psychiatrist must have good knowledge of Internal Medicine and a solid foundation in other medical specialties to dissect such a complex symptom profile.

Medical and psychiatry history is essential and must be detailed. Prior visits with mental health professionals or general practitioners for mental health complaints must be probed. Other specialist visits must be asked for, as patients might have consulted a cardiologist for palpitations, a neurologist for neural complaints, or a gastroenterologist for GI complaints, any or all of which may have been manifestations of anxiety. Obtain the history in chronological order. Specifically, ask for a history of alternative therapies such as yoga, herbal medicines, meditation, acupuncture, and any drug use (both prescription and non-prescription). These days, many patients have undergone 'counseling' or cognitive behavior therapy before seeing a psychiatrist. The name or type of therapy is not as critical, but its timeline, number of sessions, and the modalities used are essential information to gather. Sometimes, the patient might not have seen a psychiatrist or sought any remedy except plenty of self-help books, videos, or websites. Obtain a thorough medical history, too. Review the medications list thoroughly and ask for any medications that have been recommended and not taken or discontinued. These days, most doctors (regardless of their expertise) prescribe anxiolytics or mild doses of antipsychotics, which goes unnoticed. Anxiety could complicate the treatment of other medical illnesses, the most common is diabetes, where erratic treatment patterns or poor drug compliance is common. Another unique situation is epilepsy, where patients often have anxiety, and sometimes atypical manifestations of anxiety disorders and get misdiagnosed as epilepsy. Loss of consciousness must be clearly established, remember that syncope may also manifest anxiety.

Medication history is essential – medications taken for nausea, gastritis, reflux, dyspepsia, constipation, diarrhea, weight loss, or weight gain could point to some symptoms that may have existed in the past. Substance use history, including caffeine, alcohol, smoking, and street drugs must be obtained.

Family history is often positive, with similar symptoms among biological relatives of the patient. It may be related to a personality or trait cluster prone to anxiety disorders.

A personal history of separation anxiety or other types of anxiety in early childhood or adolescence must be obtained. Discussing with family members helps corroborate this aspect of history. History of avoidance-type behavior, shunning responsibilities, procrastination, missed opportunities, employment history (frequency of job change, promotions, length of each position), social history, and interpersonal relationship history are all important.

Mental status examination of a patient with anxiety ————

- General appearance and behavior - Signs of agitation (i.e., psychomotor activity) such as writhing hands, fidgeting, scratching the foot and leg, frequent swallowing, or throat movements are evident. Avoiding eye contact and sitting on the edge of the seat are typical. There may be ritualistic habits which they may try to hide.
- Affect – Fearfulness is obvious. Manifestations of fearful affect include sweating, blushing, and rapid breathing.
- Thought – 'Worrying' is common. Apprehensive expectations are a defining feature of GAD. OCD patients exhibit circumstantial and overinclusive thought forms. Remember, obsessions are disorders of thought. Suicidal ideations need to be assessed. Perceptual anomalies are not usually present.
- Insight is usually intact, although it may be temporarily lost during extreme anxiety episodes.

Diagnosis and Classification

Historically, the diagnoses of all anxiety disorders were grouped. Based on the growing body of clinical and research experience, the DSM-5 emphasizes distinction within this grouping. PTSD and acute stress disorders are grouped under trauma- and stress-related disorders, while OCD is grouped under the obsessive-compulsive and related disorders category. In addition, the DSM-5 now includes two conditions previously grouped with disorders of childhood onset, namely separation anxiety disorder and selective mutism (in recognition of the phenomenon of these disorders persisting or evolving into other anxiety disorders in adulthood). PTSD and OCD are usually associated with prominent anxiety and avoidance symptoms. Even though the ICD11 and DSM have removed OCD and stress-related disorders from anxiety disorders, they are positioned adjacent to anxiety disorders. Despite the organizational changes of the DSM-5, many textbooks cover these disorders as anxiety disorders. The diagnostic entities are practically unchanged, they are merely grouped differently.

Here, I shall discuss some general concepts related to specific forms of anxiety disorders.

Panic Attacks

The word 'panic' is derived from the Greek word 'panikos', a Greek god whose shout ushers terror into people's hearts. The word now refers to a sudden and severe episode of fear. In clinical medicine, the phrase 'panic attack' describes an acute episode of severe anxiety – the onset is abrupt, often unexpected, builds up quickly to reach its zenith (often within a matter of minutes), and then subsides gradually but completely resolves in a short time. The rapid rise to peak effect is described as the 'crescendo' phenomenon. Although the episode is short-lived, the memory of its unpleasantness lasts several hours or days. Onset is usually before age 40, and the first episode is typically unexpected and triggered by an intimidating social situation. The first episode usually creates a memorably unpleasant experience for the patient, and they may develop anxiety about future attacks. Subsequent attacks increase the anxiety about attacks even further. Gradually, the patient begins to avoid certain situations that could precipitate the attack, resulting in what we now describe as agoraphobia. Many patients report being awakened from their sleep by a panic attack. A single attack alone does not support the diagnosis of panic disorder. However, a cluster of recurrent, unexpected episodes, along with concern for consequences about future attacks leading to a change in behavior or functioning, does implicate a diagnosis of panic disorder. One attack alone does not automatically lead to a diagnosis of panic disorder. A common complication of panic disorder is depression, and it is challenging to differentiate depression as a complication of enduring panic attacks or if severe anxiety is a symptom of depression. Making two separate diagnoses requires comprehensive MSE over multiple sessions. The risk of suicide could be high, especially in men with panic disorders. Some studies report an increased risk of cardiovascular-related mortality in men with panic disorder, but not women. Another significant co-morbidity is alcoholism and substance use, found more commonly than expected in this population. Alcohol and substance use in panic disorder patients could be disastrous and associated with poor outcomes with or without treatment. Medical diagnoses commonly associated with panic disorders include thyroid dysfunctions, early pregnancy, hypoglycemia, and epilepsy. Panic disorders could be life-long and very damaging to the overall life experience. The course is that of waxing and waning, and in most countries, patients do not seek mental health attention and suffer alone throughout their lives. A key differentiating feature from a generalized anxiety disorder is the clear and well-defined discrete episodes of the anxious affective state.

Phobias

Phobias mean 'fears'. As I discussed earlier, the difference between anxiety and fear is that fear is a learned response, while anxiety is not. Fear is a learned affective-behavioral anxiety complex tagged to a specific trigger (Mananalam Clinic Experience definition). 'Phobia' is a medical term for 'abnormal fear', abnormal as in irrational, excessive, disproportionate, persistent, and disabling. The nomenclature of phobias is based on the trigger type. The trigger provokes immediate anxiety, even though the conscious brain knows that the fear is unreasonable and out of proportion; in other words, phobia patients do have insight that their fear is irrational, however, the latter realization creates a sense of 'loss of control', a feeling of helplessness about exiting the anxious state, which leads to avoidance behavior. Phobias could be associated with functional impairment. Another critical feature of phobias is anticipatory anxiety. The classic triad of the presence of a specific trigger, anticipatory anxiety, and avoidance behavior allows the clinical diagnosis of phobias (Mananalam Clinic Experience).

Phobia
- Mananalam Clinic Experience

MCE

Definition – Phobia is an irrational and excessive fear, fear being defined as a learned affective-behavioral anxiety complex associated with a specific stimulus ('trigger').

Diagnostic triad:

1. Presence of a specific identifiable trigger.
2. Anticipatory anxiety directed towards the trigger.
3. Avoidance behavior associated directly or indirectly with the trigger.

Phobias are further subtyped based on the trigger, which may be situational (heights, bridges, driving, flying, closed-in spaces like lifts, tunnels), environmental (storms, water, thunder, lightning, sounds in the environment including firecrackers, ambulance sirens), diseases ('germs', HIV, corona, etc.,) or animals. Having one phobia increases the likelihood of having another phobia of the same type. Some people have multiple types of phobias. The onset of specific phobias is in childhood, but they are transient and not brought to clinical attention. The peak age of onset is in childhood or adolescence, with a second peak in the mid-20s, and around 20 percent have spontaneous remission in adulthood. Anxiety that persists through adulthood seldom remits on its own. Specific phobias can cause considerable impairment in employment, personal time, and social life.

Agoraphobia is the fear of being in places or situations, with the anxiety of 'being trapped', 'not being able to get out', or where escape would be embarrassing. It may occur alone or with panic disorders. It causes impairment due to avoidance (which may be disabling or damaging), or they need a companion. People with agoraphobia avoid their anxiety-provoking situations, endure significant distress, or manage them only when accompanied by a phobic companion or person they feel secure with. Active avoidance of these situations may escalate to the point that they become housebound and depend on others to perform every task and activity that involves going outside. In some cases, the development of social phobia precedes agoraphobia.

Social phobia, also called 'social anxiety disorder,' is characterized by persistent fear of social interactions, being observed, or performance-type situations. There is a fear of being judged, humiliated, or embarrassed. The age of onset is usually during the teenage years when it may be considered 'shyness'. With time, it would become more pronounced, as they feel intensely self-conscious in a wide variety of rather mundane social situations such as attending meetings, gatherings, parties, conversing with superiors, approaching or talking to a person of the opposite sex, speaking to a group, or deliberating in a group. It may extend to anxiety during simple observable activities such as eating or drinking. It may lead to negative social evaluation, blushing, tachycardia, sweating, trembling, and a desire or urge to escape. They tend to achieve less than their potential at work and may end up with late marriages. Severe forms of social phobia lead to school avoidance, work avoidance, and social isolation. In India, anxiety-related isolation is mistaken for virtuousness, so do not end up consulting with a psychiatrist. However, I see many men now present for consultations with social phobia as it hampers their performance in working with teams and large corporations. Typically, social phobia is chronic, progressively worsens, and eventually becomes associated with depression. Some individuals may self-medicate with alcohol or other substances, further complicating the presentation and overall outcome.

Generalized Anxiety Disorder (GAD)

GAD is a common disorder; according to one estimate, it may account for 30-50% of all psychiatric referrals. Before the DSM III, there was no specific anxiety disorder categorization. Anxiety disorders were called 'anxiety neurosis'. A term commonly used those days was 'free-floating anxiety', a clinical entity that refers to a condition of increased 'worry', a vague sense of uneasiness, nervousness, and apprehension. Symptoms were grouped as somatic, autonomic, and cognitive. The worries were of 'minor matters' but were nevertheless challenging to control. So, it was brushed away under the umbrella term, 'anxiety neuroses'. GAD was initially thought to be a diagnosis of exclusion. Over the years, the diagnosis of GAD has evolved through the various updates of the DSM, with the most recent DSM-5 qualifying 'clearly excessive' worry for six months or more as a criterion for diagnosing GAD.

The main symptoms of GAD include restlessness, irritability, muscle tension, impaired sleep, and concentration. They report constant anxiety without discrete episodes of panic, obsessions, and compulsions. They are constantly worried about something and often use the word 'stressed' to describe their situation. Worries in GAD encompass multiple domains, typically part of routine life, like school or work performance, finances, intimate and social relationships, and health issues. These worries consume a significant amount of energy and time, interfering with the person's ability to function efficiently. Some patients will eventually get demoralized, especially when depression sets in, as it prevents them from enjoying life. Two-thirds of GAD patients are female. It can occur at any age, but the typical onset is in the early 20s. It follows a chronic indolent course with waxing and waning, with stress-induced exacerbations. A critical differential diagnosis to be ruled out is substance abuse disorder.

GAD patients typically tend to focus and complain more of the somatic complaints and explain their anxiety symptoms as being due to the somatic complaints. In the past, they may end up with multiple other specialists, such as gastroenterologists, cardiologists, neurologists, pulmonologists, and gynecologists. Most of these specialists might have extensively investigated these somatic complaints. They would have explained to the patients that their anxiety was a reasonable consequence of the undiagnosed and troublesome somatic complaint. The latter is because every physician is more comfortable making a 'physical diagnosis' rather than undergoing the uncomfortable task of revealing the possibility of a psychiatric diagnosis behind their somatic complaints. However, if GAD is left untreated, the severity of the somatic complaint is only bound to worsen and sometimes get unnecessarily worsened by treatment-associated complications arising from interventions by other specialists. The good news is that spontaneous remission (in a durable fashion) is possible in 20 to 25% of the cases. The not-so-good information is that in those who do not remit, depression becomes a common co-morbidity. Once depression sets in, the natural history of GAD becomes more chronic, associated with more functional impairment and a higher risk of suicide.

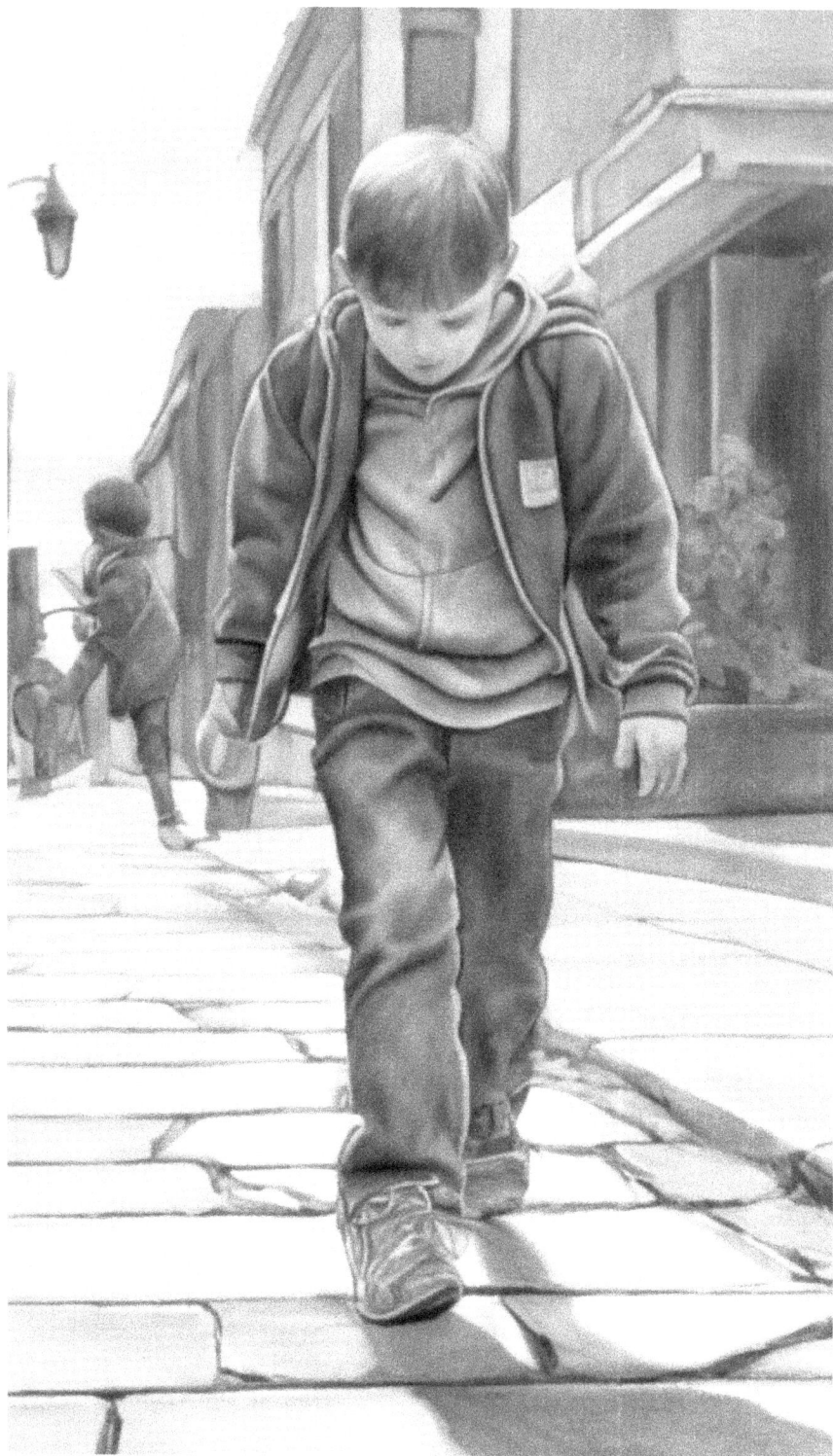

CHAPTER 11

Obsessive-Compulsive Disorder

What is an Obsession?

The word 'obsess' is derived from the root words 'ob-' and '-sess', where 'ob' refers to abnormal or wrong, and 'sess' refers to 'siege' (as in 'being captured'). Essentially, 'obsess' means to be 'captured' or 'taken siege by'. The word 'obsession' has been used in the same vein as being 'possessed', as in being taken over by another spirit. In essence, being 'obsessed' literally implies a state of being taken over by something. In the medical context, it means being taken over by a thought – a persistent thought. Let us go back to the basic concepts – The Ulan is composed of three components: mood, thought, and intellect. These components function in an inseparable amalgamation, and a change in any one component results in a change in the other components. As discussed in the earlier chapter on normality, no thought can be labeled as normal or abnormal based on its content. In the healthy state of the Ulan, any thought is 'dismissible', i.e., the self can dismiss any thought at will. If a thought becomes undismissible and persists uncontrollably, it is deemed diseased. The undismissible thought then begins to affect the other components of the Ulan, namely the mood and the intellect, causing a complex domino of effects, which are understood to be various mental disorders. The Mananalam Clinic Experience (MCE) approach is that obsession is nothing but an undismissible thought.

What is a Compulsion?

The word 'compulsion' derives from 'co-' (meaning 'with') plus '-pell' (meaning 'to drive' or 'force'). Thus, 'impulsion' implies acting through a force within, and 'compulsion' implies acting with a force. Essentially, compulsion is an urge to act in a certain way. In the medical context, it refers to a behavior brought about by an urge to do so. When the thought

component of the Ulan is disordered (i.e., when thought is undismissible),
it begins to affect the other components. The intellect component of
Ulan recognizes that an undismissible thought is present. Thus,
there is an insight into the presence of an unwanted, undismissible
thought. Whether the intellect sees this undismissible thought
as arising from within one's mind or is seen as arising from an
alien source is a matter of debate (ICD-10 approaches obsessional
thoughts as being alien, while DSM-IV views them as arising from
one's mind). The Mananalam Clinic Experience (MCE) approach is
that such differentiation is unnecessary and non-yielding.

The mood component also gets congruently affected – fear (i.e.,
anxiety) emerges due to the recognition of the presence of an undismissible
thought. As explained in an earlier chapter, anxiety is an unpleasant state,
and the intellect component of Ulan comes up with a solution to the
problem. It either comes up with a reasonable solution by employing its
intellectual faculties or by learning the conditions under which the anxiety
gets alleviated. Then, it forces the self to act in a way that brings about the
solution. This force to make the self -act in a certain way is the 'compulsion'.
For example, if the undismissible thought is that of being infected or con-
taminated, the intellect formulates washing as the solution. If the undismissible thought is about being disorganized, the intellect formulates ordering
and arranging as a solution. Performance of this act, through distraction,
creates a temporary absence of the undismissible thought, resulting in the
disappearance of anxiety, which then becomes a positive reinforcement of
the compulsive act. However, the undismissible thought recurs, progressively increasing the intensity and frequency of compulsive acts.

What is OCD?

Obsessive tendencies are common in the general population. Thoughts
of a person, a situation, a movie scene, or a musical tune may persist or 'get
stuck'. Unprovoked, constant thoughts about an ideology or philosophy are
also common. However, they are self-limiting. These obsessive tendencies
may result in some changes in people's lives but do not exert disabling
effects. Compulsions are also common – children walking on the street
back home from school may hop at every fourth step habitually or try not
to tread on the separating cracks on the pavement stones, or climb the

stairs to home taking two steps front and one backward a rhythmic fashion, or swing around a pillar twice every time before walking past it. Touching the feet of people who have been accidentally stepped on, the ritual of uttering prayer words when hearing thunder, or saluting a streetside temple while passing by it are all associated with a feeling of uneasiness when it is not done – all these are common examples of compulsive tendencies. Again, however, these are self-limiting and not disabling. In certain people, the obsessions are so severe that they become the predominant theme of their daily lives – ICD and DSM have variable definitions for identifying a threshold level, such as more than 1 hour a day or lasting for more than two weeks. Accordingly, the compulsions become a predominant theme – the individual begins to make adjustments and compromises in their otherwise normal routine to accommodate for the increasing need to satisfy the compulsions. This is when it becomes identifiable as a mental health condition, now termed as 'Obsessive-Compulsive Disorder' (OCD). Over the decades, the diagnostic criteria and assignment of OCD within the mental health diagnostic schema have varied.

Is OCD an Anxiety Disorder?

Previously, OCD was considered to be a type of anxiety disorder as anxiety was a predominant symptom in many patients. It was also often the presenting complaint that led to the diagnosis of OCD. The MCE approach is that OCD is primarily a disorder of thought, with anxiety being a complication or symptom resulting from the pathophysiology of OCD. Anxiety is 'triggered' by the presence of undismissible thought, which creates a sense of loss of control over one's own mind. The concern that the compulsions have been performed to perfection creates additional anxiety. Anxiety creates increasing compulsions and an increasing need for perfection of the compulsive acts, which in turn creates more anxiety, and hence, a vicious cycle ensues. The MCE definition is supported by the observation that treatment of anxiety does not mitigate undismissible thought.

Is OCD a Neurosis?

No. OCD has been traditionally considered and called 'obsessive-compulsive neurosis', but this was due to the observation of compulsive acts, which seemed similar to individuals with neuroses. However, the fabric of the obsessive person and the neurotic (or hysteric person) are diametrically opposite – the obsessive person is inflexible, rigid, outcome-driven, and unable to adapt; the neurotic, on the other hand, has easy, adaptable, flexible, and emotionally driven. Regarding trait clusters, the obsessive cluster is quite the opposite of the neurotic cluster.

The MCE approach to OCD is that OCD is not a neurosis but could lead to psychotic states. This approach is supported by the following observations –

- In severe exacerbations of OCD, the individual loses touch with reality and loses insight, like psychotic states.
- Compulsive symptoms are seen in other psychotic conditions. It is easily evident in the case of bipolar disorder. During times of severe illness or exacerbations of depression, the individual experiences unwanted thoughts such as cutting the skin with a sharp object or slitting the throat of a child or pet (akin to an obsessive thought) and an impulsive urge to act on it (akin to a compulsive behavior). When the severity of the illness decreases, these thoughts and compulsions disappear.
- Schizophrenic patients with catatonia may compulsively engage in mannerisms that are organized and formalized, similar to the compulsions seen in severe OCD.

Thus, the MCE approach is that OCD, in its more severe form, could be termed 'obsessive-compulsive psychosis'.

Difference Between Schizophrenia and OCD

The next natural question to the above approach is, 'If OCD is primarily a thought disorder and could lead to psychosis, how is it different than schizophrenia, which is also a primary thought disorder?'. The simplest difference is that in OCD, there is a ***single undismissible*** thought; in schizophrenia, there is a ***cluster of interconnected thoughts*** (otherwise called a 'belief system') that is undismissible. In schizophrenia, the individual experiences as if the thoughts are 'inserted' into his mind or that his thoughts are 'stolen' or 'taken away' from his mind. In other words, the

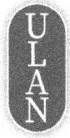

Ulan feels like it is without a fence. In OCD, no such perceptions of thought insertion or thought removal are present. Insight is typically absent in schizophrenia but may return partially with successful treatment and extensive rehabilitation. Insight is generally preserved in OCD but may become compromised during severe exacerbations. Catatonic schizophrenia patients who engage in compulsive acts like those seen in OCD report that they are engaging in these acts under external influence, with no internal capacity to resist.

The 'Obsessive Spectrum'

As mentioned above, obsessions and compulsions are not uncommon. Children playfully engage in obsessive thoughts and compulsive acts. It is common for children to enter the home in a certain way by skipping through the stairs or taking turns around the furniture while passing by it. These children would be willing to admit that these actions are nonsensical, but they would still hold some internal validity and may extrapolate these patterns to good and bad outcomes. With age, they outgrow these obsessions and compulsions. Adults also suffer through such obsessive thoughts and compulsive acts, at which point they are called 'superstitions'. Wearing a specific-colored shirt, using a particular pen, or stopping by the street temple are simple examples. Adults also extrapolate specific obsessions and compulsions to good and evil outcomes (called 'omens'). For instance, spilling salt on the table, breaking glass or mirrors, or tripping on your foot on the way out of the door are typical examples of obsessive thoughts that have evolved into bad omens and negative superstitions. These occurrences lead to fear/anxiety, and specific acts have also emerged to 'neutralize' the anxiety. For example, drinking water after a bad omen or chanting the name of a god a specified number of times have evolved as solutions to the obsessions of bad omens. These become called 'rituals'. Nevertheless, for the most part, such superstitious tendencies are self-limiting and overridden by the self when it seems unreasonable to do so. Some individuals suffer a tendency for 'persistent thinking' – they keep ruminating on rather vague or unfruitful questions (such as 'Who am I?', 'Why are men?', 'Why is black called black?', etc.). Such individuals may obsess randomly over a thought but do not feel compulsive urges. On the other hand, some individuals may feel compulsive urges without any obsessive thought patterns – these are called 'contrast ideas'. Examples include an urge to yell blasphemy in a religious setting, an urge to indulge in obscene or vulgar words or actions in a social or formal setting, an urge to throw oneself off while standing at a dangerous height, or the edge of a moving train. All these tendencies are considered within the realm of acceptable limits, do not qualify for any medical diagnosis, and form the left end of the spectrum.

To the right of the left end of the spectrum is the obsessive cluster of traits that are strong enough to dominate the individual's personality. This is the 'obsessive personality'. The obsessive cluster of traits includes rigidity, inflexibility, lack of adaptability, conscientiousness, and the love for order and discipline. The obsessive personality manifests in real life as punctuality, dependability, reliability, trustworthiness, moral scrupulousness, precision, and attention to detail. At the extremes of this trait cluster, individuals may be self-sacrificial for upholding order and principles. They are often considered 'overly ethical'. They persist and endure pursuing their target even in the face of obstacles. However, their inability to adapt and be flexible may negatively impact interpersonal and social interactions. And its persistence and endurance even in the face of obstacles. I prefer to use the word 'inertia' (not inert) to describe this personality. They are 'difficult to move' or steered away from their path.

Further to the right in the spectrum is obsessive personality disorder – where the obsessive trait cluster is so pervasive that it causes clinically identifiable distress. Use the Ulan concept of mental health here – if the personality is not causing distress to the self or others, the person is considered mentally healthy. If the personality is strong enough to cause clinical distress to self or others, then the person is not mentally healthy. At this point, the diagnosis of obsessive personality disorder becomes legitimate.

At the right end of the spectrum is OCD – a clearly identifiable disorder characterized by an undismissible thought (obsession) and an irresistible urge to act (compulsion).

The MCE approach is that obsessive nature is a spectrum and may manifest sporadically or as a trait, a personality, a personality disorder, or OCD. While obsessive traits, obsessive personality, and obsessive personality disorder are predisposing factors for OCD, OCD does occur in those without any obsessive traits or personality, too. Recent evidence shows that OCD could be drug-induced, too (as in the case of clozapine), and resolves promptly after discontinuing the drug.

Pathophysiology

The emergence of OCD is often typical – the individual is often predisposed to the condition, which gets precipitated by cumulative effects of certain factors.

The most important predisposition is the obsessive personality – in its subtle form, the obsessive personality is prone to achievement in certain career fields. The obsessive personality is orderly, disciplined, strictly adherent to rules and regulations, and generally less emotionally inclined (i.e., low in neuroticism). They are incredible assets in governmental leadership positions (such as Civil services) and law enforcement. They are the ones who function 'par excellence' and win the medals for honorable service. Obsessive personalities find themselves at home in an orderly atmosphere, and they are often the 'strict parents' who may inculcate discipline in the children. However, such personalities do not thrive well in liberal arts, and even a slight increase in obsessive traits could hamper originality and team functioning. Obsessive tendency, as a trait, does not contribute to the morbidity seen with OCD. Instead, the presence of certain other traits that occur clustered with the obsessive trait becomes the Achilles' heel. One such co-existent trait is heightened insecurity – they set high standards for their personal performance and are constantly insecure about not achieving them or not having done enough to ensure the achievement of their set standards. Sometimes, it may take the form of increased concern over their health and thus may need to be differentiated from hypochondriasis. I have also noticed that these personalities are prone to involutional depression. However, this is not to be confused with them bearing neurotic personalities – neurotic personalities are generally emotionally labile but adaptive. Obsessive individuals are typically less neurotic and have lower emotional lability than expected of neurotic personalities. Another trait that clusters with obsessive personality is rigidity/inflexibility, or the lack of adaptability – despite being overwhelmed or stressed about their performance at the target level, they would be unwilling or unable to modify their unreasonable standards for perfection. Depersonalization could also be clustered with obsessive personality – these individuals become engrossed in extreme self-criticism, ruminating intellectually, sometimes to a disabling extent. The history of depersonalized states could be seen in patients with younger onset of OCD during their premorbid years. Notably, obsessional personalities tend to raise children who end up with obsessional tendencies, too. However, it has also been observed that children with no obsessional tendencies are found in the sibship of parents with obsessive personalities. In other words, both nature and nurture play a role.

The precipitating factor is usually a circumstance that positions the obsessively predisposed individual with added responsibility or authority. The standards of perfection that they set for themselves are personally motivated and designed – so they tend to feel overwhelmed when given added responsibility or authority. Many obsessional personalities tend to have their first 'nervous breakdown' when asked to step up to additional responsibility, especially at work. This is termed 'promotion neurosis'. Sometimes, it may be additional unexpected responsibility in the family situation – such as dealing with an unexpected sickness or illness with a family member, which requires changing their rigid routines. Sometimes, the eventual death of the family member may stoke guilt in the patient that they did not do enough to save them, further ingraining their fear of not meeting standards. Thus, these obsessively predisposed individuals who are typically resistant to anxiety (more than that of an average individual) begin to experience unusual anxiety in a specific circumstance. In some instances, the anxiety may be akin to phobic conditions. This is one reason why most OCD patients end up seeking help for anxiety as the presenting symptom – explaining why OCD was initially considered as a type of anxiety disorder. The predisposing factors are endogenous, while the precipitating factors are extraneous.

Unlike the precipitating factor, which can be identified as a conspicuous event, the emergence of compulsions is insidious and hard to trace. It starts unseemingly, not raising doubts by observers, and cumulatively grows with time. The emergence of compulsions is slow enough to get 'normalized' by the patient's family and friends because the compulsive acts are firmly grounded in intellectual reasoning. For example, if there is an obsession with cleanliness, the anxiety gets warded off by handwashing (which, at the outset, seems like a laudable idea). First, a single washing of hands is enough, but the thought of uncleanliness recurs, with increasing frequency, increasing the frequency of handwashing. Eventually, the patient comes up with a blanket idea to overcome the constant anxiety of uncleanness – let's say, three handwashing acts (three feels like a magical number). Then, it becomes three handwashing acts, three times a day. Associated fears of whether the three times were counted accurately begin to arise. The patient may solicit the supervision of others (usually friends or family) to ensure the counting, and they would be happy to help them with their anxiety. However, eventually, it becomes a stress for those around the patient. Despite losses and criticism incurred during all this time, the patient cannot resist yielding to the ever-growing compulsive urges. The situation goes from bad to worse, eventually affecting major aspects of life such as work, marriage, and interpersonal relationships. It is at this stage that it becomes uncertain whether the patient is retaining insight, supporting the MCE approach to OCD as being more of a psychosis rather than the traditionally held notion of OCD being a neurosis.

Clinical Presentation

Clinical presentation is rare in the early stage of the disease. By the time the patient presents for treatment, they are middle age. However, history taking reveals that they have suffered through the symptoms since teenage or early adulthood. Intelligence is usually above average. The mean age of onset of symptoms is around 19-22 years, although clinical presentation to the psychiatrist is at a much later age. Early age of onset is typical in males and associated with a much greater severity of disease, symptoms of attention-deficit/ hyperactivity disorder, lower rates of employment, and a greater probability of being unmarried. Conversely, onset after age 40 was associated with female gender, greater frequency of precipitating factors and traumatic events, and lower odds of a positive family history of OCD. Caution must be exercised on using age at onset in predicting the outcome or course of OCD, as the criteria for identifying the onset of OCD differs across studies.

Sex differences exist, too. Men present earlier than women. There is a higher frequency of reporting sexual/religious-related complaints in men, while there is a higher frequency and severity of harm/ aggression and contamination/cleaning symptoms in women. Although the frequency of symmetry/ordering-related complaints does not differ much between the sexes, they are more severe in women.

Although OCD could occur in any socioeconomic class, patients are often not in the poorest economic class. Their occupation is usually one of orderly disposition – an office administration, clerical job, librarian, governmental office position, record keeping, or craft requiring skill. Their occupations usually do not require brisk and swift action or spontaneity. Family history is often positive for obsessional traits or personality in one or both parents or siblings, and childhood development happens in a disciplined, strict, puritanical, or religious environment. History of episodes of 'nervous breakdowns', anxiety attacks specific to a particular situation, depressive episodes, and psychosomatic complaints (usually dyspepsia, constipation) may also be positive. An 'asthenic physique' – lean, long face with an agitated conversational style is typical.

Clinical Features

OCD comes in several flavors. Depending on the predominant type of obsession, the clinical course, associated comorbidities, prognosis, and response to treatment vary. Thus, OCD is a multidimensional disease. The Yale-Brown Obsessive–Compulsive Scale (Y-BOCS) identifies at least four distinct dimensions; other scales have identified more. However, nearly 80% of OCD patients report symptoms across multiple dimensions. I shall now discuss the salient aspects of each OCD type.

The 'Neat OCD'

The obsessional thought is that there is a 'lack of order', which may pertain to objects, ideas, or actions. The patient has an undismissible thought that there is some mistake or defect in how objects, ideas, or actions are ordered. It commonly manifests as a lack of symmetry. The compulsion is resetting or arranging things, ideas, or activities back in order. According to some studies, this is not the most common type of OCD symptom. When the psychiatrist performs community outreach and increases awareness among referring doctors and the community about this type of OCD, the psychiatrist would notice that symmetry/order OCD is probably the most common type. Often, minor forms of this obsession are welcomed as good ones, such as the perfectionist tendency, and are not brought to the clinic unless it is of disabling severity. These patients typically obsess over things 'not being just right' or that objects such as books or pencils are improperly arranged. They would like to be 'symmetrical'. During school years, they might feel like the schoolwork is never done correctly or perfectly, always making repeated rewritings or additions. Clothes have to be perfectly folded, put only in assigned places, and ordered in a certain way; table covers have to be hanging at perfectly symmetrical lengths, pictures have to be centered and aligned in the perfect center, or symmetrical images have to be placed, particular objects or furniture must be placed in special places, books and objects have to be 'put back in its right place', or 'put back where it was taken from', geometrically arranging things are all examples of obsessions. These symptoms are often not voluntarily reported as a presenting complaint – the presenting complaint may be irritability, anxiety, or rage at children, family, or co-workers when objects are not put back in their place or if furniture or objects are moved. They may be distressed if pens or the pen tray are not symmetrically arranged in the clinic waiting room. Sometimes, the compulsions are in the form of a specific act or sequence of acts – tapping the spoon on the table every time it is picked up, touching the edges of the sofa chair before leaving home, switching the lights on/off three times before bed. In the West, they are sometimes called the *'neat freak'*.

Early age of onset is usually related to order-type OCD. There may be a history of traumatic incidents in the past. With time, the need for order could result in increasing time to task completion of the compulsive act. Patients could take hours to complete a simple task, such as cooking a simple meal or shaving. They may take 'forever' in the bathroom to finish the toilet routine or 'hours' in the prayer room with rituals, often due to the volitional slowing of the act to ensure perfectness. This is called *'compulsive slowing'*.

This type of OCD could be associated with a higher risk of suicidal ideation, ADHD, alcohol dependence, or bulimia nervosa. This type of OCD is often disabling, resulting in many missed opportunities for a successful and enjoyable life, but it often goes unnoticed. In other words, it is probably the most common, earliest in onset, but is brought to clinical attention only in the late and severe stages.

The 'Clean OCD'

This is the classic type of OCD with the most awareness among the general public and non-psychiatrist physicians. The undismissible thought is 'dirty' or 'impurity'. It spans a wide variety of contamination concerns, involving dirtiness on oneself or about objects. The most common form of compulsion is handwashing, and it may extend to cleaning the whole body (such as bathing, showering, colonic cleansing with laxatives or enemas, excessive brushing, and gargling the mouth) and extensive cleaning of objects or surfaces. This may extend to unavoidable situations (such as urination, defecation, or sexual acts), which may become disabling. There is a sense of incompleteness despite extensive cleaning and a sense of disgust, even with minor infractions with dust. The cleaning acts begin to take the form of a ritual with specific maneuvers repeated a specific number of times in a specific order. The rituals tend to get more complex with time.

Studies have shown that the clean-OCD patient's compulsions are not specifically associated with any cognitive pattern. Separation anxiety in their siblings is often elicited during MSE. The patient might have been known as a *'clean freak'* among friends and family. These patients could be misdiagnosed as hypochondriasis. The clean-OCD typically follows a chronic course and is associated with impairments in leisurely and social activities and a lower quality of life. More severe forms of the clean OCD are associated with poorer insight.

The 'Moral OCD'

In this type of OCD, the obsession pertains to an undismissible thought considered forbidden or immoral. It could be of three kinds – aggression/violent, sexual, or religious. Examples of aggression/violence-type obsessions include thoughts of harm or acting aggressively towards a person or living being, object, or situation, such as slapping, spitting at, kicking, stabbing, cutting, slitting, bleeding, or torturing. Sexual-type obsessions may include thoughts of sexual violation of various kinds, and religious-type symptoms include yelling blasphemous utterances in a religious setting, performing a sinful act like defiling a place of worship or religious symbol, or acting like the devil. Essentially, the patient is obsessed with something considered *'forbidden',* such as a taboo or stigma. Often, such a thought is related to something they believe to be of high value, making it highly distressful for the patient. For example, I have examined a young man who has been an enthusiastic fan of a famous movie actor that he adores but had an undismissible thought of spitting at an image of him. Sometimes, it is a thought of a sexual violation towards a parent or family member. There is intense fear and shame in disclosing these thoughts to others, even to seek help. Initially, the patient begins engaging in avoidance behavior to avoid situations where such thoughts might occur. However, the patient soon realizes that thoughts may persist, and that avoidance behavior may be impractical or ineffective. There is an emergence of compulsive acts through some form of magical thinking – such as praying or self-harm (such as pinching oneself or slapping oneself) to 'punish' or 'neutralize' the lousy thought. Other compulsions include checking if the feared outcomes of not having committed perfectly to the compulsion have happened, compensatory acts such as cleaning, washing, or rituals, and avoidance behavior that may result in social isolation or shunning of responsibilities. They may overcompensate with extraordinarily moral behavior in other domains or overindulge in moral policing of themselves or those around them. They are the 'good freaks'.

Typically, this type of OCD is not seen in the clinical scenario as much as it should be due to shame related to discussing these thoughts. It is also challenging to convince the community that these thoughts are simply a harmless mental condition, not an expression of evilness or poor character. The caretakers of the patient and the community tend to distance themselves from patients with this type of OCD due to the stigma attached to this category of thoughts. The natural history of this type of OCD is usually chronic and fluctuating and is associated sporadically with suicidal ideation. Other associated comorbidities include mood disorders, panic disorders (typically agoraphobia), social phobia, separation anxiety disorder, nonparaphilic sexual disorders, somatoform disorders, body dysmorphic disorder, and tic disorders. Aggression thoughts in this OCD are associated with PTSD, impulse control disorders, and excoriation-type compulsions.

Although some research has suggested that forbidden thoughts may be associated with higher overall OCD severity, the course fluctuates between better and worse times and relatively less commonly irreversibly deteriorating, with higher odds of OCD remission with time (especially with harm-related obsessions).

The 'Doubt OCD'

The undismissible thought here is some form of 'doubt' - a specific thought of constant query. For example, when sitting in a room, there is a constant thought about whether the wall on the patient's right side is the west wall or the east wall. The patient gets plagued by this single question, unable to perform or focus on any other mental or physical task. The question persists even after the patient solves the question by finding the direction. If the patient leaves the room and walks in again, the solved problem recurs. If the patient walks to the room on the other side of the wall, the query occurs again despite the obvious answer that it is in the opposite direction of the solved question. A variant of this type is an undismissible thought that some harm might happen, and repeated checking could occur to confirm that the harm had not happened. Compulsions may not exist or be severely disabling, such as walking around the home multiple times to check if all doors are locked, checking every tap to ensure even a slow dripping of water is not present, repeated rechecking of the oven or stoves, etc. Other compulsions, such as washing or arranging, may be associated with this type of OCD.

Tic-Related OCD

Tics (i.e., rapid and recurrent purposeless movements or sounds) deserve special mention. The prevalence of tics in the OCD population is high, roughly 24% in adults and 30-50% in younger age groups. Tics could be simple (such as blinking eyes, jerking limbs, grunting, squeaking) or complex (rubbing, touching, picking mannerisms). Complex tics may give the appearance of being purposeful to the untrained eye. Tic-related OCD was more common in men, associated with earlier onset, greater OCD severity, higher rate of comorbid disorders, and lower overall efficacy of SSRIs and cognitive behavioral therapy and characterized by a higher proportion of males, an earlier onset of OCD, and possibly with greater OCD severity and higher rates of some comorbid disorders. Due to the research that suggests that tics may be associated with distinctive clinical features, tic-related OCD was added as a specifier to the DSM-5, and tic disorders were cross-referenced with OCD in the ICD-11.

Other OCD Types

Hoarding is a compulsion. The hoarding OCD is a consequence of an un-dismissible thought of some possible harm arising from deficient resources. The 'what if' thoughts and the associated fear make people hoard. In India, a common manifestation is the hoarding of temple offerings ('prasadams') or leftovers of religious rituals.

Insight in OCD

Insight is relatively well preserved in OCD. Research suggests insight may be impaired in approximately 9-22% of OCD patients. The extent to which insight is impaired is variable. For the most part, OCD patients recognize and realize that their obsessions and compulsions are unreason-able and do not need convincing that the non-performance of compulsion will not harm them. They also acknowledge that they have some form of magical thinking (such as the specific power of a number - washing 'three' times is required). They do realize that their thought pertaining to the obsession is illogical. Nevertheless, they are unable to dismiss the thought or resist the compulsion. Insight, when impaired, is called 'delusional OCD' – but this term is a misnomer. Insight is usually impaired only in relation to the specific undismissible thought and its associated compulsion. Delusional OCD is not a psychotic state – this needs to be kept in mind, as delusional OCD responds appropriately to OCD-type treatment rather than the treatments directed towards psychotic conditions.

Impaired insight in OCD is associated with earlier onset, greater OCD severity, lower remission rates, and the need for multiple medication trials. Impaired sight could complicate psychotherapy – therapists must modify therapy content to the level of insight. Educating the patient on insight across multiple sessions is helpful.

Folie Du Doute

Apart from the primary undismissible thought, there is often another recurring pathological thought pattern –a thought of doubt about whether the compulsion was performed correctly. It is not that the compulsive act was not completed the correct number of times, but a doubt of whether it was performed correctly or performed at all. This phenomenon is called 'folie de doute', which means 'madness of doubt' in French. The Merriam-Webster dictionary describes this term as 'pathological indecisiveness' when pertaining to ordinary matters. In OCD, it refers to endless recheckings. The bookkeeper or accountant checks, checks, rechecks, and rechecks the addition of columns and labels; the clerk constantly rechecks if the letters have been placed in the correct envelopes; the sweeping of the mailbox multiple times to make sure no letter was left behind, or the simple act of locking turns into multiple unlockings and lockings to ensure it was locked. One of my physician colleagues had the habit of repeatedly asking the details of dog bites to make sure rabies was not missed in the differential diagnoses. His patients complained that dog bites were more tolerable than the doctor's. The doctor would diligently check and recheck the prescription endlessly to ensure it was correctly written, resulting in undue patient waiting times. I had also dealt with a male OCD patient who had folie de doute with masturbation – he felt compelled to observe every slightest movement and sensation, so much that no other fantasy would occur. Nearly always, he felt 'failed' by having missed something and had to wait with tremendous anxiety until the next day when his sexual powers recuperated sufficiently for another attempt.

Ritual Compulsions

Typically, patients complain of having 'doubts'. They complain about constantly being in doubt about whether something is dirty, disorganized, etc. If these so-called 'doubts' are critically analyzed, it will become apparent that these are not actually doubts but repeated occurrences of a single offending thought. Usually, patients say that they have doubts. Nobody will recognize it as repeated thoughts, and they do not feel it was enough thinking about it. They do not feel 'finished' with that line of thought. It goes like a loop. These patients do ***not*** have doubts – they are absolutely sure that they have enacted the compulsion. They are indeed sure that they have cleaned thoroughly, and everything is locked. Despite this knowledge, they get repeated thoughts of uncleanliness or something left unlocked. So, they feel the urge to enact the compulsive behavior again. This intellect component of the Ulan adjusts to this disrupted thought pattern by rationalizing it as a 'doubt' of whether the initial compulsive act was performed to perfection. The real doubt happens in psychotic states – the patient doubts others or the happenings in the environment and is pervasive. The so-called 'doubts' of OCD patients are not directed at others or the environment. The 'doubts' of OCD patients pertain only to the perfection of their compulsive acts and are not pervasive. Psychotic patients feel like things are not 'okay' around them. OCD patients know that everything is okay. They are just not satisfied with their actions. They end up complicating their compulsive behavior to achieve satisfaction, but in vain. These complicated compulsions, which take the form of repeating a specific number of times or a particular sequence of events, are called 'rituals'. The word 'ritual' comes from the word 'rite', which means to count or observe carefully. The intellect component of the Ulan comes up with an explanation for this ritual, which makes sense only to the patient. Hence, it is referred to as 'magical thinking'. For example, washing three times or five times may be required because some magical thinking is associated with the number 3 or 5. Rituals often mean that the pathology has already existed for a while, and the obsessional-compulsive sequence has become firmly established in the patient's Ulan.

Phobioids (Mananalam Clinic Experience)

The OCD patient could present with many 'fears' that have led to the patient's social isolation. These fears are associated with anxiety and could be misdiagnosed as anxiety disorders or phobias. However, they are not real phobias but phobioids (i.e., phobia-like fears). Phobia, in the truest sense, refers to a pathological fear triggered by an external situation. The trigger is real. In OCD, the trigger or object of fear is not real but imaginary. The OCD patient undergoes some form of rationalization or magical thinking, either primarily or to cope with the undismissible thought, resulting in an imagined situation, which is then feared. For example, I have treated a woman who was avoiding traveling by public train transport that she needed to use to get to work, as she was afraid of traveling on the train. At the outset, it may seem like agoraphobia or claustrophobia in the metro train, but during MSE, she revealed that she was afraid that she would gaze at male trousers and see impressions of male genitalia, which caused her immense distress. Another male patient I had encountered had a constant fear that his nose would 'go red' in public. Sometimes, he would excuse himself from a meeting or a gathering to a lonely place where he would excessively rub his nose to 'rub off the redness'. These are imagined fears, not real ones. Another clue to differentiate phobias from phobioids is that phobia patients typically possess neurotic traits; the fear is sudden, fleeting, and progressively pervasive. OCD patients with phobioids are typically devoid of pre-morbid neurotic trait patterns; the fear is usually specific to a particular situation that 'might happen' and associated with some form of irrational or magical thinking.

Ruminations

Obsessional ruminations is the term used to describe the phenomenon of undismissible circular thought processes, often irrelevant to practical and immediate living needs. Typically, they start in the form of 'contrast ideas', i.e., an idea that is the very contrast to what is required by the context of the situation. For example, a blasphemous thought inside a place of worship, a sexual thought in a family setting, a thought of violence towards an innocent or dependent, an idea of yelling in an area of quiet, an idea of jumping off the train when standing close to the edge, etc. It is the diametrical opposite of the idea that is appropriate. Starting as contrast ideas, they evolve into circular, unending questions that the individual incessantly ruminates. They are unable to dismiss this thought even when called to attend to a matter of urgency or timely importance. The latter may deal with a cascading disruption of the day's duties and schedule, leading to overworking, less rest, and sometimes sleep loss. In times of exacerbations of these ruminations, depersonalization or derealization may occur. Ruminations may take the form of hypochondriacal preoccupations as well. OCD ruminations are disabling, and the patient gets hamstrung by an undismissible query that paralyzes the rest of the thinking processes. They lose spontaneity, resulting in uncomfortable social experiences, leading to isolation that increases the rumination. Frequently, these ruminations may take a pseudo-philosophical flavor, with persistent thoughts like 'Who made the world? Who created God? How fast is the fastness of light? How many substances are there in the universe?' Though intellectual and lofty-sounding, these questions are irrelevant to daily living, and when such irrelevant thoughts are persistent enough to paralyze daily activities, they become easily distinguishable as pathological phenomena. A common type of rumination is numbers – some patients feel compelled to memorize or investigate the nature of every number they come across. This may become pervasive enough to include every license plate number of the vehicles seen on the street, every barcode number in a shopping product, every receipt or confirmation number on a bus or train ticket, etc. They may start solving arithmetic problems using these numbers as well. Another common type of obsessional rumination is ideas of death – a constant fear of 'running out of time', where they feel that life has passed with every tick of the clock. I have known many famous people affected by this type of rumination.

Academic circles have disagreed on whether there is any deeper meaning or symbolism to the content of the ruminant thought or OCD type. Does an obsession with a certain number have a deeper meaning or symbolism? Is the question that is unable to be dismissed a signal about an underlying disorder? Disciples of Freud and proponents of the psychoanalytic doctrine have supported the notion that there is a meaning to the content of obsession or compulsion, while others have dismissed such notions. The MCE stance is that there is validity to obsessional symbolism. However, it is valid only for the individual patient and the patient-specific history and traits. After a thorough MSE, a psychological conflict may be identifiable as the origin of the content of the obsessional thought (or compulsive act). However, I would exercise caution in drawing generalized conclusions on symbolisms based on the content of the undismissible thought – not infrequently, I have seen patients have one type of OCD (such as cleaning or washing) undergo impressive remission and return to an otherwise mentally healthy life, and then represent years later with a different kind of OCD. I have also noted that the obsessions and compulsions may not be logically related – for example, the patient may clap several times (instead of washing) for an obsession about contamination. OCD compulsions may pre-exist obsessional thoughts and shift from one type of compulsion to another.

Diagnosis

The DSM and ICD are good resources to rely on for diagnosis. They are not perfect, but they are pretty utilitarian. In the Mananalam clinic, I emphasize the following criteria for the diagnosis of OCD.

Diagnosis of OCD
- Mananalam Clinic Experience   **MCE**

The diagnosis of OCD requires *all* of the following criteria

- Presence of an undismissible thought (the obsession).
- Absence of psychotic state* (no distortions of perceptions of reality).
- Evidence of a remedy** to the undismissible thought (the compulsion).
- Functional impairment.***

*Use the MCE definition of psychotic state
** Remedy is self-made by the patient and may be in the evolving or fully formed stage.
*** May range from mild to severe

Note- if an enduring psychotic state exists, a comorbid psychotic state to OCD or a differential diagnosis to OCD must be considered.

Ask yourself these questions: ' Does the patient suffer from an undismissible thought?' If yes, then there is evidence of a thought disorder. Next, 'does the patient maintain the ability to see reality and unreality apart?' If yes, then there is no psychosis. The latter implies that there is a thought disorder that is not pervasive enough to qualify as a psychotic state. Next, 'is there an evolving or fully formed remedy the patient employs to antagonize the undismissible thought? If yes, then there is evidence of the presence of a compulsion. An obsessional thought disorder, accompanied by a compulsion to antagonize the obsessional thought but does not constitute psychosis, essentially fits the disease paradigm of OCD. Finally, ask the question, 'Is there evidence of impact or impairment to the functioning of the patient?' If so, the disease paradigm is now understood as an active disease state. The functional impairment may be in the form of excessive worries, ruminations, phobioids, folie de doute, disruption to the planned day or schedule, missed opportunities, evidence of compulsive slowing, delinquencies, shunning of escalating responsibilities, and social isolation. The prevailing diagnostic criteria elsewhere note that obsessions and compulsions could exist without the other. However, they coexist nearly 99% of the time; hence, the MCE approach has been to view them as necessary to make a diagnosis.

Other clues to OCD are the history of past or current tics, family history of OCD, or OCD spectrum of disorders, i.e., hoarding, trichotillomania (hair pulling), onychophagia (nail biting), excoriation (skin picking), Body Dysmorphic Disorder (BDD).

As per the Ulan concept of Mental Health, the OCD patient satisfies the first and second criteria for mental health but not the third criteria, which is that all actions of the self must not be non-detrimental to self or others. In the case of OCD, the patient's compulsions or state of the Ulan is such that their actions are not non-detrimental; hence, they are not mentally healthy. OCD initially causes distress to the patient (when the patient is in the mentally not healthy part of the mental health spectrum) but then progresses to a state where the compulsions involve others having to cooperate with reconciling the perfect execution of the compulsions, at which time the patient moves to the worse end of the mental health spectrum – the mentally unhealthy state.

Differential Diagnoses

The critical differential diagnoses are schizophrenia, specific phobias (or other anxiety disorders), major depressive disorder, and personality disorders.

OCD, especially delusional OCD (discussed above), may be misdiagnosed as schizophrenia. The key differentiating feature is the presence of a psychotic state in schizophrenia and the absence of the same in OCD. Unlike schizophrenia, insight is largely preserved in OCD, except in severe or exacerbated conditions.

OCD is differentiated from specific phobias by an undismissible thought (which occurs without a trigger), unlike phobias, which are essentially an affective state of fear with an identifiable trigger. The thoughts in specific phobias are mood-congruent, while the thoughts in OCD are recognized as autonomous, incongruent, or irrespective of the prevailing mood/affective state. Fears in specific phobias are real but excessive, while fears in OCD are not necessarily excessive but unreal and imaginative (i.e., phobioids).

Major depressive disorder could present with ruminations, different from OCD ruminations. MDD ruminations are mood-congruent and non-specific. For example, the patient is depressed, and the depressed mood brings about thoughts congruent with the depressed mood. They keep worrying about 'something or the other'. They usually worry about various thoughts, although one may be more prominent than others. OCD ruminations are not mood-congruent and are specific to the content of the obsessional thought. The patient may eventually get depressed due to suffering from untreated OCD, but depression does not precede obsessions unless MDD exists as a comorbid psychiatric condition.

Clinical Course and Prognosis

In most cases in routine clinical practice, where there are obsessional states, the obsession or compulsion are not the presenting symptoms. In most cases, neither the intensity of the obsession nor the impact of the compulsion is disabling. Obsession and compulsion reach a 'steady state' and stay there for an extended period, sometimes years, without worsening. The patient develops successful adaptation techniques to accommodate the increased need for time or flexibility in the day's schedule that their compulsions may necessitate. Missed opportunities for success in careers or relationships are often forgotten, and they begin to normalize their steady state periods as the 'new normal'. However, during these periods, there could be episodes of increased anxiety (without associated increases in OCD severity), involutional depression, or disruptive exacerbations of their pre-morbid personality disorders or psychiatric conditions, which then pushes them to seek psychiatric help. OCD may be unseemingly uncovered and diagnosed in these patients. Symptomatic or standard symptomatic treatment for these depressive, anxious, or psychotic states may suffice, and the short-term prognosis of OCD is predictably favorable in these patients. Periods of increased anxiety may lead to increased severity of compulsions, but they are transient and subside after the resolution of anxiety. Psychotherapy (of no intensive kind) focusing on the explanation and feedback of the symptoms, reassurance, and constant education would suffice, provided the therapist's aim is not too high enough to work on removing every obsessional thought). Social and environmental adjustments, even minor ones, may benefit symptom control.

Medical treatment has mainly focused on sedative restitution. If OCD of this variety is not treated promptly and allowed to fester, chronicity ensues. According to one study, nearly two-thirds of patients treated for a present illness of OCD had a history of prior OCD episodes. Chronic OCD is less likely to undergo complete and durable remission.

Ripe OCD

The other clinical subset of OCD patients is the 'ripe OCD'. The obsessional state is firmly established and enduring. The compulsions are prominent enough to push the impact of coexistent depressive and anxiety symptoms to the sidelines. History would suggest chronicity, going back years in time to the onset. The course of the illness was gradually ingravescent, with a progressive elaboration of rituals, the establishment of rationalization (in the form of magical thinking) to explain the rituals and an increasing incapacity to disjunct oneself from the abnormal patterns of behavior and social isolation. The patient often clearly recognizes the irrationality in their rituals and the deleterious impact of the OCD on their functioning but is still unable to resist the obsession or compulsions. Pharmacological therapy is beneficial only for symptomatic control of anxiety, and at the cost of worsening OCD severity eventually. Social and environmental adjustments provide minor, if not negligible, benefits. Psychotherapy may prevent or slow down further clinical deterioration but often fails to reverse the pathology. Leucotomy may help. Prognosis depends on the chronicity and severity of OCD before clinical diagnosis – in patients where a clear undeviating progression of the disease is elicitable, prognosis is guarded. The best possible outcome in such patients would be the prevention of further deterioration. The patient's family must be counseled clearly that the minimum goal of therapy is maintaining the status quo. The value of psychotherapy is solely keeping up beneficial activity as much as possible. Here, it is essential to remember that chronic OCD must be distinguished from cyclical obsessional conditions, which are typically rapid in onset, occur in the background of a non-obsessional and labile (or cycloid) personality, and bring forth a history of satisfactory prompt recovery (within weeks or months) from prior episodes of 'breakdown'. Long-term follow-up (13-20 years) studies suggest that distinct clinical improvement occurs in about 25% of patients, with the rest showing minor to no improvement. An obsessive personality in the pre-morbid life, history

of childhood anxiety, unmarried/single status, and severe clinical derange-
ment at the time of first hospitalization are poor prognostic signs.

Psychiatric comorbidity

Psychiatric comorbidity is very common (~90%), the most common
categories being anxiety disorders (~70%), mood disorders (~60%),
impulse-control disorders (~35-50%), and tic disorders (~25%). When
analyzed as individual diagnoses, common comorbidities are major
depressive disorder (~40-50%), social phobia (~30-40%), specific phobia
(~30-40%), separation anxiety disorder (~30%), alcohol use disorder and
generalized anxiety disorder.

Functional impairment

Functional impairment with OCD is significant, especially in social and
interpersonal relationships. Studies on marital status in the context of
mental health suggest that OCD is associated with one of the highest risks
of staying single/unmarried. This could be due to the inability of OCD
individuals to engage in social relationships or potential mates finding
OCD individuals unsuitable for long-term fulfilling relationships. The
families of untreated OCD individuals are significantly affected – spouses
or family members of OCD individuals would get pulled into OCD
compulsions such as washing, cleaning, and arranging. They might have
to change their life routines to accommodate their loved one's indulgences
in compulsions. In general, OCD individuals are embarrassed by their
thoughts and compulsions and try to keep it secretive. Families, especially
in Asian and Middle Eastern communities, try to go along with it and
sometimes augment the compulsions to enable the secrecy.

Suicidality

Suicidality has been reported to be common in OCDs, with ~60% of
OCD patients reporting ideas of life not worth living, ~20% having suicidal
plans, and roughly 10% having attempted suicide. However, I have noticed
that although thoughts of questioning the worthiness of their lives are
common, isolated OCD diagnosis is often not associated with high suicidal
risk, especially if they are under the care of a psychiatrist. The classic
thinking patterns of high suicidal risk, such as constriction and psychache,

are not brought about by OCD but by other coexistent psychiatric comorbidities. Thus, if high suicidality is discovered in an OCD patient, repeat thorough MSE is needed to look for other diagnoses.

In a nutshell, the natural history of OCD is typically chronic, with a low (~15%) rate of durable remission. There may be a partial relapse in another ~20%, with a relapse rate close to ~ 60%. Also, remember that aging itself has a tempering effect on the severity of OCD.

Before the 1950s, the prevalence of OCD was considered low (approximately 0.5%); however, with a widening understanding and expansion of diagnostic criteria, the prevalence is estimated to be higher, in the order of 2-3%. From my experience, I glean that the actual prevalence is even higher.

Key Concepts in Treatment

Treatment aspects of OCD include pharmacological intervention, environmental readjustments, psychotherapy, electroconvulsive therapy, and surgery. A comprehensive discussion of various treatment strategies is beyond the scope of this chapter. Here, I shall go through some key principles in OCD management, as learned from the plentiful experience with OCD patients at the Mananalam clinic.

- **The offending 'thought' cannot be removed** - The patient complains of the undismissible thought and expects the doctor to remove the thought. The latter is not possible. Clearly articulate this in simple words to the patient. The patient struggles to block the thought and inevitably fails. Repeated failures contribute to worsening anxiety, adding to the misery brought about by compulsions and functional impairment. The repeated failures of the patient to remove the undismissible thought makes the patient feel helpless and under control of the thought. Exposure and response prevention strategies are also not helpful. Psychoanalysis and discussing the symbolic meaning of the obsessions is not beneficial either. Sigmund Freud himself alluded that obsessional states respond poorly to psychoanalysis. Instead, work on strategies for not reacting to the thought – i.e., cognitive therapy to impress that the thought is harmless and that 'it is okay' to have such thoughts. Anxiety dissipates gradually when the patient realizes that the thought can exist harmlessly, and it is possible not to yield to the thought in the form of rumination or compulsion. Thereby, the vicious cycle of anxiety catalyzing the mutual worsening of the obsession and the compulsion by the other gets disrupted. Unless the psychiatrist explicitly and directly verbalizes that the offending thought cannot be removed, the patient may have unrealistic expectations about the outcome of therapy. It must also be clearly articulated that remissions may occur, and the offending thought may cease to recur – but this is not a predictable outcome of the psychiatric intervention.

- **Minimize or refrain from sedative or anxiolytic medications** – Use of sedatives or anxiolytics may result in immediate and impressive relief of the obsessional thought and compulsion. The patient and the family may see this as an impressive success and may tempt the psychiatrist to use more of these medications. However, this is a flawed strategy – as mentioned before, OCD is not an anxiety disorder. It is a thought disorder. The thought does not stop, nor does the psychopathology get disrupted by sedation. I have noticed that using anxiolytics and sedatives worsens the overall severity of OCD, and the patient feels very overwhelmed, albeit in a fatigued state with the obsessions and inability to execute the compulsions due to sedation. Alcohol abuse could have similarly disastrous consequences in OCD individuals. So, use anxiolytics or sedatives only when needed and judiciously.

- **Clomipramine helps symptom control** – even when there is no evidence of depressive illness, in about 15-20% of the patients (the proportion of patients responding to imipramine may vary with the type of practice and the population studied). Full doses in the 200- 250 mg range may be needed in the initial stages and then may be subject to dose reduction.

- **ECT is beneficial in OCD with depressive symptoms** – Depression in the obsessive personality patient, OCD with depressive symptoms or depression, OCD with coexisting MDD, and OCD with minimal reactive depression all respond very well and nearly always to electroconvulsive therapy. Patients with hypochondriacal and neurasthenic features may benefit from ECT, too. Do not hesitate to consider ECT when OCD and depression are seen together (unless absolute contraindications exist).

- **Treat aggressively in the early stages of OCD** – The general tendency of doctors is to make the treatment proportionally more aggressive to the severity of the disease. With OCD, such an approach would be counterproductive. Shorter previous history of OCD symptoms is a good prognostic sign. Educate your community and refer physicians about heightened awareness to detect OCD in the early stages. When the disease pathology gets well established, pharmacological treatments and environmental readjustments will be less beneficial, and reversal of the disease process to the point of return to premorbid functioning is unlikely. I have noticed that well-established OCD pathology of 5-10 years before the first psychiatric consultation could be prevented by continuing medical and community education.

- **Surgery is beneficial** – Making a surgical lesion that interrupts the neuronal tracts in certain areas of the brain (prefrontal cortex, cingulate region, etc.) is associated with improvement of symptoms in OCD and other psychiatric disorders. However, with the advent of multiple pharmacological therapies, surgery has become less used. Nevertheless, surgery for OCD is still an option. Limbic leucotomy and anterior capsulotomy could provide impressive outcomes in about 60% of the patients. Patients who have undergone surgery typically report that thoughts may exist but do not feel as compelling as they did before. Extensive rituals may be seen to resolve impressively after surgery. However, surgery is not without adverse effects, including a small risk of mortality. Postsurgical patients continue to need ongoing educative and rehabilitative therapy.

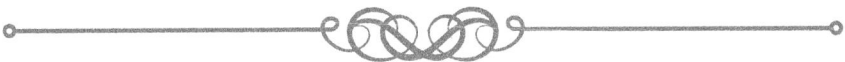

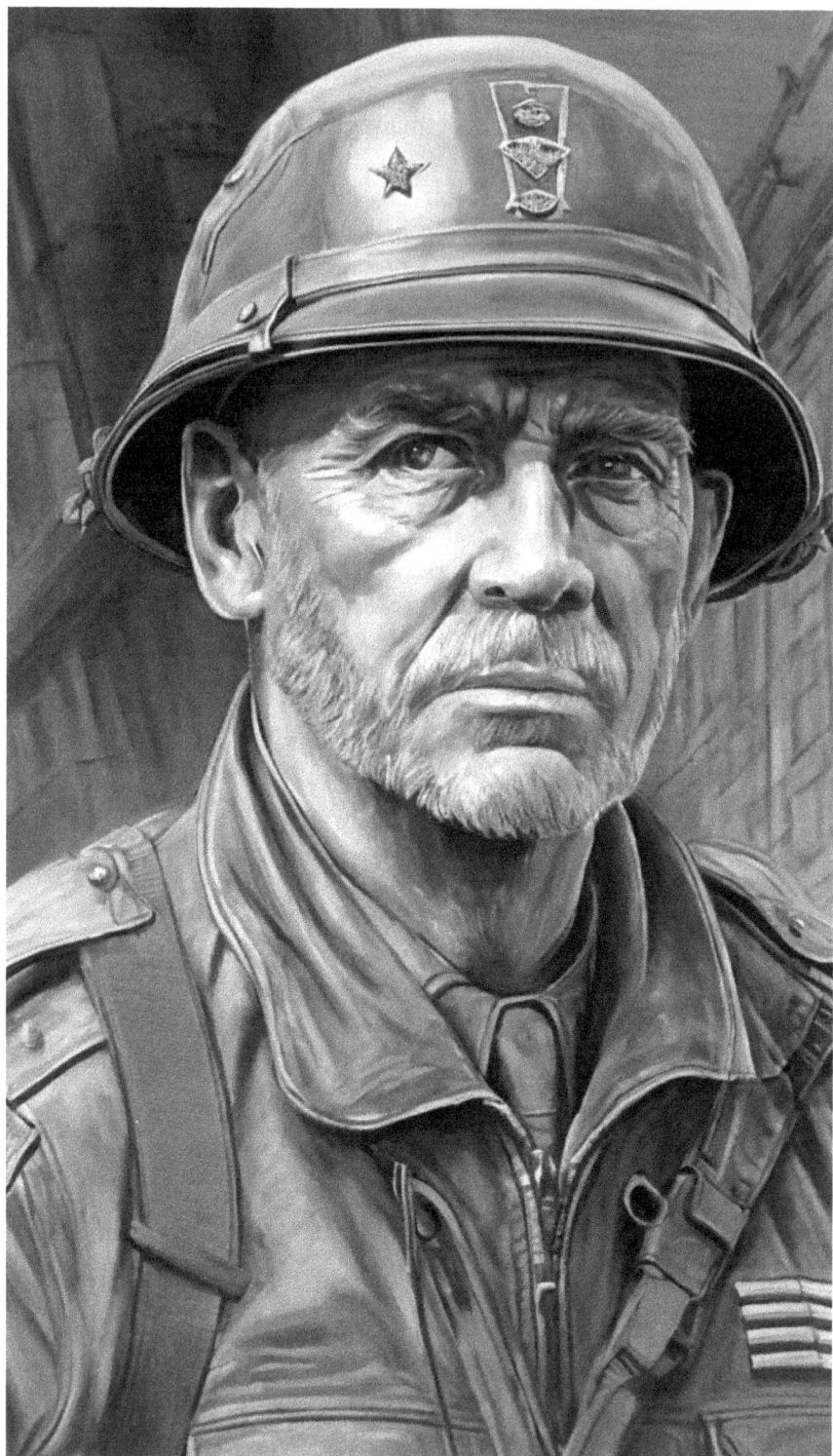

CHAPTER 12

Post-Traumatic Stress Disorder

Fundamentally, Post Traumatic Stress Disorder (PTSD) is an anxiety disorder. However, it deserves a special mention and study for several nuanced reasons, the most important being the presence of a qualifying and identifiable 'traumatic event', considered the etiological factor in this diagnosis. I shall devote this chapter to discussing some of these nuances.

What is Trauma?

The word 'trauma' arises from the Latin root '-tere', which means to twist, lacerate, or tear. The word trauma was initially used to describe a disturbing or distressing experience. In due course, it became used in medicine to refer to physical injuries as well. Physical trauma could cause mental trauma, and the effects of severe mental trauma can be manifest through physical symptoms. Post-traumatic mental symptoms have been described in history in various literary works. However, its introduction into psychiatry has been relatively new.

It is essential to understand specific terms used when discussing post-traumatic disorders (Mananalam Clinic Experience), and caution must be exercised in not using these words interchangeably.

Nomenclature related to Post-traumatic disorders MCE
– Mananalam Clinic Experience

- Traumatic *event* – Refers to what happened *within the sensory environment* of the patient. It is an objective account. The event must have occurred (not imagined), be identifiable and verifiable, should have happened to the patient, and be timed before the onset of the post-traumatic disorder. For example, a life-threatening event that happened to the patient, such as attempted murder, brutal violence, sexual assault, etc., is a traumatic event. The attributes of the event (such as severity) are non-modifiable and not patient-related. Bad news read in the newspaper or heard from someone else is not a traumatic event.

- Traumatic *experience*-- Refers to what happened *within the patient's Ulan* in response to the traumatic event. It is a subjective account and is self-reported. It is not verifiable, except partially through detailed behavioral assessment and comprehensive and prospective mental status examination of the patient across a period. The attributes of the event are patient-related and variable across individuals who have experienced the same traumatic event. The traumatic experience is primarily the affective response to the traumatic event.
- Traumatic *trigger* – Refers to a stimulus *within the sensory environment* of the patient that reproduces the traumatic experience, in whole or in part, after the onset of the post-traumatic disorder. The trigger is objective and verifiable, but the account of the traumatic re-experience is a subjective, self-reported account.

General physiology is that after any traumatic injury (physical or mental), the injured entity undergoes a reparative healing process to restore optimal functioning. The hypothetical pathophysiology of post-traumatic syndromes is that the traumatic event has evoked a traumatic experience severe enough to exceed the threshold of permanent mental recovery, leading to enduring traumatic re-experiences, which further leads to functional disability.

The Mananalam Clinic Experience working hypothesis is that the traumatic event injures the mood component of the Ulan so severely in susceptible individuals, resulting in enduring neurochemical or anatomic disruptions in brain functioning, which leads to malfunctioning of the other components of the Ulan.

Now, let us discuss each of these terms in more detail.

The Traumatic Event

The idea that events could be traumatic to the mind is not new. Philosophers and psychologists have long recognized that traumatic events produce enduring and permanent memories that shape behavior, learning, and personality. My schoolteacher used to say that a student tends to more effectively retain, recall, and apply knowledge learned from questions answered incorrectly compared to knowledge learned from questions answered correctly.

The impact of traumatic events on psychology was best recognized by the lasting effects of traumatic events in childhood correlating with psychological changes in adulthood. Hence, the adage 'child is the father of man'. Sigmund Freud also noted that trauma, particularly childhood trauma, could predispose the individual to psychiatric symptoms later in life – he went on to postulate that hysterical symptoms reflected the individual's subconscious attempts to deal with repressed memories of childhood trauma. However, after accumulating experience with psychotherapy, he concluded that many of these traumatic memories were imagined (i.e., fantasies or fears) rather than actual events. In other words, he shifted emphasis from the traumatic event to the reconstructed traumatic experience, which then became the source of psychological conflict. Freud's shift impacted the whole of psychiatric thinking in the later period – it began to shift the emphasis of psychological distress to the patient factors rather than the traumatic event. While he was correct in part, it is also true that the severity of the traumatic event has a bearing on the causation of symptoms.

The importance of the traumatic event in causing psychological manifestations came to light in 1871 when an American physician, Dr. Jacob DaCosta (1833-1900), described an anxiety disorder with cardiac manifestations in soldiers. It was described as 'irritable heart', 'soldier's heart', or 'DaCosta syndrome'. Later, during World War I, military doctors observed a similar constellation of symptoms. The British described it as a 'disordered action of the heart', while the Americans called it 'shell shock'. The latter description reflected the presumption that those symptoms were attributed to the trauma of shelling and explosions on the battlefield.

During the years around World War II, the existence of an anxiety symptom complex due to mental trauma became obvious, assuming a newer name, 'combat neurosis'. Apart from the combat veterans and soldiers, such a disorder was increasingly recognized among civilians who had undergone higher than usual levels of mental trauma. Around the same time, in 1942, a massive fire in a packed nightclub in Boston during the Thanksgiving holiday ended in a mass casualty of 492 people and received much attention from the American health system, press, and public (the 'Cocoanut Grove fire'). Some of the exit doors of the club were reportedly locked to prevent re-entry, and it was a traumatic experience to escape the fire. Austrian-American neurologist and daughter of the famous Freudian psychiatrist Dr. Alfred Adler, Dr. Alexandra Adler, studied more than 500 survivors of this fire accident and observed the presence of increased anxiety in more than 50% of them. Furthermore, survivors of Nazi concentration camps were observed to experience symptoms of anxiety, motor restlessness, hypervigilance, insomnia, nightmares, and phobic avoidance of situations that resembled their traumatic experience, along with persistent, intrusive, and painful recollections of their experiences. The prevalence of this constellation of symptoms, later came to be called 'concentration camp syndrome' was so high among the survivors of these camps (75%) that it had to be concluded that the traumatic event was the causative factor and that these were not merely an exaggerated anxiety response to trauma in susceptible individuals. Survivors of the atomic bombing in Hiroshima and Nagasaki were also noted to have similar symptoms, providing corroborating evidence from the Eastern hemisphere for the phenomenon of a mental trauma-induced anxiety disorder.

Due to such growing evidence for a trauma-related mental disorder, the DSM-I published in 1952 included a diagnosis of 'gross stress reaction', which was described as a transient and self-limiting change in an individual's personality in response to stress. In the DSM-II published in 1968, this diagnosis was dropped, and another diagnosis called 'adjustment reaction to adult life' was introduced.

The Vietnam War (1955-1970) contributed more information about this disorder - many veterans displayed a characteristic syndrome that included anxiety symptoms, emotional numbness, and intrusive thoughts of re-experiencing the trauma. Many veterans petitioned for benefits but did not fit into a formal diagnostic category.

During the 1970s, more trauma-related mental disorders in abused children and women (such as rape trauma syndrome and abused child syndrome) began to be recognized and recorded. All the latter accumulating evidence led to the consolidation of the first description of Post-Traumatic Stress Disorder (PTSD) in the DSM-III published in 1980. The diagnosis was placed in the anxiety disorders category, and some commentators have argued that we would be better off returning to the earlier perspective of a 'stress disorder'.

The DSM-III recognized an acute and chronic type of PTSD based on whether the onset of symptoms and duration was within or later than six months after the traumatic event. In the DSM-III editions, the nature of the traumatic event was understood to be so severe that it was 'outside the range of usual human experience', i.e., an event that would be expected to be profoundly stressful or distressing to almost anyone.

However, in the subsequent DSMs, the scope of events to be considered traumatic was widened. Nevertheless, the occurrence of a traumatic event continues to be a necessary criterion, often referred to as 'Criterion A' in academic discourse. The DSM-5 implies exposure, threat, or experience related to death, severe injury, and sexual assault as traumatic events.

Use your discretion in the clinic based on local, cultural, and societal norms on whether the patient experienced a severe traumatic event. Classically, the most common traumatic event is combat trauma for men and sexual trauma for women. But over the years, other forms of traumatic experience such as violent personal assault like kidnapping, physical battery, rape, torture, violent accidents like motor vehicle accidents, falling from a building, cliff or extreme heights, fire accidents, crush injuries from heavy machinery, disasters (natural or artificial), military combat, hostile situations such detainment in a concentration camp, or as a prisoner of war, being taken hostage, mass shootings or diagnosis with an acute life-threatening illness are increasingly considered as qualifying traumatic events. Witnessing a violent injury or death or unexpectedly seeing a dead body or dismembered body parts is also being qualified as a traumatic event. Non-violent events like watching a scary movie, being fired from a job, or being served with divorce papers are not considered qualifying events.

Some stressors are milder but more chronic. For example, marital discord, divorce-related stress, job loss, employment-related harassment, and financial stressors can be traumatic and, when persisting over a more extended period, may result in a similar anxiety complex. Still, it is wiser not to include them in the PTSD diagnostic basket. Generally, the more severe the stressor, the larger the proportion of individuals exposed to the same stressor would develop PTSD. However, since many people exposed to extreme stress do not develop PTSD, at least an enduring and disabling form of it, the presence of a traumatic event is a necessary but insufficient criterion for the clinical label of PTSD. The likelihood of developing trauma-related mental disorders weighs in more with the severity of the traumatic event in the case of severe stressors and more with patient-related factors in the case of stress disorders in the case of minor stressors.

The Traumatic Experience

Is severe trauma, one that could qualify as Criterion A, rare? The simple answer is no. Epidemiological research from the World Mental Health Survey Consortium suggests that nearly 70% of the population has been exposed to a traumatic event. In some studies, it could be as high as 90%. However, the overall lifetime prevalence of PTSD in the general population is estimated to be much lower, in the 1-3% range. An additional 5-15% may have experienced some symptoms of PTSD without meeting diagnostic criteria (which again depends on the criteria used). Regardless, the lifetime risk of developing PTSD after a traumatic event is estimated to be about 25% (subject to variation depending on the study population). Thus, only a fraction of those exposed to trauma develop PTSD, and accounting for that fraction depends predominantly on how PTSD is defined. A similar pattern of statistics is seen in women exposed to sexual trauma. In one community sampling study, about 75% of women reported having undergone at least one victimization through crimes, and many women reported multiple experiences of victimization. There is also another statistic from a nationwide survey of college women in the USA which demonstrated that nearly 50% reported sexual victimization in some form, with 15% of them meeting the legal definition of rape. Another study done through a telephone survey suggested that 27% of women and 15% of men reported a history of childhood sexual abuse. Suppose we include other traumatic experiences such as the tragic death of a loved one, major traffic accidents, robbery, assault, mugging, etc. In that case, it can be concluded that not being exposed to a significant traumatic event would be a rarity rather than a norm.

So, how do we understand these numbers? Trauma elicits a stress response, and most exposed individuals would experience psychological symptoms – but these symptoms may be anxiety-type symptoms, grief or depression-type reactions, changes in personality, or other psychiatric complications such as alcohol/drug use, worsening of pre-existing substance use, psychotic states, etc. When a relatively new set of anxiety-type symptoms emerge but do not persist for more than four weeks, it becomes labeled as a self-limiting condition, called 'acute stress disorder'. According to one study, up to 50% of individuals exposed to significant trauma may develop acute stress disorder. In some patients, symptoms may persist beyond four weeks but not to the extent or severity to qualify for PTSD diagnosis. In the remainder of individuals, a characteristic symptom complex (mostly related to an anxious affect) becomes consolidated. At this point, PTSD becomes a legitimate differential diagnosis – the actual diagnosis then depends on the country you practice in and the diagnostic criteria you use.

The recent DSM criteria make it necessary for the patient to have experienced 'intense fear, helplessness or horror' – essentially an extreme affective state of fear. In those who receive a diagnosis of PTSD, it is labeled as *'acute PTSD'* if onset and duration are within six months of the traumatic event and *'chronic PTSD'* if it is beyond or more than six months. **Delayed PTSD** (onset greater than one year after the traumatic event) occurs without a preceding acute stress disorder and is a rare type of this disorder. It may occur after extreme natural calamities like earthquakes, tsunamis, etc.

In essence, a given traumatic event may evoke a rainbow array of psychiatric sequelae, implying the strong influence of patient factors in developing PTSD. This inference corroborates with the data that when PTSD does occur (in the fraction of those exposed to the traumatic event), it rarely occurs alone – nearly 75% of PTSD patients have other psychiatric comorbidities. Psychiatric conditions like major depressive disorder, alcohol/substance abuse and dependence, and phobias occur at least twice as often in victims of sexual abuse than in the general population.

Thus, it becomes evident that the initial traumatic experience evoked by the traumatic event depends on the patient's Ulan – and the most reliable predictor of the patient's vulnerability would be the initial traumatic experience. The experience must be horrific for the patient – the DSM has labeled it as 'Criterion A2' and has described it as 'intense fear, helplessness or horror'. In clinical practice, ask the patient to describe the experience – descriptions suggesting a sense of being trapped or caught in a situation with no exit or escape, i.e., powerlessness or helplessness, are typical of the traumatic experience that leads to PTSD. The latter descriptions of the traumatic experience by the patient are essentially perceptions (i.e., thoughts) that bring about an intensely fearful affect.

The more severe the traumatic event, the higher the probability of feeling powerless. For example, combat veterans are more likely to experience PTSD when they have been exposed to witnessing or experiencing 'great' danger, cruel atrocities, mass casualties, or death or dismemberment of friends. Among rape victims, those exposed to physical force, the display of a weapon, or a bodily injury are risk factors for a traumatic experience that could lead to PTSD.

A critical patient factor that predisposes patients to PTSD is the history of prior traumatic events. History of child abuse, previous sexual abuse, exposure to domestic violence, and history of battery or physical abuse are important risk factors. It seems like the damage brought about by the trauma is cumulative – prior severe traumas, although recovered from, make the patient more susceptible to psychological damage by future minor traumas (akin to the 'kindling hypotheses' proposed for mood disorders). Childhood trauma, especially one that has been repeated or chronic, may have contributed to personality disorders (such as borderline PD), including trust issues, fragile self -esteem and increased vulnerability to anxiety. These individuals are more likely to feel powerless or helpless in response to trauma.

The Traumatic Trigger

The traumatic event produces a traumatic experience – however, this alone is insufficient to diagnose PTSD. The patient begins to 're-experience' the traumatic experience without the initial traumatic event. These re-experiences are intensely unpleasant and noxious experiences. The re-experiences may be spontaneous or associated with a trigger. The longer a PTSD patient is observed, the more it would become apparent that there are predictable times or situations associated with these re-experiences. Such predictors are referred to as 'triggers'. The triggers may be so innocuous that these re-experiences may be considered spontaneous. These triggers bring about the following effects –

- avoidance of these triggers.
- emotional numbing.
- increased baseline arousal state ('hyperarousal').

As discussed in the Ulan chapter earlier in this book, mood, thought, and intellect are inseparably amalgamated components of the Ulan, and changes in one component cause changes in the other. The affective state of fear causes changes in thought patterns, cognition, and eventually impairment in functioning. The most profound thought disturbance is the inability to control the thoughts. Thoughts of the traumatic event penetrate the Ulan in the form of vivid visual imagery, flashbacks, reliving, or dissociation. The individual feels like these painful thoughts break into their Ulan, like intruders in their home. Hence, the description 'intrusive' is used for the memories and thoughts experienced by the PTSD patient.

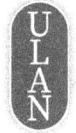

The patient begins to avoid situations evenly remotely connected to the emergence of these re-experiences, sometimes going out of the way to avoid these situations. The avoidance behavior could extend pervasively to limit the patient's recovery significantly. For example, a woman who has undergone sexual assault or rape may begin to avoid her husband or other family members, who are vital to her support situation. Some patients isolate themselves from family and friends, erecting the so-called 'trauma membrane'. Typically, they allow only those who have 'been through it themselves' (such as in the case of sexual abuse) or those who have 'been there' (as in the case of combat veterans) across the trauma membrane. Avoidance directed at close family and friends introduces guilt in these family members and friends for 'not having been there' and hence not feeling 'good enough' to suggest remedies. This leads to distancing the patient from their support system. Essentially, PTSD patients profile who can and cannot approach them and handpick who is eligible to interact with them. Often, the physician is not on the favorable side of the trauma membrane and is met with hostility and mistrust. Hence, group therapy is an excellent place to start engaging these patients.

Further effects on the affective component of the Ulan as a response to repeated re-experiences include emotional numbing – i.e., a restricted range of emotional expression, loss of interest in enjoyable activities, and feelings of detachment. Essentially, it mimics the onset of depression and decreased psychomotor activity. The patient is unable to rest – there is a hyperarousal state manifested as insomnia, increased startle response, and hypervigilant behavior. Intrusive thoughts and hyperarousal are more common symptoms of PTSD, and avoidance behavior and emotional numbness signify a more severe pathology.

Triggers are typically those that re-introduce thoughts related to the traumatic event. Physical injuries to the body due to the traumatic event are enduring triggers and may cause the patient to seek treatment for chronic pain or reconstructive surgeries. The patient's daily living environment is the source of most triggers, and modification of the environment is necessary to facilitate recovery.

Pathophysiology

So, how exactly does trauma cause mental disorders? The simplest and most reliable pathophysiological explanation is Pavlovian – i.e., PTSD is a learned response and behavior. A severe traumatic event (an unconditioned stimulus) is initially associated with an intense traumatic experience (the unconditioned response). The latter reaction, being an extreme affective response and a robust autonomic response, then gets 'tagged' to or progressively generalized to other stimuli (i.e., triggers) in the environment, which causes re-experience of the toxic reaction. The response is noxious, so the individual seeks to avoid it. Initial avoidance is beneficial, so avoidance behavior patterns are quickly reinforced. Sequelae further downstream, including affective changes (such as emotional numbing), thought disturbances (intrusive memories, flashbacks, vivid imagery), and functional impairment (such as cognitive disturbances), are best explained by the amalgamation aspect of the Ulan concept.

The closest animal model to PTSD is the ***'learned helplessness' paradigm*** - an animal subject to repeated trauma (electrical shocks) in an inescapable environment makes the animal not attempt escape even when the environment is made escapable. Learned helplessness is a learned behavioral complex characterized by passivity, diminished responsiveness to environmental stimuli, and an inability to act on opportunities to escape stress. Interestingly, the propensity to develop this syndrome varies among strains of mice raised under the same circumstances, suggesting the importance of genetic factors. The neurochemical mechanism behind learned helplessness is the initial hypersecretion of brain norepinephrine (during the initial traumatic events), which leads to subsequent depletion of norepinephrine stores. Administration of tricyclic antidepressants (which raise brain norepinephrine and serotonin levels) improves learned helplessness, corroborating this explanation.

Heritable biological factors also play an essential role. Family studies suggest that genetic factors account for a significant percentage of the variance in whether Vietnam veterans exposed to trauma did or did not develop PTSD. Another proposed mechanism is limbic kindling, which is that repeated minor traumas or a single major trauma in the past have caused 'sensitization' of the response circuit, which gets relatively easily activated by future minor traumas. Such a sensitized emergency response system means that the emergency response metabolism is constantly 'on', with higher than usual levels of glucocorticoids or adrenaline exposures, which in turn may lead to autonomic hyperarousal, as evidenced through higher resting heart rates, elevated blood pressures and higher urinary epinephrine levels in PTSD patients compared to control patients. Such heightened adrenergic levels could be neurotoxic, resulting in brain damage. The hippocampus (related to memory function) is particularly susceptible to such injury – volumetric magnetic resonance brain imaging studies have shown losses in hippocampal volume in the brains of patients with PTSD or major depressive disorder. This finding correlates with memory complaints at times of acute stress faced by patients with known PTSD or major depressive disorder. Generally, coordinated activity along specific brain circuits is necessary for the arousal response required for adaptation to acute stress or danger. When these circuits get overwhelmed or 'burnt' by traumatic events, the network may get activated with lower firing thresholds, resulting in 'replaying' of the activities in the circuit upon exposure to triggers. The latter implies increased noradrenergic activity at the locus coeruleus, the region involved in stress responses. Thus, there is a possibility of heightened activity along pathways linking the locus coerule-us to the hippocampus and amygdala, which may explain symptoms such as arousal, flashbacks, and nightmares.

Another possible explanation could be dysregulation of the hypotha-lamic-pituitary-adrenal axis. Our understanding of the role of serotonin in PTSD is not comprehensive. Nevertheless, serotonin is involved in impulse control and affect regulation. Thus, decreased serotonergic activity in certain pathways may be linked to increased irritability, depressed mood, and heightened anxiety.

Another interesting explanation is the ***endorphin hypothesis,*** which turns the conventional explanation of PTSD psychopathology on its head. Trauma is also associated with endorphin (a type of opioid) release, which creates a sense of gratification after stress exposure (like euphoria after exercise) and pain tolerance. Perhaps individuals with repeated exposures to trauma may have gotten 'addicted' to the experience of trauma, and the absence of trauma produces a withdrawal response (i.e., symptoms of PTSD). The argument for this hypothesis is based on two findings – first, the symptoms of PTSD are those of hyperarousal, which is similar to opioid withdrawal (sympathetic arousal, anxiety, emotional numbness, and dysphoria), and the intrusive thoughts of trauma are similar to the psychological cravings replaying the intoxication experience; second, administration of naloxone (opioid antagonist) reduces analgesia in PTSD patients after exposure to a trigger event. While this hypothesis may not explain all of PTSD psychopathology, it may explain some of it and co-exist with the noradrenergic pathway-based explanations discussed above. The latter explanation is corroborated by known neurobiology, that norepinephrine and endorphin networks are interconnected. For example, clonidine, an a-2 receptor agonist that decreases neuronal norepinephrine release, helps reduce autonomic hyperarousal symptoms seen with opioid withdrawal. Interestingly, animals with learned helplessness behavior also demonstrated improvement in their analgesia with naloxone, thereby suggesting that learned helplessness behavior may be associated with increased endorphin activity. Another interesting corroborative finding for the endorphin hypothesis is the observation that war veterans and survivors seek out higher-risk jobs (such as flying airplanes or fast vehicles such as ambulances), perhaps to seek the experience of greater arousal.

In summary, trauma does impact the complex neurological systems in the brain, and a domino of events (that we have not clearly understood) gets put in place, leading to a progressive disturbance of the functioning of the arousal system. Treatment aims at interrupting this progressive disturbance at multiple points and enabling the ability of the patient to function in life at the best possible level alongside these disturbances.

Politics of PTSD

All psychiatric diagnosis attracts politics, but PTSD is extra special in this regard. Historically, there has been skepticism and antagonism towards mental health care. Mental disorders were considered a sign of personal weakness, lack of integrity, absence of moral strength, or being forsaken by God. The stigma attached to mental illnesses is evident and strong. Throughout history, life stressors have been used to explain mental diseases, but the patient still bore the bulk of the burden of the mental illness. The formulation of the concept that trauma causes mental illness has caused a paradigm shift in the age-old approach to mental illnesses. If someone caused physical injury or bodily harm, the victim could legally make the causer of the injury liable for damages. With the formulation of PTSD, the victim of mental injury could make the cause of the injury liable for damages, too.

Furthermore, PTSD has shifted the 'blame' of the illness from the patient to a life stressor, allowing the patient to collect compensation for these damages. So, PTSD has become a 'preferred diagnosis' for patients due to reduced stigma and for trial lawyers due to the increased scope of representing the patient's interest for damages. It is not unreasonable to expect that those looking for compensation may also prefer to get diagnosed with PTSD. In the 1980s, when the Veterans Administration in the USA authorized compensation and service-related benefits for veterans with delayed-onset PTSD, it was rapidly flooded with claims. There was concern that some of these veterans presented for their psychiatric evaluations, citing every classic PTSD symptom described in the textbook.

It has also caused a shift in how a symptom complex is approached clinically. For example, a patient experiencing depressive and anxiety symptoms may also have work-related personal conflicts with colleagues or employers. The available facts of the situation could be arranged in multiple ways – employment-related stressors could have caused, contributed to, or exacerbated mental health problems in the patient...or mental health problems could have caused difficulties in interpersonal relationships at work. In both cases, one could worsen the other, and a vicious cycle may ensue. Whether the symptoms were present before or after an event at work and the relative impact of the events on the patient's mental status are impossible to verify. So, various clinical diagnoses, including PTSD, could be made.

With the criteria for PTSD evolving through the years and the differences between the professional societies drafting these criteria, there is a wide range of play left for the clinician and the patient to manipulate. For example, suppose an employee sues the employer for punishment and damages on the grounds of harassment that results in depression and anxiety. In that case, the employer may argue that depression or anxiety are mental illnesses with an endogenous biological basis and not necessarily due to the employer's actions. However, if the employee sues the employer for having caused PTSD due to employment-related stressors, the employer's case weakens.

The medical community has absolved the burden of the causal link between the stressor and disease through its use of a diagnosis of PTSD. The scope of what qualifies as a traumatic event or stressor is constantly increasing, and what constitutes a traumatic experience is becoming increasingly subjective and unverifiable. We are left with the only option of believing the patient's word, as the benefit of the doubt has to be given to the 'victim'. Suppose the traumatic event claimed to have caused the illness is unverifiable. In that case, the diagnosis of PTSD cluster of symptoms ends up being offered as 'proof' that the event must have been of extreme severity. In other words, because the diagnosis is 'incident specific', the presence of PTSD could be used for prosecuting an incident for damages. Dr. Alan Abraham Stone (1929-2022), a forensic psychiatrist and former president of the American Psychiatric Association, commented in 1993, "No diagnosis in the history of American psychiatry has had a more dramatic and pervasive impact on law and social justice than post-traumatic stress disorder". So, it is hard to dismiss all the critics skeptical of this diagnosis category, and the controversy might only worsen with the ever-changing definitions and diagnostic criteria.

In the clinic, focus on the patient's symptoms, their correlation to trauma, and triggers causing re-experience. The basic principles of dealing with anxiety disorders still hold good for these patients, with the presence of specific nuances, of course. Also, it is essential not to be carried away by the skeptic arguments, as PTSD is indeed a terrible and disabling diagnosis. These patients might have suffered permanent brain damage and need long-term care and rehabilitation. Earning their trust and working with them is also not easy. Again, as with other complex psychiatric problems, it is always wise to seek the help and guidance of experienced and senior psychiatrists while dealing with these patients.

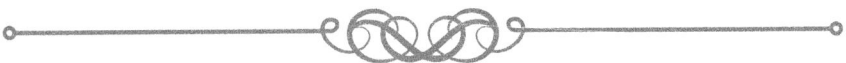

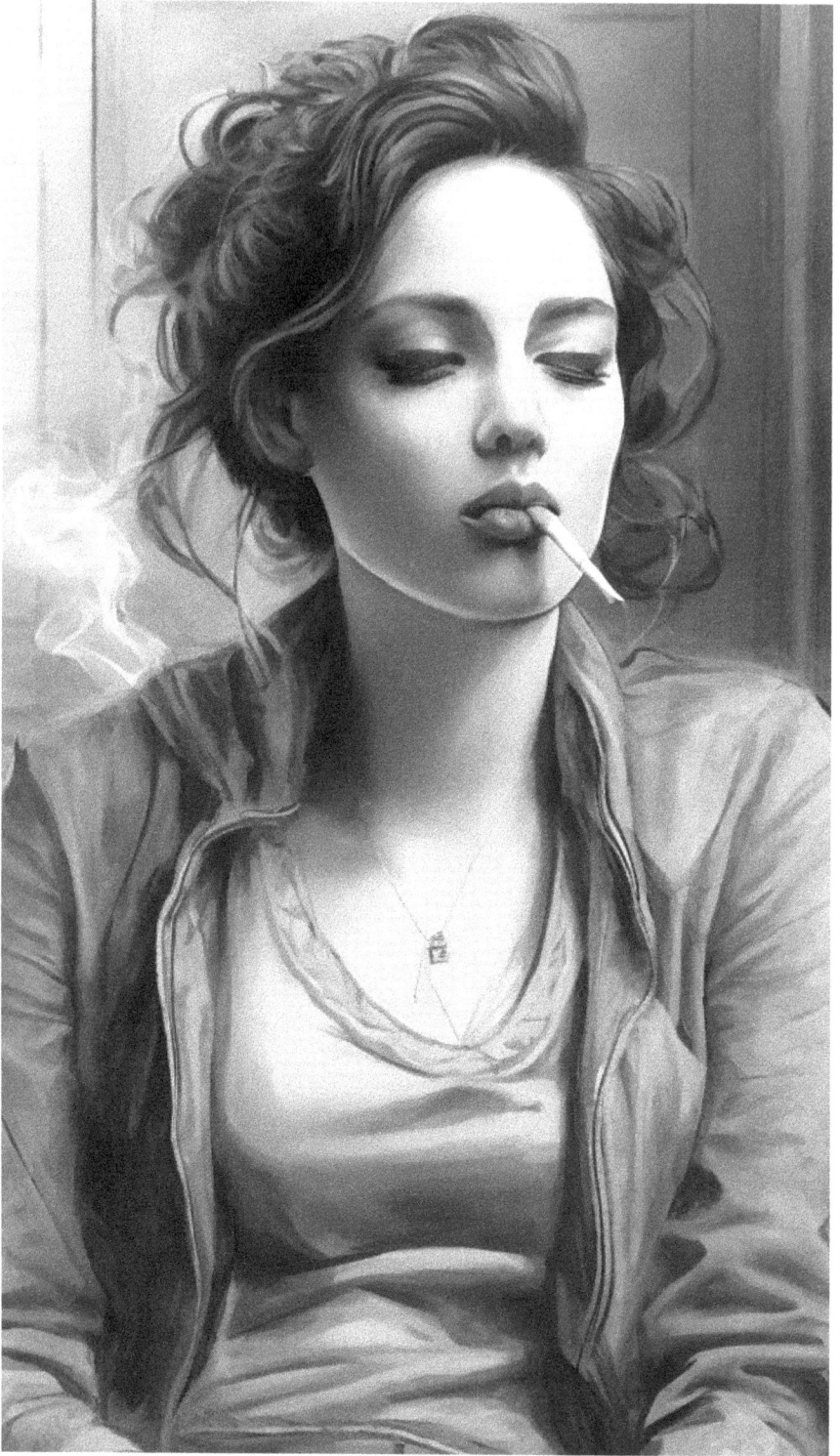

CHAPTER 13

Addiction and Substance Abuse

Addiction, more accurately termed 'addictive behavior', and substance use are broad and overlapping topics. Based on the substance consumed, there are specific differences in the clinical approach, but there are some fundamental principles underlying all forms of substance abuse and addictive behaviors. This chapter will focus on such basic principles, and I have devoted two more chapters with additional focus, one on alcoholism and the other on internet/gaming addiction.

Let's begin by asking some broad conceptual questions. Is using a substance a disease/illness? If so, why? And why is it a psychiatric illness? Why can't the internal medical specialist deal with it? What is the difference between use and abuse? Do alcohol and other drugs fall into the same category of illness? What is addiction? Is it a medical or psychiatric illness? What are the criteria to identify addiction? Can a person be 'cured' of substance use or addiction?

Use vs Abuse

One of the fundamental axioms in medicine is that health is a homeostatic physiologic state, i.e., a dynamic equilibrium between constantly opposing mechanisms (Please refer to earlier chapters of this book, where homeostasis has been discussed at length). In other words, health is not a static state which can be unilaterally shifted. Instead, it is a state of dynamic equilibrium between two or more opposing forces that are constantly operating. Thus, health can and does exist without any external intervention. When the equilibrium of these opposing forces is disturbed, the resulting non-homeostatic state is referred to as 'disease', which results in the deterioration of bodily processes resulting in discomfort and misery to the individual. In these situations, it is essential to intervene with the physiological process by using certain substances that can either correct the disturbed physiological process and restore homeostasis or alleviate human suffering. When substances (or chemicals) are intentionally introduced into the human body for a 'positive effect' on health to prevent illness when risk factors exist or to treat diseases, it is called 'use'. On the other hand, if a substance is introduced into the human body other than for the latter indication of restoring health or treating illness but to alter the mental state, it is called 'abuse'. A more accurate term would be 'substance abuse'. However, due to the stigma attached to the word 'abuse', the term 'substance use disorder' has replaced the latter term.

In summary, other than a wholesome diet and clean drinking water, no other chemical substances are needed for a healthy state. No artificial 'enhancers' need to be consumed for better health. Any chemical intro-duced in the body to 'enhance' the physical or mental state will eventually disturb homeostasis and cause illnesses – physical, psychiatric, or both. Nearly all substances consumed that end up being on the list of substance use disorders are initially intended to directly or indirectly 'enhance' the sense of physical or mental well-being. Any substance can result in such disorder, including but not limited to coffee, sugar, alcohol, opioids and other sedative/hypnotics, amphetamine, cocaine and other stimulants, hallucinogens, etc. Any experience that is 'consumed', i.e., non-substances, such as the internet, games/gambling, shopping, sex, food, etc., can also result in similar disorders that eventually lead to addiction.

Is Substance use a Medical or Psychiatric Condition?

No. Using or consuming a substance is not a medical condition. There are some substances whose use may be illegal depending on the laws of the land. Still, from a medical standpoint, using any substance alone does not qualify as a diagnosable condition or illness. However, the health consequences (physical and psychiatric) resulting from substance use are a disease state. Simply put, not the use but the abuse of the substance leads to a disease state. In a state of health homeostasis, an individual must be able to modify/control one's behavior related to substance consumption to prevent a disease state. Any inability to do so is also a health consequence of prior substance usage – i.e., the inability of an individual to control abuse is a disease state arising from previous use (i.e., abuse) of the substance. At this point, it becomes qualifiable as a diagnosable condition.

In summary, using a substance is not a medical condition, but the health effects from the use of the substance are a medical condition, and the inability of the individual to reverse or mitigate such a medical condition by appropriately controlling or modifying the behavior related to the usage of the substance is also a medical condition.

Since substance abuse is primarily intended to alter the mental state, and the underlying cause is related to behavior (i.e., using and controlling use), substance abuse or substance use-related disorders fall within the realm of psychiatry.

As mentioned in the prior chapter of this book, mental health is defined by three criteria, one of which is that all actions must benefit oneself. Substance abuse disturbs mental health; hence, individuals with substance abuse are not considered mentally healthy. They are best treated by a well-trained psychiatrist.

For example, an individual unable to limit alcohol usage, intoxicated by alcohol, causes a motor vehicle collision and sustains a fracture. An orthopedic surgeon fixes the fracture and discharges the patient. In the realm of orthopedic surgery, the diagnosis is a fractured bone, the etiology of the fracture is trauma, the treatment is a surgical fixation of the bone, and adequate healing of the surgical site and return to pre-trauma function is measured as a good outcome. However, in the context of the overall health of the patient, the diagnosis is substance use disorder, the etiological agent being alcohol; the risk factors include genetic, psychological, and social elements; the complication of this disease is the fracture, orthopedic surgery is the treatment for the fracture alone, and the overall treatment is detoxication and de-addiction to alcohol. The patient refraining from further alcohol use is the best medical outcome.

How to Approach a Patient with Substance Abuse?

There are two categorically different ways in which substance abuse can be approached. They are the moral model and the medical model.

Moral model - As mentioned above, using or consuming a substance is a behavior. All behavior is initiated by the individual. Therefore, it was traditionally believed that substance use disorders and addictive behaviors are related to a patient's will, self-control, morality, or 'strength of character'. The patient was expected to discontinue or modify the behavior. If they failed to do so, the approach relied on admitting patients to 'correctional facilities' where behavior modification techniques were imposed. Sometimes, they were summoned to religious commitments such as amplifying religious conviction, increased praying, and ritualistic penances. Failure to de-addict or refrain from substance use was viewed as a 'weak character' or 'lack of Good' in the person. Addiction-afflicted individuals were perceived as evil or deviant, 'falling to temptations' of the evil forces. Addiction was viewed as an inability to resist the temptations of the devil. This model created a stigma associated with substance use disorders, resulting in patients and their families trying to conceal their behavior and delay seeking professional help. This model solely blamed the patient for the health conditions, discouraged public discourse and education, and resulted in late presentations, low treatment rates, chronicity, and plenty of medical complications (such as liver dysfunction) due to resistance to seeking medical care.

Medical model – In this model, substance use disorder is viewed as a medical condition within the psychiatry subspecialty. Substance use disorder is considered to be due to physiological and psychological alterations arising from the first or continuous use of the substance, which sets a particular psychopathology in motion, resulting in the inability of the individual to modify the use of the substance at the required promptness to avert or mitigate health consequences. A significant advantage of the medical model is that once a particular condition is brought within the realm of medical diagnoses, it becomes approached through all the robust, time-tested logical and rational principles already existent in clinical medicine. In modern medicine, the doctor approaches any disease by looking into the basics first. The latter includes the relevant anatomy, biochemistry, genetics, risk factors, natural history, etc. Once substance abuse began to be approached through the medical model, doctors started looking into the anatomical parts of the brain affected by substances, the relevant biochemistry and metabolism, the genetics associated with increased risk of developing addictive behaviors, etc. Further, the fundamental principles of clinical medicine, such as 'first do no harm', 'do not blame the patient', 'measure before and after treating', etc., became to be applied while formulating treatment plans. It also subjected treatment plans to peer review and garnered the weight of knowledge available already in clinical medicine to be applied to benefit these patients. More importantly, this model shifts the onus of treatment success from the patient to the treating physician. An advantage of this model is that it has spurred enormous scientific research through the techniques commonly used and mastered for the study of medical illnesses for centuries, leading to abundant knowledge about these illnesses within a relatively shorter period. Furthermore, it has tempered the stigma, increased public discourse, and led to earlier presentations, more effective treatments, and better outcomes. Another tangible benefit of this model is that it has allowed for earlier detection and treatment of substance use-related organ damage. For example, the medical model approach to alcoholism has led to more and earlier detection of alcohol-related liver damage, cirrhosis, malignancies associated with alcohol and substance abuse, etc.

Natural History and Psychopathology

Any substance consumed by the individual has a specific effect on the physiological processes. When the effect is beneficial in disease states to restore health, then it is prescribed in calculated doses by trained physicians. These substances are called pharmacological agents, medications, or drugs. When the effect caused by the consumption of the substance is not intended for restoring health in disease states, it becomes consumed in uncalibrated doses, resulting in detrimental effects on physiology. In these cases, they are called 'toxins' or 'poisons' and hence the term 'toxicology screen' for the tests used to detect substance abuse or the word 'detoxification' for managing adverse effects from substance abuse.

Essentially, these substances are consumed for experiencing a positive or enjoyable mental state – called a 'high'. This delightful mental state is transient, and after the first use, the individual experiences satisfaction, i.e., a feeling of 'enough', i.e., satiety with the substance. The mental state then returns to baseline. This phase in substance use is called the *'contact phase'*. The contact phase usually is an overall positive experience – a transient enjoyable high can be attained with predictable certainty effortlessly, merely by consuming a substance, followed by satiety, and then returning to sobriety. 'It is *perfect*' is what it feels like for the individual after the first high; hence the use of the term 'euphoria' to describe the high. Due to the sensation of reward felt due to the usage of the substance, the user begins to repeat using the substance to re-experience the pleasure or increase the pleasure.

With time, the individual starts to use the substance to increase pleasure at positive circumstances (such as birthday parties, family events, etc.) or to blunt frustration or dullness of negative events (such as a bad day at work, emotional stress, loneliness, loss of employment, etc). At this stage, there is a rapidly increasing dosage and frequency of substance use. This phase is called the *'user phase'* or, more accurately, the *'habitual user phase'.*

With time, it leads to an enduring change in behavior patterns. By this, I mean that the individual's overall nature would appear to have transformed. They may invite trouble or get into bad situations. They find or manipulate the environment to seek opportunities to use the substance. This phase is called the *'problem user phase'.* The biochemical mechanism underlying this phase is that the neurochemical changes related to the euphoria from the initial substance use create a reward circuit reinforcing the behavior. At the same time, the brain's sensitivity to the substance decreases over time, leading to increasing amounts of the substance required to feel the 'high'. This phenomenon is called *'tolerance',* which results in the individual not feeling enough.

Quite rapidly during the problem user phase, the patient begins to lose the sense of satiety after experiencing euphoria. The individual starts **chasing the first incredible high** by constantly increasing the dosage and frequency of the substance. The individual never experiences the 'perfectness' felt during the contact phase but does not stop chasing it due to a strongly reinforced reward circuit. However, during this time, the constant introduction of the substance into the body begins to durably alter the physiological process in the body to create a new state of equilibrium that incorporates a steady state of the bioavailability of the substance. In other words, the absence of the substance in the body results in a breakdown of the body's physiological equilibrium. This stage is called the *'dependence phase',* wherein the lack of constant bioavailability results in negative or painful physical and psychological experiences. These noxious experiences triggered by refraining from substance abuse create a punishment circuit – i.e., the individual is punished if the substance is not consumed. As we know from Pavlovian psychology, the punishment circuits are more potent than the reward circuit, which further reinforces substance use. The consumption of the substance has interfered with the physiology, psychology, and sociology of the person, resulting in complications in each aspect of life. At this point, the individual is suffering from substance use and hence becomes a diagnosable disease state.

As mentioned in the Ulan chapter, mood, thought, and intellect always function in unison. Thus, all faculties of Ulan, including the thought and the intellect, deploy its infrastructure to ensure the substance's bioavailability. Essentially, the individual becomes pre-occupied with the substance – procuring it, storing it, saving it in excess, economizing its usage, protecting it, etc., In other words, the substance enacts a pervasive takeover of the individual's life and behavior. This phase is the most severe stage of the pathophysiological process and is called the *'addictive phase.'*

What is Addiction?

The word 'addiction' is derived from a Latin term implying 'to devote oneself to'. Practically, it means 'giving up oneself completely to'. In Tamil, it translates as 'becoming a slave to'. Essentially, addiction is a physiological state characterized by a distinct set of behaviors that occur during the addictive phase of the substance abuse history mentioned above. However, in the clinical setting, it is difficult to demarcate the onset of addictive behavior. In my experience, I use three criteria, called the 'Addiction triad' for diagnosing addiction objectively (see table next)

Criteria for Diagnosing Addiction – *the 'Addiction Triad'* - Mananalam Clinic Experience — MCE

Addiction is diagnosed when *all* three following criteria are met –

- *'Urge'* – refers to an irresistible impulse to physically perform the act of consuming the substance. For example, holding a cigarette, lighting it, and blowing the smoke in smoking addiction, handling the bottle and mixing the drink in alcohol addiction, strapping the tourniquet, and injecting in the case of IV drug use. Playing a card, rolling the dice, buying a lottery ticket, and booking a bet in a race are all examples of urges in gambling addiction.

- *'Craving'* – refers to an irresistible desire to mentally experience the consequences of the act of using the substance. For example, the feeling of warmth and anxiety-dissipation with cigarette smoking, the sense of buzz with alcohol, or the feeling of somnolence and analgesia with sedative/hypnotic *drugs.*
- *'Denial'* – refers to a thought abnormality wherein the individual recognizes the ill effects of substance abuse in general but strongly believes it will not occur to them.

Let us review the rationale for this triad of manifestations of addiction. As discussed earlier, a strong positive reinforcement is brought about by the euphoric experience of the substance used. This positive reinforcement (i.e., reward) sets a learning pattern that associates the behavior associated with substance use (i.e., the physical act or series of actions during the procurement and consumption of the substance) with the euphoric experience. With time, the mere act of procuring and consuming the substance gives pleasure, signifying the development of the 'urge'. This is readily evident with cigarette smokers, who have the urge to inhale or blow smoke; the more smoke they blow, the better they feel about it. The biochemical changes related directly or indirectly to the bioavailability of the substance are also associated with the euphoric physical and mental experience. 'Craving' refers to the irresistible desire or impulse to experience that euphoric/ecstatic experience resulting from achieving the required bioavailability of the substance. In essence, the urge is satisfied without the bioavailability of the substance, while craving is satisfied only with the bioavailability of the substance. The urge can be satisfied by substitute substances, while craving is not.

Both urge and craving result in markedly abnormal experiences and behaviors, intensifying slowly over time – addiction does not happen overnight! During this protracted period of deteriorating health, individuals can recognize their worsening situation and seek help. Alternatively, friends and family notice their worsening problem use and enable them to seek help. In most cases, the latter does happen, and the individual is able to cut back on the habit or abstain from it willingly. However, this corrective mechanism does not deploy in a fraction of users. Somehow, their habit continues unabated, leading to a theme of devoting themselves to the pursuit of satisfying their urge and craving. Invariably, this is due to a thought abnormality – although the individual can cognitively recognize the ill effects of substance abuse, they believe that it will not happen to them. They are in denial of experiencing the ill effects of substance abuse. This denial is the hallmark sign of addiction. Denial is subtle but strong. The individual may agree verbally or appear to agree that they are suffering from the substance but would behave otherwise. ***Denial is not retrieved through interrogation but through elicitation.***

It is important to note that the nature of the substance consumed is not a deciding factor for the presence of addiction. The traditional mainstream school of thought was that the neurochemical effects of the substance are responsible for the euphoric experience and, hence, the potential for addiction. The chemical nature of the substance does not matter while applying the Mananalam Clinic Experience criteria. Any substance or anything that is consumed could lead to addiction. For example, abuse of non-substances such as gambling, shopping, sex, internet use, gaming, etc., could also lead to addictive behavior. In essence, addiction is a behavior phenomenon that could result from substance abuse or a non-substance.

Why Must Substance Abuse and Addiction be Handled by a Psychiatrist?

As outlined above, there is a solid medical and, more specifically, a psychiatric background to the evolution of substance abuse into addictive behavior and organ damage. The nature of addiction is such that the individual is 'caught' or 'trapped' in a situation from which self-extraction is impossible. The use of the word 'hooked' is apt for this purpose. A hook is a tool with a curve designed to prevent the escape of any trapped object. When patients or their families try to extricate the patient from the addictive spiral, it is unsuccessful, if not even more damaging.

Only a portion of the general population consumes substances. Most people who consume a substance for the first time do not end up becoming habitual or problem users. Only a fraction of them does, and only a fraction of that fraction ends up with addictive behavior. Thus, the development of substance use-related disorders and addiction are not entirely due to the substance but due to biological and psychological determinants inherent to everyone. Recent studies have also supported the biological and psychological etiologies, shifting focus away from individual morality or strength of character. In brief, substance abuse-related disorders and addiction are medical illnesses.

Management by a psychiatrist with focused training in substance abuse and addictive behavior, or at least a well-trained physician, is essential. Patients and their families must be educated that non-medical approaches for substance abuse and addiction could delay care, late presentation, organ damage, and overall poor outcomes.

Understanding the Terminology

I have found that the loose and interchangeable use of language in the this field of psychiatry by non-medical and medical people alike has contributed to much confusion, stigma, and controversies. So, let us review the accurate use of some often-used terms in this field.

- **Substance use disorder (SUD) –** Refers to the recurring use of the substance despite adverse consequences. For example, recurring use to the point of failure to fulfill major obligations at work, school, or home, recurring use in hazardous situations, recurring use resulting in legal problems, social and interpersonal problems, and recurring use resulting in significant functional impairment or distress. Tolerance and withdrawal are signs of problem use. SUD may lead to addictive behaviors, but addiction is not a requisite for SUD.

- **Substance-induced disorder (SID) –** Refers to psychological or behavioral changes because of the substance on the nervous system. These changes could be acute or chronic and may exist in the absence of SUD. The symptoms of SID may overlap with other psychiatric diagnoses, such as affective disorders, thought disorders, cognitive dysfunction, etc.

- **Stimulants –** refers to substances that produce heightened awareness or wakefulness. Examples include cocaine, amphetamine, and methamphetamine.

- **Opioids –** It is a generic term to describe opium and its derivative/class of drugs. They belong to the sedative-hypnotic class of drugs. Intoxication is a less common presentation. Overdose is a more common presentation and is life-threatening. Intravenous heroin/opioid use produces an intense spike of 'high', often likened to a sexual orgasm, and dissipates slowly after hours. These contrasting high and low experiences are referred to as a 'roller coaster' effect, which is responsible for reinforcing recurring use. Opioid withdrawal is characterized by depressed mood, nausea, vomiting, muscle aches, lachrymation, rhinorrhoea, pupillary dilation, piloerection, sweating, diarrhea, yawning, insomnia, and fever.

- **Cannabis –** commonly used to refer to marijuana class of drugs and used interchangeably with cannabinoids and THC. Intoxication is common and may present with conjunctival injection, dry mouth, tachycardia, increased appetite, craving for sugary foods, altered sense of time or distance, and intensified sensory perceptions. Prolonged inhalational use can cause COPD. Withdrawal is characterized by sleep disturbances, vivid dreams, depressed mood, decreased appetite, irritability, anger, restlessness, aggressiveness, flu-like symptoms, and anxiety.

- **Polysubstance abuse –** Refers to the use of more than one substance and is an increasing occurrence in contemporary times. Caffeine, energy drinks, and tobacco/nicotine are the commonly used co-substances to the dominant substance, usually alcohol or marijuana.

- **Tolerance –** refers to an ongoing physiological phenomenon wherein the prior dose of a substance does not produce the previous euphoric experience or desired effect, thereby requiring increasing doses of the substance.

- **Dependence –** refers to a clinical state requiring a certain level of bioavailability of the substance to avoid distressing physical or mental experiences. In other words, the substance is no longer needed for a positive experience but to prevent a negative experience. Dependence is associated with significant functional impairment in daily life and risk of withdrawal if abrupt discontinuation of substance is attempted. Dependence often requires intense psychiatric management, including hospitalization. Polysubstance dependence is also becoming more common recently.

- **Intoxication** – refers to a state of acute marked deterioration of physical and mental abilities caused by the substance. Essentially implying being 'poisoned' by the substance. Symptoms depend on the substance used and may include but are not limited to manic state, paranoia, delusions, hallucinations, and panic/anxiety. Intoxication is often accompanied by physical signs such as dilated/constricted pupils, tachycardia/arrhythmias, hypotension/hypertension, perspiration, chills, rigors, nausea, emesis, dystonia, dyskinesias, altered mental state/confusion, seizures, coma, weight changes, appetite changes, speech disorders, sleep disorders, etc. Stigmata of substance use, such as needle tracks, septal erosion in nares, burns in mucous membranes, etc., may be found.

- **Recreational drugs** – is a broad term referring to all chemical substances consumed for non-medicinal uses. They are typically obtained without a prescription. Often referred to as 'party use' or 'party drugs. Local or national laws differ in what constitutes recreational usage and the drugs permitted for such usage.

- **Overdose** – Often referred to as 'OD', it implies a toxic level of bioavailability of a substance, resulting in life-threatening or fatal outcomes. Overdose is a medical emergency arising from ingesting a lethal dose of a substance. The dosage is typically not intended for suicide and is due to accidental dosing errors or due to the use of high doses due to tolerance. Polysubstance abuse (such as alcohol with prescription narcotics benzodiazepines) is common in lethal overdose.

- **Withdrawal** – refers to a clinical state characterized by physiological and psychological disturbances causing bodily and mental harm due to abrupt discontinuation of the bioavailability of the substance. Withdrawal can be life-threatening and lethal if not managed promptly and appropriately.

- **'Crash'** – a term often used to refer to a stimulant withdrawal characterized by exhaustion, anhedonia, lack of energy, depressed mood, fatigue, vivid yet unpleasant dreams, psychomotor agitation, or retardation. Depression is common during withdrawal, hence the risk of deliberate self-harm during the crash.

- **Recreational drug use –** Refers to chemical substances for purposes of experiencing a particular mental or bodily experience. This description is used to specifically differentiate non-prescription or medicinal intentions for the use of the substance. The list of legally approved substances for recreational use differs between countries. Recreational use is a gateway for habitual use, leading to problem use and addiction.

In general, the effects of a substance depend on both pharmacokinetic and pharmacodynamic properties and the route of administration (inhalational, snorting, sniffing, smoking, oral, aboral, intramuscular, or intravenous use). Smoking and IV use have shorter onset action times for euphoric effects than oral use. Typically, IV use and smoking effects are immediate (in seconds), while snorting takes minutes. Dependency, especially chemical dependency, happens quicker with intravenous opioid use than marijuana or cocaine.

Approach to Patients with Addictive Behavior

- **Identify the stage of use –** As mentioned above, the individual progresses through the following phases – contact phase, habitual user phase, problem user phase, dependence phase, and addiction phase. There is an overlap between these stages. The individual may persist in a stage for a long time or may fall back to an earlier stage. Not all patients progress to addiction, so the treatment strategy needs to be individualized on a case-by-case basis. The phase at which clinical presentation first happens also varies significantly – while private mental health clinics usually receive individuals in the problem user or dependent phases, general hospitals and tertiary care centers handle patients presenting with overdose, withdrawal, or addiction. Financial resources required for durable long-term treatment for relapse prevention is also a commonly encountered factor determining outcomes.

- **Detoxification –** Refers to the phase of treatment to support or correct a patient's physiological and psychiatric state, starting from the discontinuation of the substance until the return to acceptable functioning without bioavailability of the substance. This phase of treatment involves both the treatment of organ damage and the psychiatric aspects of care. It can be conceptualized into the following five components:
  - Discontinuing the substance.

- Management of withdrawal.
- Treatment of physical and organ-damage-related complications
- Supportive care to improve the overall general condition of the individual.
- Management of any psychological complications.

- **De-addiction** – Refers to the phase of treatment of the patient who has discontinued use to address the etiological factors for substance use and prevent relapse. It can be conceptualized into five components:
  - Comprehensive mental status examination to understand the motivation, temperament, personality traits, and environmental factors that have contributed to the addictive behavior.
  - Individualized treatment protocol for de-addiction.
  - Strategies to prevent relapse.
  - Rehabilitation.
  - Termination of treatment.

- **Doctor-patient relationship** – Establishing a trusting doctor-patient relationship with substance abuse/addiction patients is challenging, as they could be disrespectful, dishonest, non-compliant, and lacking trust. The latter are sequelae of the psychopathology of their illness and substance use, not an indictment of their character. The doctor must navigate these challenges non-judgmentally, with restraint exercised during communication with the patient and family. Being open-minded, non-critical, and non-judgmental could go a long way in forging a durable bond with the patient. A confrontational line of questioning could be counterproductive. Express sincerity and empathy.

- **Client's reliability** – As a general principle in psychiatry, substance abuse must be within the differential diagnosis when a patient resists or is hesitant about collaborating history with the spouse or other family members. The psychopathology of substance abuse and addiction is such that the individual becomes allegiant only to the substance. As a result, the victims behave in any manner that serves their purpose for the time being. They make lofty promises that they forget to keep or deny their responsibilities and liabilities. They are often stricken with guilt and shame and may become hostile, evasive, or belligerent when confronted. They attempt to hide or weather down the severity of their complaints and functional impairments. In other words, the client is unreliable. Gender, socioeconomic factors, and cultural differences further complicate the situation. For example, in Asian societies, women with substance abuse suffer a severe social stigma, so these women do not bring their substance abuse habits and troubles to medical attention. They may also resist involving their spouse, parents, children, or in-laws in the discussion or treatment strategies. This factor must be kept in mind, and the psychiatrist must establish rapport and trust by navigating the interrogation and discussion nuancedly.

- **Doctor's approach** - I have noticed that the physician's attitudes toward substance abuse strongly influence their approach to such patients. The doctor must cautiously introspect and consciously work to avoid such bias. Their prior distasteful firsthand experiences with people using substances may make them sensitive to the belligerence and unreliability of the clients. Such physicians may turn unknowingly punitive or harsh towards the patients, which must also be avoided. If substance abuse is suspected, but the client vehemently denies it, keep amicably engaging the client and re-explore substance abuse at another visit. Neither dismiss nor accept the client's denial of use readily. If you are not a substance abuse and addiction specialist, do not hesitate to refer the patient to such a specialist or seek advice and ongoing guidance from trained experts. There is a tendency among physicians to consider other medical and psychiatric diagnoses as the predominant problem and consider substance abuse as a 'minor' or 'additional' issue that could be dealt with later. The latter is an erroneous and potentially dangerous assumption.

- **Stigma** - There is a robust stigma attached to substance abuse and addiction that transcends geographical and cultural differences. Substance abuse also has legal implications, which exacerbates the stigma. The stigma associated with substance abuse is that they would be considered 'weak in willpower', 'unable to exercise moral restraint', 'unreliable', 'immoral', 'powerless', 'deceitful', and 'untrustworthy'. In South Asian communities, families abet in the concealment of their substance abuse behavior and functional impairment. Beliefs that substance abuse could be severed successfully through religious conviction or pilgrimage, or if the patient is 'married away', are commonplace in South Asian societies as well. In the West, significant legal implications of substance abuse, such as divorce, loss of employment, and non-employability, also exacerbate the stigma.

- **Adolescents and children with substance use** – In this age group, the most reliable symptom of psychoactive substance abuse is marked behavioral change, deteriorating academic performance, severance of relationships with old friends, changes in personality, and sleep and appetite disturbances. Indicators that must make the psychiatrist suspect undiscovered substance abuse in this age group are listed below –

Indicators for substance abuse in children/ adolescents – Mananalam Clinic Experience **MCE**

- Perceived peer approval for drug use.
- Perceived parental approval for drug use.
- School absenteeism.
- Truancy.
- Poor academic performance.
- Distrusting teachers and parents.
- Low aspirations for achievement and competitiveness.
- Emotional distress.
- Observed adult drug use.
- Dissatisfaction with life.
- Little to no religious commitment.
- Altered sleep pattern.
- Missing appointments /assignments.

- **Elderly/Geriatric patients** – The first contact with the substance usually happens in adolescence or early adulthood, progressing over several years, and persists into late adulthood. However, new onset in late adulthood is also possible, although uncommon. Advancing age increases susceptibility to substance abuse. New onset in this age group may go unnoticed due to increased autonomy with growing age or diagnostic confusion of functional impairment due to neurocognitive deterioration with age. Risk factors for substance abuse in this age group include loss/death of friends, loss/death of spouse, loss of employment, retirement, failing health, and disability.

Key Aspects in History and Clinical Examination

In addition to the usual comprehensive mental status examination, the following aspects must be explored in cases of substance abuse.

- **Use details** – Includes age at first contact with substance, age of onset of regular use, pattern of current use, including frequency, amount of substance and route(s) or consumption, use of paraphernalia, periods of heaviest use, last substance use, periods of abstinence, history of overdose, intoxication, and treatment for substance abuse. Often, the patient downplays the amount/dose of substance used. Collaborative history is essential to confirm the actual doses.

- **Client perception of use and insight** – The perception and insight of the patient about the severity of their use, the positive and negative consequences of use, and the need for discontinuation or change must be explored.

- **Examination and laboratory analysis** – Physical examination must be completed to identify signs of substance use (such as nasal erosion, needle tracks, etc.) and organ damage (COPD, bronchitis, jaundice, cirrhosis, neurological examination). Laboratory analysis of serum and urine samples for a toxicology screen is helpful.

- **Social history** – This patient's social, economic, and personal relationship factors strongly influence the psychopathology of substance abuse. Details to be gathered include the history of personal, physical, emotional, or sexual abuse, history of being a victim of violence or neglect, living situation with other substance users and non-users, obstacles to sobriety or abstinence, significant relationship problems, employment-related stressors, and means of income. These details aid in understanding the precipitators of substance abuse and the obstacles to be tackled while planning an individualized treatment strategy for de-addiction and relapse prevention.

- **Legal history** – Details include arrests for driving under the influence of alcohol or other drugs, misdemeanors and infractions related to intoxication in public, holding, selling, or peddling substances, disorderly conduct, and petty crimes. Adverse legal history must also be documented.

- **Chronological storyline** – After gathering all relevant data, a chronological 'storyline' and any other psychiatric diagnoses that may co-exist must be built. The latter provides a broader idea of the overall clinical situation and the treatment strategy required.

Patient Education and Counseling

I use the analogy of a banyan tree to counsel patients about substance abuse and addiction. A banyan tree has a main trunk, giving off multiple branches that drop accessory roots to the ground. These accessory roots may become bulkier and more prominent with time than the primary trunk. Similarly, substance abuse is the primary trunk of the clinical conundrum, which gives off branches (such as affective disorders, self-harm, anxiety, cognitive dysfunction, organ damage, and legal and social dysfunction), which in turn may root itself so deeply, to cause diagnostic bias as to which constitutes the primary etiology to the clinical problem. Substance abuse, no matter how subtle, must be given due importance amidst other comorbid physical and psychiatric diagnoses in the overall treatment strategy.

Patients and their families must be educated that substance abuse disorders and addictive behaviors are treatable conditions with durable and appreciable improved clinical outcomes and overall quality and quantity of life. They should be warned against the dangers of withholding medical attention and treatment due to stigma.

Terminating substance abuse is relatively easy - users can 'stop' using any number of times without the intervention of a mental health professional. However, 'not restarting' almost always requires external help, best provided by a trained psychiatrist. Relapse is very common, and individuals cannot remain sober without treatment. Active ongoing treatment is necessary to prevent relapse.

Public outreach and awareness programs are also needed to increase public awareness about this mental health condition.

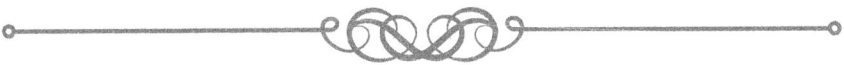

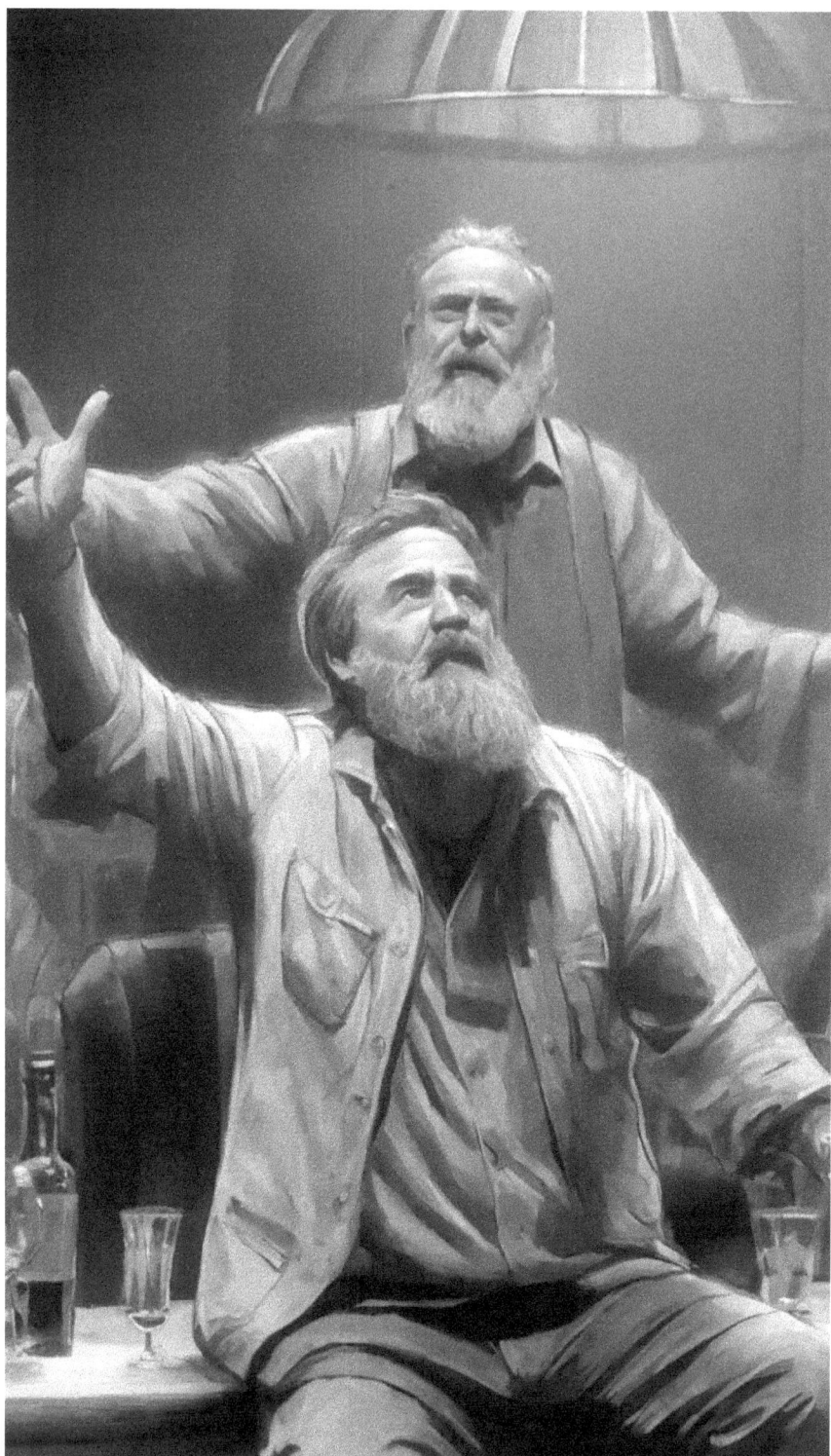

CHAPTER 14

Alcohol Use and Addiction

Alcohol is by far the most used and abused chemical substance world-wide. It is widely available, even over the counter, in grocery stores in some countries and is also considered a household substance. It is a restaurant menu staple and served on the table during family dinner. It is used as a gift in many societies and as an ingredient for religious rituals. The presence and use of alcohol is ubiquitous. Understanding the impact of alcohol use in the evolution of various psychiatric disorders as a comorbid factor versus its evolution as the primary psychiatric diagnosis is a sophisticated task.

At the most superficial level, it is easy to perceive alcohol as harmless. It facilitates socializing behavior, augments a feeling of well-being and ease, and is viewed as a 'relaxer' after a long day of work. In the lower socioeconomic strata of the population and among those who indulge in physical labor, alcohol is believed to be an antidote to fatigue and stress. In modern medicine, the detrimental effects of alcohol in terms of organ damage, morbidity, and mortality are well documented through research. Thus, there is a stunning gap between the undisputed medical ill-effects of alcohol and its yet unchallenged, unbridled widespread usage. To my knowledge, there has and is not any substance that is so detrimental to health but widely permitted for everyday usage. Due to this mismatch between knowledge and practice, alcohol use disorders are still widely ignored, overlooked, underestimated, underdiagnosed, and under-treated. In many cases, they are misdiagnosed and mistreated too.

First, I shall review some of the basics of alcohol as a pharmaco-chemical substance. Alcohol is consumed orally and rapidly absorbed from the gastrointestinal tract. Absorption of alcohol into systemic circulation begins as proximal as the mucous membranes of the oral cavity. Alcohol is an irritant to the GI mucosa. After absorption from the intestine, it is carried through the portal venous circulation to the liver, where it is metabolized, and then carried through the hepatic veins to the inferior vena cava and then to the pulmonary circulation, which is responsible for the 'odor in the breath' after alcohol consumption. It leaves the lungs through the pulmonary veins, which return to the left heart, from where it reaches systemic circulation through the aorta and its branches and through the latter, to the brain and other organs. Blood alcohol reaches peak levels approximately 2 hours after ingestion. Alcohol is excreted unchanged through the lungs and kidneys. The typical 'alcohol breath' odor is caused by the volatile metabolites of alcohol and is a reasonable but inaccurate estimate of the alcohol consumed. One of the effects of alcohol is peripheral vasodilation, which creates the feeling of 'warmth' (appreciated in colder climates) and a feeling of 'relaxation'.

Understanding the Drinking Episode

The 'drinking episode' refers to a single period in time from the start of the first drink until discontinuation that leads to sobriety. The drinking episode must not be confused with the customary habits associated with the drinking behavior of a patient. The neuropsychological effects of alcohol during the drinking episode are universally 'depressive' or 'inhibitory'. However, this depressive effect occurs differentially, affecting certain faculties of mentation first and others later, and certain faculties more durably than others. The experience and behavior of an individual while alcohol is in the systemic circulation is a net effect of these differential effects on the brain and somatic functions.

The immediate effects of alcohol ingestion are dose-related and can be understood in three phases. Alcohol exerts its effect (an inhibitory effect) on the 'higher' centers first (phase 1) and the 'lower' centers next (phase 2). By 'higher' centers, I mean the parts of the brain that are essential for regulating and disciplining impulsive behavior. Thus, during phase 1 after alcohol ingestion, behavior becomes less inhibited, more instinctive, more primitive, and more spontaneous, giving the experience of boosted confidence and relief from worry or anxiety. During this phase, introverted or tongue-tied people may become more verbose and articulate, facilitating socializing behavior. It is also the reason why alcohol is permitted and encouraged in social occasions, festivals, celebrations, and parties. It is this transient phase which is often mistaken for the aphrodisiac effect of alcohol. Nevertheless, these effects are short-lived (lasting for minutes) and occur at the expense of alertness, best judgment, and self-awareness. Even small quantities of alcohol impair intelligence, memory, attention, and judgment, as the latter faculties are also the functions of the 'higher centers'.

In essence, the ***intellect component of the Ulan is the first to get dulled.*** During phase 2, there is more global slowing of neural and mental faculties. Neuromuscular functioning, motor function and coordination, response times, visual-spatial skills, pharyngeal dysfunction, balance, gait, and speech become impaired. Mood changes (often depression), somnolence, and lethargy also become evident. Emotional spikes, including aggressive behavior, self-harm, suicidal thoughts, and risky behavior, may get precipitated in some individuals, especially in those with other psychiatric comorbidities.

Phase 3 is characterized by abnormalities in vital signs, such as heart rate, blood pressure, respiratory depression, cerebral edema, and profound dehydration. If alcohol consumption is not promptly stopped around phase 2, phase 3 is characterized by intoxication and overdose-related morbidity or mortalities. It could lead to alcoholic coma, which can be identified through hypothermia, stertorous respiration, feeble and thready pulse, pupillary abnormalities, pallor, clammy skin, and severe alcoholic breath odor. Differential diagnoses include, but are not limited to head injury, epilepsy, and hypoglycemia. Acute alcoholic intoxication and alcoholic coma could be lethal. In these situations where the latter does not happen, there are delayed physiological effects of alcohol resulting in somatic and psychological effects lasting for hours or days after the drinking episode, colloquially referred to as a 'hangover'.

It is essential to understand that the elimination of alcohol from the systemic circulation is relatively slower than its absorption process. Hence, the effects of such absorption are maximal several minutes or hours later. Slow and smaller portion consumption of alcohol could permit disruption of the drinking episode before an individual reaches phase 2. The disruption of the drinking episode is much more effective when people are around to terminate the drinking after phase 1. If alcohol is consumed in larger amounts within a short period, phase 1 becomes much faster and inevitably progresses to phase 2. Drinking alone also leads to unmonitored higher initial doses and is a potentially risky behavior.

Psychosocial behavior is affected while being under the influence of

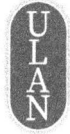

alcohol. The feeling of inner pleasure is associated with deceptive self-confidence, disappearance of feelings of fatigue, moral laxity, intellectual looseness, and overall descent to lower values due to lack of restraint. It could lead to indiscriminate behavior, i.e., an individual begins to treat everything equally. Hilarity with an aura of fellowship and brotherhood or self-pity with an aura of despair and dejection could also occur. After sobriety, most individuals regret their behavior and actions committed while under the influence of alcohol. ***Failure to abstain from alcohol after such regret is an early sign of evolving alcoholism.***

Special Terminology

Specific terminologies are often used in alcohol-related literature that deserve special mention. It is paramount that healthcare providers understand these terms and avoid inaccurate usage.

- **'Compulsive drinking'** – Refers to a behavior where an individual who has started a drinking episode is unable to stop it for a reasonable length of time. The individual could continue drinking until intoxication or coma or continue drinking for days until the money supply runs out or is removed forcibly from access to alcohol by others who find the activity disruptive. These individuals display high chemical tolerance to alcohol and experience cravings.

- **'Symptomatic alcoholic'** – Refers to an individual resorting to alcohol consumption as a result of another psychiatric or organic illness, i.e., alcoholism is a symptom secondary to another disease. These individuals report seeking alcohol to 'ward off anxiety' or that alcohol 'helps deal with their mental issues'.

- **Binge drinking** – Refers to bouts of consumption of large amounts of alcohol, with long phases of abstinence or sobriety in between. Individuals may drink socially during these so-called 'intervals' between binges. No stress or trigger may be identifiable for such binges. They may be 'weekend drinkers'. Binge drinking is harmful to liver health and has serious long-term effects.

- **Harmful use** – A term used in medical literature to refer to persistent use despite evident and apparent ill effects on physical and mental health.

Natural History

In the previous chapter on substance abuse and addiction, I discussed the natural history of substance abuse in multiple phases, namely the contact phase, the problem user phase, the dependence phase, and the addictive phase. In brief, the ***contact phase*** is characterized by the 'first high', an enjoyable euphoric experience that becomes the principal incentive to pursue repetitive exposure. The next phase, the ***problem user phase,*** is the phase of rapidly increasing frequency of substance usage, resulting in lifestyle and behavior changes. The ***dependence phase*** is characterized by behavioral changes in the individual to promote circumstances to maintain constant bioavailability of the substance actively. The last phase, the addictive phase, is characterized by pervasive behavior affecting all spheres of the individual's life solely to maintain substance consumption. The natural history of alcohol use follows these same phases of evolution. One could remember these phases as a ***good drinker, bad drinker, sad drinker,*** and ***mad drinker,*** respectively.

Quantifying Alcohol Use

The National Institute of Alcohol Abuse and Alcoholism (NIAA), established in 1970, drafted specific guidelines to quantify alcohol use. Generally, 14 grams or 0.6 ounces (one ounce is approximately 30 ml) of 100% alcohol is considered 'one standard drink'. Thus, 12 ounces of a 5% alcohol drink (such as beer), 5 ounces of a 12% alcohol drink (such as wine), or 1.5 ounces of distilled spirit, i.e., 40% alcohol drinks (such as whiskey), is considered a standard drink. However, the definition of a standard drink differs between countries.

There is a widespread perception that alcoholism is defined by the amount of alcohol consumed. Alcohol use disorder (AUD) is independent of the amount of alcohol consumed. In other words, AUD can occur even in individuals who consume low amounts of alcohol, such as one standard drink a day. However, the risk of AUD is directly related to the amount of alcohol consumed. Accordingly, the NIAA has identified 'low-risk drinking' defined as no more than three drinks on any day, or no more than seven drinks within a week for a woman, and no more than four drinks on any day, or no more than 14 drinks in a week for men, is associated with less than 2% risk of AUD. However, as per the NIAA, *'even within these limits, people can have problems if they drink too quickly or have other health issues'.*

Binge drinking is defined as drinking that raises BAC (Blood Alcohol Concentration) to 0.08 g/dL (0.08%) or higher, also considered the legal guide for driving in the USA. Typically, 4-5 drinks within a 2-hour time frame could lead to such high levels. Drinking patterns that lead to BAC 2 times or higher than binge drinking levels are called 'heavy drinking'.

Generally, the threshold for safe drinking is lower for women than men, and no amount of alcohol consumed over time is 100% safe.

Causative and Risk Factors

Exploring the causative and risk factors is essential in examining a patient with alcohol use disorder. Several professional bodies (medical and non-medical) have come up with multiple explanations for alcoholism and have classified it variously. The ICD-8 identifies alcoholism as one of the 'other non-psychotic mental disorders', while the ICD-9 identifies it as 'alcohol dependence syndrome'. Alcoholism is approached as a personality disorder in the DSM I and DSM II, as a substance abuse disorder in the DSM III and DSM IV, and as a substance-related disorder in the DSM 5. In essence, the condition of alcoholism has remained the same over centuries or millennia, but it is perceived and understood differently over time.

Alcohol (or substance) addiction results from the interaction of a unique and complex set of biological, psychological, and social factors. These factors only confer susceptibility for addiction and do not predestine the individual to addiction. Ultimately, it is an individual's choice to explore the consumption of alcohol (or another substance) for the first time that could set off an inevitable train of events that results in addiction.

Biological factors

Biological factors play a crucial role. Genetic factors determine the type of experience (pleasurable vs repulsive) undergone by the individual after consuming alcohol (or the substance). The ability to metabolize alcohol is genetically determined, and hence, the dose required for euphoria, satiety, and dependency are also impacted by genetic factors. A family history of alcohol or substance use disorders is therefore essential during the initial clinical examination.

Psychological factors

Psychological factors include personality traits such as impulsivity, novelty seeking, risk-taking, tendency to seek immediate gratification, etc., which confer increased vulnerability to try alcohol or other chemical substances. Earlier, I had discussed the natural history of the evolution of alcoholism, from the contact phase to the problem user and then to dependency. An individual's cognitive and behavioral framework determines if an individual will have insight into this progression and work to actively reverse it or be a victim of the natural progression of the disease. At least in part, the passage through these phases is learned behavior – it is modeled through observation of others and rehearsed over time, even over several years. In those individuals where it continues to progress, the initial experience with alcohol has been exclusively positive. It hence acts as a positive reinforcement to attempt repetitive consumption, which then leads to a state of physiological and psychological dependency, after which lack of alcohol results in a negative experience, which further reinforces the behavior promoting alcohol consumption. Environmental factors such as peer groups that consume alcohol (college parties, work parties), events or activities where alcohol consumption is typical (like concerts and birthday parties), and paraphernalia become strongly associated with the euphoric experience and may trigger urges and cravings. An increasing body of literature suggests genetic/biological explanations for personality traits and cognitive abilities, which suggest that these psychological factors may manifest yet unstudied biological factors.

Social factors include cultural acceptance of alcohol, the nature of the peer groups, availability of alcohol, family situation, etc. Poverty, lower education level, manual labor, and being involved with the supply or trade of recreational substances are other note-worthy risk factors.

Screening tests

The following are helpful adjuncts during the mental status examination of an individual with alcohol use disorder or alcoholism -

- CAGE (need to **C**ut down on alcohol, **A**nnoyed by criticism about drinking, **G**uilt, and use of alcohol as **E**ye opener) criteria is a simple and rapid test. It minimizes the effect of patient denial, and any positive response to any criteria must be considered significant.
- AUDIT (Alcohol Use Identification Test) – a brief 10-item, self-reported test that could be administered within minutes. Eight items are scored on a 0-5 scale, while two others are scored as 0, 2, or 4. A score of 8 or more indicates hazardous levels of drinking.
- MAST (Michigan Alcoholism Screening Test) is a 25-item test that screens for problematic alcohol use and could be obtained through self-reporting or administered by the clinician.
- SMAST (Short Michigan Alcoholism Screening Test) is a shorter, 10-item version of the above MAST method.
- DAST (Drug Abuse Screening Test) is a self-reported 20-item instrument used to screen for non-alcohol substance abuse or dependence.

Clinical Approach to Alcohol Related Disorders

Individuals with alcohol or substance use problems are generally defensive and sensitive to judgment or criticism. Shifting the blame or cause away from them and objectifying it as a 'problem' rather than a disease helps forge a better relationship with the psychiatrist. Hence, it is preferable to address these individuals as 'clients' rather than as 'patients.

Alcohol-related disorders (AUD and alcohol addiction) run a chronic, progressive course, with waxing and waning use, interspersed with periods of relative sobriety or abstinence and binge drinking. While some clients display a slower and indolent course over several decades, others may rapidly decline. Usually, most clients have had some level of introspection into their drinking problem when it is past the problem user phase. Introspection alone does not help in recovery – the critical factor is the level of motivation to get better. Whether motivation is a non-modifiable trait or a transient state of mind is uncertain. Social support affects motivation to get better positively. The pre-morbid level of functioning, comorbid psychiatric diagnoses, and a positive doctor-client relationship are other factors that affect the overall outcome of psychiatric intervention.

Clients are usually in one of many stages in their response to the drinking problem. The transtheoretical model (TTM) of behavior change could be applied to alcoholism clients as a guide to understanding the readiness of the client to change. A client who does not consider their drinking as a problem is in the pre-contemplation stage. A client who has experienced thoughts or ideas of modifying drinking behavior is in the contemplation stage. Ambivalence about the need to make changes, yet openness to suggestions and advice, is seen in this stage. Doctors play a crucial role in moving the patient to the next stage, called the 'preparatory stage,' which involves acquiring resources and a cognitive schema necessary to effect the contemplated changes. Planning strategies to avoid exposure to triggers that precipitate alcohol consumption is essential to this stage. The next stage is the 'action stage', where these plans are implemented. Successful implementation could result in the termination of drinking, at which point the client enters the last yet most complex and challenging stage – the 'maintenance stage'. Abstinence from alcohol is a constant struggle and challenge that requires tremendous effort. Failure to sustain abstinence leads to relapse. The psychiatrist's expertise lies in preventing such relapses and, more so, in managing relapses. Relapses are discouraging for the client and the psychiatrist. Clients tend to withdraw from treatment, and keeping the relapsed client compliant within the care of the treating psychiatrist is challenging.

As mentioned earlier, motivation for change is the key to a good prognosis in alcoholism. Objective assessment of motivation and its augmentation can be achieved as follows –

- Assess the relevance of the change in the client's life. In what way is the drinking problem affecting the client's life? Can a change be shown to be relevant to their overall well-being? Verbalizing and framing the relevance of a change in drinking behavior in making the client more efficient, productive, and confident can bring about motivation.
- Next, explore the tangible rewards of terminating alcohol use. This step is often overlooked in clinical practice and replaced by a 'to-do' advice style of making changes that

limit the patient's autonomy. If offered a to-do list or advisory monologues, ambivalent clients may withdraw from treatment rather than embrace it.

- Explore the possible risks of making changes to the client's life. Many measures required to curtail the drinking habit limit the client's freedom of movement and choice and may affect their professional and social routines. Stay ahead of the client by identifying and verbalizing those risks before they bring them up as arguments against changing their behavior. The psychiatrist must create a contrasting vision of the paths ahead – one without changing the drinking problem and the other after making a change successfully. Such contrasting visions, when well-articulated by the mental health provider in a non-judgmental and non-threatening fashion, can forge a cognitive schema that sets the patient on a path to abstinence.

- Gauge the possible roadblocks to the client's successfully and durably implementing the strategies to terminate drinking and maintaining abstinence. Anticipate these roadblocks and brainstorm possible solutions proactively. These roadblocks could cause regression of the action phase to the pre-contemplation or contemplation stages. Articulate the potential roadblocks to the client before they happen and provide solutions if they were to happen.

- Repeat the process each time the client is unmotivated about the process!

The above method, dubbed the **'5Rs'** (*Relevance, Rewards, Risks, Roadblocks, and Repetition),* could be a helpful guide for clients with alcohol, tobacco, and other substance use disorders.

Take Home Points

The impact of alcohol on the population is vast, with a million shades of grey. The available diagnostic criteria do not accommodate all the variations and severities of alcohol use-related disorders. There is a general tendency to consider addiction alone as the only form of this disorder requiring intervention, thereby approaching alcohol-related issues as an all-or-none phenomenon. Most alcohol use disorders are overlooked and neglected. Community programs designed for alcohol-related problems tend to focus on early-stage users more. There is also a tendency to implement non-evidence-based measures in alcohol-related service programs.

My message is simple. ***Don't try alcohol.*** It is impractical to predict accurately who might turn into an addict. There is no known advantage to alcohol consumption; even if there are any, the risks far outweigh the benefits. It is wiser to avoid alcohol altogether, as it is an entirely preventable form of self-injury.

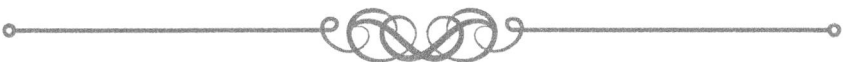

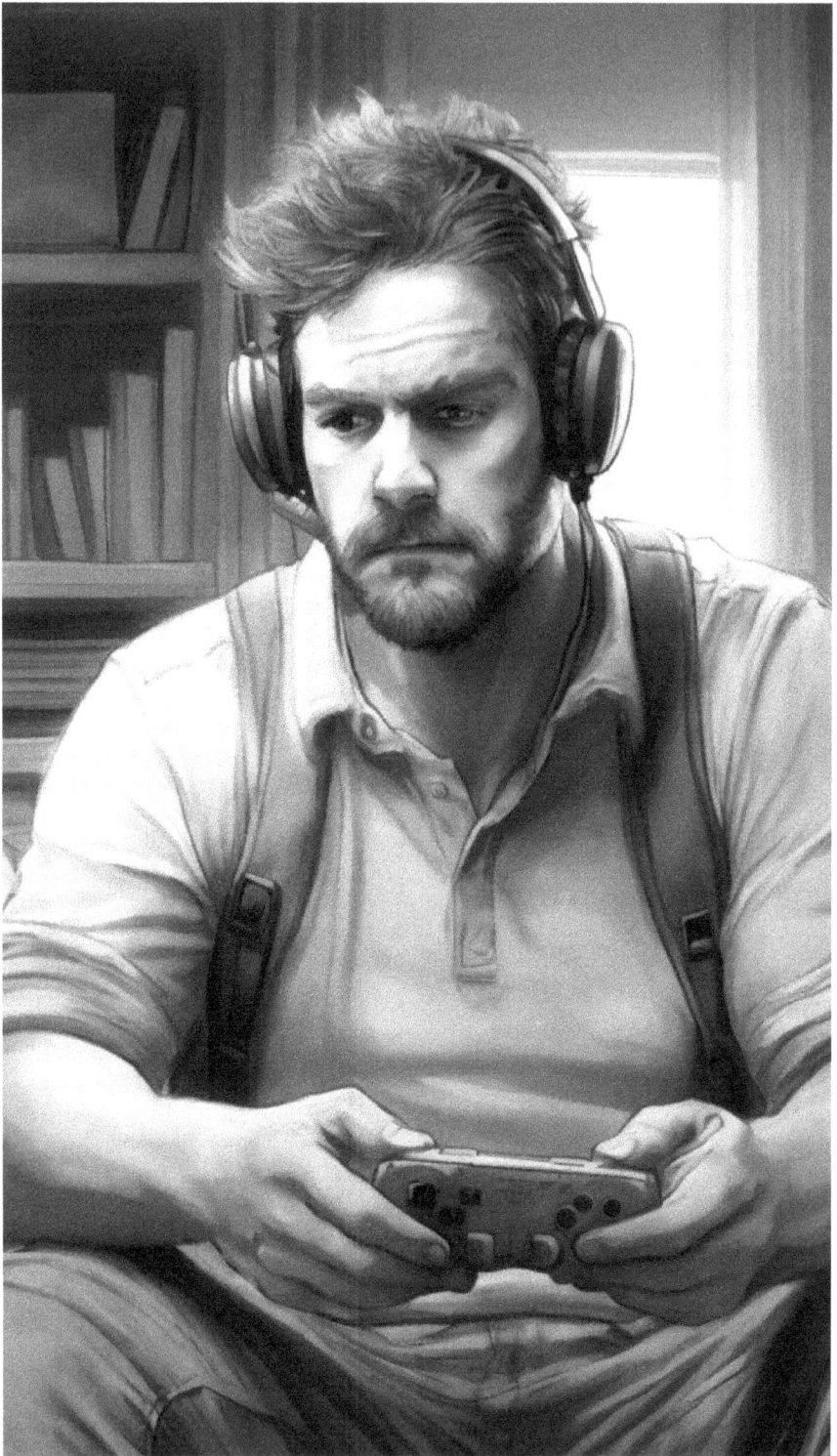

CHAPTER 15

Gaming and Internet-Related Disorders

There is an increasing trend toward identifying psychological disorders around gaming and internet-related activities, leading to a subset of psychiatric literature. The basic concepts underlying addictive behavior apply to this subset of non-substance-related abuse disorders. However, some terminologies and nuances are specific to this field, where the data is evolving, vague, and challenging to the practicing psychiatrist. Hence, I have devoted a separate chapter to preparing the clinician with the fundamental concepts to build further expertise in this field.

What is Gaming?

The word 'game' refers to the form of a competition or contest among individuals conducted in a controlled setting. In nature, organisms within a given species constantly compete with each other, resulting in various dominance hierarchies that constitute their societies. Winning or losing the competition decides an individual's position within the group, regulating access to resources available for the group. The latter includes but is not limited to access to food, safe and convenient shelter, mates of the opposite gender, and power within the group. Complex neurological pathways have evolved within the brains of organisms to make them fitter in this competition for survival. Ethics, morals, values, and virtues have evolved to deal with how to go about this competition. Based on progression within these contests, an individual's social position, recognition, and 'roles' keep changing. Winners of conflicts are respected, admired, and accepted as role models in society, while losing tendency is considered an unfavorable trait. Losers are often stripped of their responsibilities and their roles downgraded. Contests between competing individuals are constantly observed and followed by the rest of society with keen interest.

A 'game' is an artificially constructed contest within a controlled setting – by which I mean a specific context defining the conditions in which the competition is conducted, rules, regulations, and a judge or arbitrator to decide the winner and loser. A game is a miniature,'toy form' of a real-life contest. They are often confined to one or few specific skill sets (mental or physical) and arbitrated by a deciding authority. Winning and losing are clearly defined (more clearly defined than in real life), with several rewards and punishments made available with certainty (also with more confidence than in real life). Dominance hierarchies are developed for the winners, and losers are ejected from the games. Games are often watched, recorded, and relayed to the public.

Games have been present since time immemorial. Recent advances in technology have resulted in games played on a screen (graphic interface), and amplified communication abilities with people across the world through the internet have pushed the nature of the gaming world into uncharted territory.

Gaming vs Gambling

Gambling is also a form of a game, with two specific differences. First, the outcome of the game is primarily determined by an element of random chance (i.e., 'luck') rather than the skill set of the individual; second, the rewards and punishments relate to gaining or losing monetary or other valuable possessions, leading to an exaggerated positive or negative experience. For these purposes, gaming must not be confused with gambling addiction.

Benefits of Gaming

Games have been known to man since immemorial and are part of human nature. Children themselves design their games, decide their own rules of the games, choose their arbitrator or judge, cooperate, and voluntarily abide by their own rules to make the game happen. They learn the fundamentals of social interaction within a society, compete without hurting, and team building. They gradually learn how to react, cope with successes and failures, enjoy rewards, and tolerate punishments. Adult games, athletics, and sports are extensions of this behavior pattern built during childhood. Games are also a ripe and opportune setting to educate children on motivation, skill development, discipline, ethics, and values.

Video games (online or offline) are a subset of games where an individual interacts with a graphic interface on a screen. Skill abilities are mostly mental (visual-spatial, attention, multitasking, pattern recognition, etc.), with a lesser proportion of physical/musculoskeletal skill development. The player's identity is anonymous, and the player's appearance to other players can be edited and tailored to the player's preference. In other words, the player can choose how others see the player's identity (called the 'avatar'). Players could choose their skin color, gender, facial appearance, emotion, garb, and posture, allowing them to gain confidence and self-esteem. Games allow players to select the specific skill (i.e., game) in which they can flourish, allowing them an alternate space to nurture positive emotions and experience. Online games are a magnet to attract people of similar interests across various ages, allowing for reinforcing online friendships that reduce feelings of loneliness. Online rewards such as badges, exclusive gadgetry or weaponry, life energies, and treasures can be used to further progression in the game, leading to promotions in one's rank and status in the online society. A sense of kinship, guild, and clan also develops, which allows players to nourish interpersonal bonding. Furthermore, constant exposure to specific visual interfaces may promote visual-spatial skills, cognitive abilities, and multitasking. A minority of academic researchers and psychologists have echoed the above arguments as being the benefits of video gaming despite most of the literature focusing on the ill effects of video games.

Risks of Video Gaming

Video gaming is essentially a computer software-based technology and thus allows for a level of certainty in reward and punishment that is impossible in real-world games. Rewards and losses are clearly defined. Furthermore, the effort-to-stimulus time is foreshortened to a few seconds, allowing instant gratification or pain, exposing the brain's reward circuits to reinforcement strengths unavailable in the real world. Instant gratification through instant rewards and the certainty of those reward patterns quickly reinforces gaming behavior.

Online video gaming allows social interaction while maintaining anonymity, which is impossible in the real world. Anonymity shields players from sociological controls that limit unfavorable behavior towards self and others. Online gaming communities provide a diverse set of highly unique niches to nourish a pattern of behavior that one might find hard to sustain in the real world – thereby shifting the player's involvement from the real world to the virtual world. The ability to role-play is another potential reason for players shunning real-world social interaction.

Social interaction in the real world is possible only with a handful of individuals. Online gaming allows thousands, if not millions, of players to interact simultaneously. These games, termed Massively Multiplayer Online Role-Playing Games (MMORPG), are created with an online world called the 'persistent world', which keeps running indefinitely, into which any player can log on at any time. In other words, the game environment never ends.

These extraordinary environmental situations, being drastically different from real-world scenarios, pose potential risks for nurturing behavior patterns that may cause suffering to the individual in the real world.

During the last few decades, video game availability has increased through regular home computers, laptops, tablets, and phones. Thus, more people are playing video games than ever before. Screen time of young children and adolescents has increased to 8-11 hours per day, i.e., 30-50% of the day or more than 50% of the waking hours. In other words, screen time has consumed time that would otherwise be spent with family, friends, or teachers. As a potentially enjoyable and stimulating activity, individuals with intra- and interpersonal issues tend to gravitate to computer gaming to avoid confronting such problems.

Computer gaming may, therefore, be visualized as a spectrum ranging from an enjoyable pastime, coping strategy, pathological use, and addiction.

Definition of Gaming Disorder

Being a relatively new field of study, there are plenty of overlapping terms and definitions describing gaming- and internet-related disorders. Some of the terms used are Internet Gaming Disorder (IGD), Internet addiction, Technology-based addiction, Pathological technology use, Pathological video gaming, Pathological Internet use, Computer addiction, Screen addiction,

Addictions to video games and Online role-playing games, Game overuse, Video game addiction, Smartphone addiction, Cyber relationship addiction, Net compulsions, etc. I have used the term Internet Gaming Disorder (IGD) for this chapter.

In 2013, IGD was provided a provisional status in the DSM-5, and in 2019, the World Health Organization (WHO) officially adopted the diagnosis within the ICD-11.

As per the DSM-5, diagnosis of IGD requires 5 of the following nine diagnostic criteria over a 12-month period –

- Preoccupation with internet games has become the dominant activity in daily life.
- Withdrawal symptoms (such as irritability, anxiety, or sadness) on removal of internet.
- Tolerance, i.e., need to spend more time with Internet gaming (tolerance).
- Lacking control over the Internet.
- Loss of interest in hobbies and entertainment previously enjoyed.
- Continued (i.e., ongoing) excessive use despite knowledge of psychosocial problems.
- Deception (as in willful deception or misleading) of family members, therapists, or others about the amount (i.e., time spent) of Internet gaming.
- Escape from or relief of negative mood (e.g., feeling helpless, guilty, anxious), i.e., using gaming as a coping mechanism.
- Loss of important aspects of life (e.g., significant relationships, jobs, or educational/career opportunities).

As per the ICD-11, an individual may be diagnosed with gaming disorder if they experience the following –

- Impaired control over behavior.
- Increased priority given to video gaming-related activities to the point of assuming precedence over other life interests and daily activities.
- Continued gaming behavior despite adverse consequences (i.e., significant impairment in personal, familial, social, and other vital areas of functioning).

Thus, the key differentiating factor between the DSM-5 and ICD-11 classifications is that, unlike the DSM-5, the ICD-11 requires significant functional impairment as a criterion. Thus, the ICD-11 diagnostic approach may capture a more severe form of gaming and internet-related disorders than the DSM-5 framework. Prior to the provisional DSM-5 criteria, researchers would often adapt the criteria of other disorders (e.g., pathological gambling in the DSM IV-TR) for use in gaming and internet-related disorders (Fisher, 1994; Griffiths & Hunt, 1998).

Etiology

The etiology of IGD is complex and not fully understood. From what we know, it helps to think of the factors associated with ICD as internal or external factors. External factors may be family-, social- or game-related factors.

- **Internal factors** – include psychological archetypes and behavior patterns that could predispose affiliation to games and internet usage. These factors include deficient self-regulatory abilities, impaired decision-making due to dysexecutive problems, mood dysregulation, reward system dysregulation, avoidant behavior patterns (such as escapism, deficient coping with negative emotions), low self-esteem, poor self-efficacy, and psychiatric comorbidities.

- **Family-related factors** – include poor relationships with parents and peers, absence of parental control, negative role models, and positive parental attitude towards adolescent substance abuse. Ignorant, oppressive, and hostile parental environments, single-parent families, and 'broken' family environments are associated with increased screen time for adolescents.

- **Social factors** – Individuals who suffer an unenriching social life in the real world tend to gravitate towards gaming environments where socialization happens. Shy and isolated children may find the virtual gaming environment a safe and rewarding way of interacting with others. Team aspects of gaming are also positive experiences that reinforce gaming interests. Like-minded players may begin to interact outside the virtual environments as well. The ability to tailor the avatar skin instills social confidence in the virtual environment. To some extent, individuals who find meaningful interactions in the virtual world tend to feel less loneliness and boredom.

- **Game-related factors** – Structural characteristics of a specific game genre could contribute to pathological gaming behavior. Internet gaming is more strongly associated with gaming disorders than offline gaming. Role-playing structures could promote addictive behavior as well. Certain features of MMORPGs, such as the never-ending game design, the possibility of acquiring more 'power', glory, immunity or invincibility, and achievement of power or gain that is typically forbidden in the real world (the 'forbidden fruit hypothesis'), a progression through a hierarchical social organization, regular membership benefits, narrative elements, realistic graphical quality, and fast loading times are some of the features that promote gaming attachment. Commercial factors such as monetarization and obligation to purchase items (that were initially free-to-play) are other factors. Curiosity, role-playing, belonging, obligation, reward, and escapism could predict MMORPG addiction.

Relevant Neurobiology

Some literature suggests that reward deficiency, reduced impulse control mechanisms, impaired decision-making, and impulsivity are associated with IGD. Executive control networks in ADHD may increase the susceptibility to IGD. Like depression, IGD may be ameliorated by treating dysfunctional connectivity between emotional and executive control mechanisms. Associations between excessive use of social media or screen time and IGD remain to be explored in more granular detail.

Craving-related changes in the brain are identifiable through functional magnetic resonance imaging in patients with IGD but not in subjects with recreational game use (RGU). Cue-induced craving is assumed to be important in maintaining addictive behavior and producing relapse. Although cue-induced craving was much more robust in Internet addicts, craving symptoms in nonaddicted internet users have also been described.

Psychopathology and Symptomatology

The psychopathological pathways involved in developing IGD are not yet fully understood. From my understanding of the available literature and clinical experience, I surmise that the basic concepts of substance abuse disorders and addiction are applicable here as well, the difference being that the substance consumed is the gaming experience rather than a chemical substance. The gaming experience can mimic chemical substance use and hijack reward and punishment circuits. The rewards and punishments are predictably certain and are obtained instantly. In disorders where individuals tend to be looked down upon and ostracized in most real-time social environments, gaming offers an opportunity to rise in a social dominance hierarchy. In essence, growing within a social dominance hierarchy, a highly gratifying reward experience that may be difficult to attain for many individuals in the real world becomes a more achievable target for most individuals in the virtual world. With increasing gaming activity, the user becomes/begins to seek 'quicker' response times to rewards and punishments. In due course, several of the following symptoms begin to emerge.

- **Increasing screen time** – The user begins to spend more and more time in the gaming environment. After exhaustion of free time, weekend and holiday time begin to be used, resulting in dropping out of other pleasurable and leisure activities in the real world. However, I caution clinicians against using screen time alone as a yardstick for identifying a gaming disorder.

- **Preoccupation** – The gamer becomes occupied with game-related thinking or preparation for the game, thereby spending non-gaming time indirectly towards the gaming activity. Preoccupation is essential to identify in the clinical setting, as these hours (not just screen time) are also time lost towards the gaming activity.

- **Salience** – Refers to a state where gaming becomes the most important activity in one's life. i.e., the gamer plays games to the exclusion of other activities, resulting in missed life opportunities, interference with usual routine, neglect of essential self-care (such as sleep, eating, and personal hygiene), shunning real-world social interactions (such as at school, work, family related activities), and delinquencies with duties for the family or work. Salience can be identified through the gamer's perceived 'loss of control' over their life, being consumed by gaming and seeming unable to regulate their time with the game. Salience is recognized as a core feature of gaming addiction in many studies.

- **Tolerance** – refers to the need for increasing gaming activity by the user.

It is an essential symptom of gaming disorder, but it is hard to identify. Screen time alone cannot be used to identify tolerance, as the user may switch to games that provide quicker or stronger rewards to compensate for growing tolerance. Most games are designed to battle the user's expected tolerance by providing a more rewarding experience, progressing them through various 'stages' in the game, or providing 'bonus rounds'. Furthermore, the inability to increase access to the gaming environment or equipment influences screen time – another reason for screen time being an inaccurate surrogate for measuring tolerance.

- **Craving and withdrawal** – Craving refers to an irresistible mental impulsion to undergo the gaming experience. It is often associated with a negative experience when the individual is not gaming, i.e., withdrawal. Craving and withdrawal are more subtle with gaming disorders than with chemical substance use and hence are only variably included in studies as a criterion for diagnosis of these disorders.

- **Conflictuosness** – or 'conflictedness' is a state of harboring opposing emotions and will towards a particular issue. In other words, they are ambivalent in judgment towards their gaming activity. The presence of conflicts implies that the individual has begun to suffer from gaming activity (i.e., pathological gaming has already started) and is considered a core symptom of gaming disorders by certain researchers.

- **Mood imbalance** – includes sadness, irritability, and anxiety related to gaming activity. Feelings of guilt and depression may occur, usually in response to the perceived loss of control over gaming. Thus, psychiatric comorbidities should be evaluated through a thorough MSE in patients assessed for gaming-related disorders.

- **Relapse** – refers to the resurgence of gaming-related disorderly conduct or behavior after abstinence/remission. It is pretty clinching of the diagnosis, differentiating it from recreational game use.

As with other disorders, there is much variability within patients presenting with gaming-related disorders, and understanding the broad types of patients helps the clinician construct an individualized treatment strategy. One classification of online gamers that I find helpful, as proposed by Billieux et al., groups gamers into five subtypes – two problematic and the rest non-problematic. They are –

- Regulated Recreational Gamer (Non-problematic): low impulsivity trait, high self-esteem.
- Regulated Social Role-Player (Non-problematic): low impulsivity, low self-esteem, motivated towards gaming by social interactions and role-playing.
- Unregulated achievers (Problematic): high impulsivity, primarily motivated by achievements in the game.
- Unregulated escapers (Problematic): low achievements, poor self-esteem, high escapism.
- Hardcore gamers (Highly problematic): typically suffer adverse consequences of excessive involvement in gaming.

Complications

Somatic complications of excessive media use or screen time include sleep disturbances, auditory hallucinations, enuresis, encopresis, musculo-skeletal injuries (wrist, neck, elbow pains, tendosynovitis – 'nintendinitis'), obesity, skin blisters, calluses, hand arm vibration syndrome, and peripheral neuropathy.

Psychological complications include increased association with depression, anxiety, suicidal ideation, and suicidal planning. The effects are more emphatic in gamers who spend several hours gaming, typically more than 5 hours daily.

Social complications include decreased academic performance, leading to low self-esteem and confidence. Employment loss, disruptive behavior at work, financial losses, interpersonal relationship breakdown, and overall reduced quality of life.

Screening and Assessment Tools

Gaming, an inherently harmless activity not involving a chemical substance, being used primarily and widely for recreational purposes, poses a tough challenge for the clinician. As mentioned earlier in the book, no screening tool or diagnostic checklist should be solely relied on. However, some of the below-mentioned screening tools could be useful –

- **Internet Gaming Disorder Test (IGD-20)** – The IGD-20 consists of 20 five-point Likert scale items developed by Pontes, Király, Demetrovics, and Griffiths (2014) to evaluate IGD, incorporating the DSM-5 diagnostic criteria and the six dimensions of the Griffiths addiction model (2005), namely salience, mood modification, tolerance, withdrawal, conflict, and relapse. The study measures online and offline gaming activity during the previous 12 months and has been validated.

- **Internet Gaming Disorder Scale Short Form (IGDS9-SF)** – This brief instrument developed by Pontes and Griffiths (2015) consists of 9 five-point Likert scale items, incorporating the nine DSM-5 diagnostic criteria to assess the severity of IGD and its harmful effects by evaluating online and offline gaming activities during the previous 12 months. The objective of the instrument is not to diagnose IGD but to evaluate its severity and harmful effects on the gamer's life, with a cut-off established at 36 points to differentiate between gamers with and without the disorder. This instrument has been validated in English, Portuguese, Slovenian, Italian, Persian, Turkish and Polish.

- **Problematic Online Gaming Questionnaire (POGQ)** – Demetrovics et al. (2012) developed this instrument of twenty-six 5-point Likert scale items to detect problems related to online gaming. Of the original 26 items, 18 were retained and organized in six dimensions: preoccupation, overuse, immersion, social isolation, interpersonal conflicts, and withdrawal symptoms. Four types of gamers were identified: gamers with below-average use, gamers with low risk of problematic use, gamers with medium risk of problematic use, and gamers with high risk of problematic use. This instrument has demonstrated a sensitivity of 96% and a specificity of 100%.

- **Problematic Online Gaming Questionnaire Short Form (POGQ-SF)** – Papay et al. (2013) developed an abbreviated form of the POGQ by selecting the two items with the highest load of each factor. Thus, the POGQ-SF comprises 12 five-point Likert items covering the six POGQ dimensions.

- **Video Game Addiction Test (VAT)** – The VAT is a direct adaptation of the items on the Compulsive Internet Use Scale (CIUS), focusing on online video game playing. It consists of fourteen 5-point Likert scale items with the following components: loss of control, conflict, preoccu-pation/ salience, coping/mood modification, and withdrawal symptoms.

- **Clinical Video Game Addiction Test (C-VAT 2.0) –** The C-VAT 2.0 is a clinician-administered test for use in the clinical setting. It consists of 11 yes-no items about IGD symptoms within the last year and three more questions on gaming habits. It is also based on the DSM-5 criteria but probes into craving and other symptoms. This instrument also includes a short table of recommendations for identifying comorbid problems.

- **Internet Gaming Disorder Scale (IGDS) –** Lemmens, Valkenburg, and Gentile (2015) developed this twenty-seven 6-item German-language instrument based on the DSM criteria, expanding each criterion into multiple questions.

Generally, the instruments with the broadest acceptance internationally are those developed in the United Kingdom. The IGDS 9-SF is the most widely used, with the most translations to other languages and validations, although a more complete study of its psychometric qualities is lacking. Moreover, most of its validations do not identify the different player types. The IGD-20 has the advantage of analyzing various gamer profiles. Still, it lacks non-Spanish cross-linguistic validations, is long, and is ambiguous with certain negative-ended statements (for example, "I never play video games to feel better").

These instruments are merely a guide for the clinician, who must learn the basic principles of dealing with addictive disorders as explained in the previous chapters and then modify them accordingly for gaming-related diseases. It is also wise to seek advice and guidance from experienced psychiatrists while dealing with gaming-related disorders.

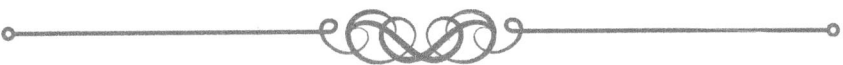

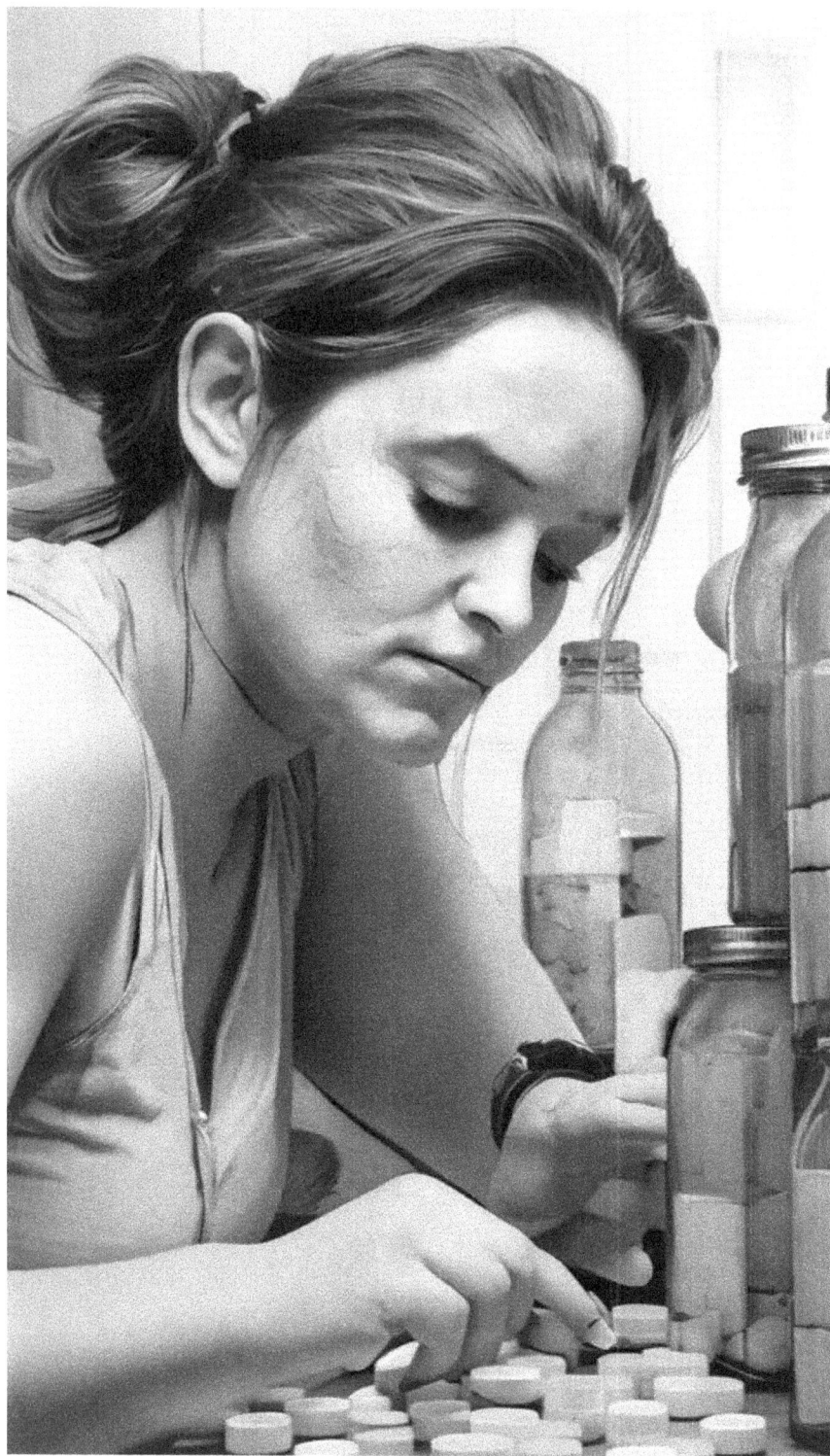

CHAPTER 16

Somatoform Disorders

Psychiatric illnesses have existed as long as humanity itself, and for the overwhelming majority of its time in the history of medicine, has been a condemned branch of medicine. Nevertheless, it was never an unpopular field. It continued to attract the attention of the public and medical professionals through its dealing with 'hysteria'. Sigmund Freud gained attention and popularity by dealing with 'conversion' and 'dissociation' related conditions. Even today, labeling any medical condition or symptom unexplained by mainstream internal medicine as "psychological" is extremely common.

I have found the management of somatoform disorders to be truly rewarding in terms of both professional satisfaction and revenue growth. Educating your community's physicians and referral doctors about this group of disorders would dramatically increase the influx of patients to your practice. If managed correctly, these patients would do very well and appreciate the psychiatrist in bettering their lives.

Background

It behooves a student of medicine to be well-read on philosophy, as most of philosophy is psychology and has affected the schools of thought of medicine in general and psychiatry more so. One such philosophical school of thought that has exerted profound influence on mainstream medical thought is dualism. Propounded by Edmund Descartes, later known as Cartesian dualism, this school of philosophy views all entities or matters of concern as originating in one of two spheres – the real world or the mental world. These spheres were considered mutually exclusive – i.e., any entity or matter of concern could be ascribed to only one of these words, and its presence in one implied exclusion from the other. There was supposed to be no overlap or crossover.

Cartesian dualism's influence on medical thinking dichotomized human illnesses into two such spheres – the body and the mind. To date, this dualistic thought pattern stiffly influences medical education and the conceptualization of illnesses. The diseases of the body are considered 'medical diagnoses' and understood through dysfunctions of the bodily structure or functioning (i.e., 'pathology'), are evident through visualization objective measurements of bodily parameters (i.e., 'investigations'), enumerated in the International Classification of Disorders (ICD), and treated by physicians. The diseases of the mind are considered to be 'psychiatric diagnoses', understood through dysfunctions of the mental process (i.e., psychopathology), are evident only through the patient's self-report or interpretational report of the psychiatrist (i.e., 'elicitation'), enumerated in an entirely separate manual called the Diagnostic and Statistical Manual (DSM), and are treated by psychiatrists. No other specialty is more wholesome yet distinct from mainstream medicine than psychiatry. While all medical specialties are housed under the same roof of a hospital, psychiatry is often housed under a separate building and sometimes in an entirely different campus with restricted access – not for the same reasons a children's hospital or a cancer hospital would exist separately, but for a reason which has existed since the history of psychiatry itself - the dualistic school of thought in medicine – mind vs body.

Dualism has had its advantages. It recognized the mind (what we better understand as 'Ulan' now) as the equal half of all matters of life and worthy of special mention while placing everything else in a single basket to share the other half. It has been recognized that matters of the mind are of a fundamentally different domain and substrate. However, the pitfall of Cartesian dualism is the belief that the mind and body are exclusive and that there is no crossover. There is plenty of crossover – physical illnesses affect the mind and may manifest purely through psychiatric symptoms, and complications of these illnesses may also be psychiatric. The treatment of such physical illnesses may be psychiatric in nature, too. Conversely, psychiatric conditions affect the physical body, manifest purely through physical symptoms without identifiable psychiatric symptoms or signs, and produce physical complications. Failure to understand the complex intertwined pathophysiology of medical and psychiatric illnesses has been the most significant deficiency (in my opinion) of the modern scientific mainstream medical school of thought. This school of thought has been so deeply embedded in academic medicine that we have now trained generations of doctors who think of symptoms in the binary (medical vs psychiatric). Medical students get the attitude that they need to understand the basics of all specialties, except psychiatry, which they tend to ignore unless they contemplate becoming a psychiatrist. Conversely, students who want to become a psychiatrist often do not attempt to deep-dive and develop expertise in other medical and surgical specialties. Thus, the medical community is in two silos – non-psychiatrists and psychiatrists.

As mentioned above, there is plenty of crossover between the clinical spectrum of medical and psychiatric disorders. Psychiatric disorders may manifest solely through bodily symptoms. This phenomenon wherein disturbances in the functioning of the Ulan are manifested as physical symptoms is called 'somatization' (as 'soma' means 'body'). A vast proportion of complaints presented by patients visiting the general medical clinic are somatization disorders.

Non-psychiatrists who encounter such somatic symptoms tend not to consider somatization disorders in their differential diagnosis and plunge the patient into investigations, some of which are expensive and redundant. Often, an incidental finding is picked up on these investigations, further expanding the investigational search. The patient may end up being recommended unneeded treatments and suffer from treatment-related adverse effects. On the other hand, if the investigations do not yield any diagnosis within their specialty boundaries, the specialist labels it as 'all in the mind' without considering the possibility of having an undiscovered, legitimately non-psychiatric diagnosis. The best examples are autoimmune disorders, inflammatory bowel disorders (Crohn's disease and ulcerative colitis), and porphyria. For several centuries, patients with these disorders were labeled as 'mad' due to a lack of explanation of the symptoms that did not fit the existing medical diagnostic categories of those times. It is also common for non-psychiatrists to prescribe medications after labeling the disorders as 'all in the mind'. Multivitamin tablets, pain killers, NSAIDs, H2 blockers, proton pump inhibitors, muscle relaxants, antacids, and dietary changes are commonly prescribed unnecessary medications for somatoform disorders *after* having dismissed these symptoms as psychological in origin. Such unnecessary investigations and medications further add to the confusion in the patient's mind. In essence, psychiatric disorders may present with purely somatic symptoms, and non-psychiatric conditions may present with purely psychological symptoms. The absence of a medical diagnosis does not mean that the cause of the problem is psychological – in other words, the ***conclusion that a disorder is psychiatric must not be a diagnosis of exclusion.*** The inclination to consider a psychiatric diagnosis only and when a medical diagnosis is not possible is a consequence of the cartesian dualism in medical education (***'it's either the body or mind and if it is not one, it is the other'*** kind of thinking).

Now that we have established that psychiatric disorders may present through purely somatic symptoms (i.e., somatization), we must recognize that psychological symptoms (such as anxiety, insomnia, depression, thought disturbances, cognitive disturbances, etc.) can coexist with these somatic symptoms. Let us take it a bit further – there are conditions where the patient willfully lies or feigns a medical illness – i.e., fakes it. Their complaints are not real. Are they considered psychiatric/medical diagnoses, too? The simple answer is yes. The reason is that the person, though feigning the illness or complaints, is doing so because they genuinely suffer from an underlying psychiatric disorder. Their faking of the complaints is a maladaptive method to seek help or attention and is a consequence of the underlying psychiatric illness. Doctors (psychiatrists and non-psychiatrists) are in the business of relieving suffering. The word 'pathology' comes from 'pathos', which means 'suffering'. All sufferings are within our realm. Patients with factitious disorders also suffer, and they are indeed pathologies. They are patients, too, and not criminals.

Disease vs Illness

As mentioned above, ambiguous physical symptoms are insufficient to merit classification as a psychiatric disorder. Patients may present with multiple somatic complaints across various organ systems, which various specialists have treated with a hodgepodge of medications. How must the psychiatrist approach such a complex situation? Here, it is essential to understand certain fundamental concepts, namely ***disease, illness, and illness behavior.***

Any dysfunction in the body or mind produces a state of altered or abnormal functioning. Such an altered state of functioning is termed 'pathology' (from the root word 'pathos' meaning 'suffering', as the altered state of functioning creates or may potentially create suffering). The pathological condition causes the patient to present with various symptoms. These symptoms may be physical or mental, or both. The umbrella term for the conglomeration of presenting symptoms is called 'illness'. In other words, ***illness is patient-defined.***

The illness then invokes a particular reaction pattern within the affected individual, resulting in additional symptoms. For example, cancer may cause pain. How the patient reacts to the diagnosis of cancer could result in anxiety, insomnia, excessive crying, hypersensitivity to pain, etc. All of which are not initially a part of the cancer itself but a consequence of the cancer. This reaction pattern and the symptoms of the condition are called 'illness behavior'. Illness behavior is patient-specific and a spectrum, ranging from very subtle to overly exaggerated.

Diseases are man-made conceptual frameworks designed to understand, categorize, and predict pathological processes to facilitate diagnosis and treatment. Simply put, ***diseases are physician-defined.*** Pathologies, symptoms, and illnesses do not have to fit disease definitions – instead, diseases must be defined and manipulated to accommodate pathologies, symptoms, and conditions.

Therefore, any symptom could be a manifestation of the disease, an illness, an illness behavior, or an atypical illness behavior. For example, a headache could be due to a disease (such as refractory errors, sinus infections, or brain tumors), an illness (such as somatization disorders), or an atypical illness behavior (such as a headache due to insomnia or crying because of another condition).

Patients with somatization disorders often present with many symptoms involving multiple organ systems and may be undergoing treatments by various specialists. Some of these symptoms may be due to actual disease, while others may be a part of the illness or illness behavior or maybe a side effect of a treatment. The psychiatrist must dissect the symptoms and under-stand the positioning of the symptoms from the disease perspective versus the illness perspective. This requires thorough medical knowledge across multiple specialties to be able to aid in this symptom dissection. This is another reason I stress that general medical knowledge and a strong founda-tion in the principles of all specialties are a prerequisite to being an excellent clinical psychiatrist. Medical students who contemplate a post-graduation or residency in psychiatry must expend more time and effort in acquiring deep knowledge in multiple specialties during their medical school.

Identifying Somatoform Symptoms

Somatic complaints, unexplained by non-psychiatric medical diagnoses, account for 40-75% of medical practitioner visits. Many of these may get referred to a psychiatrist, and most of these patients might have coexistent somatoform disorders, other psychiatric disorders, and medical (non-psychiatric) diagnoses. So, how can the psychiatrist tell if the symptom is of somatoform etiology or otherwise? I use the following criteria -

---

Clues to identifying a somatoform etiology of symptom - Mananalam Clinic Experience

MCE

- Experience of somatic distress – the patient does experience distress in some form identifiably somatic or of bodily concern. The distress is real.
- Cognitive association of the symptom – The patient ascribes a particular cognitive explanation to the occurrence of the symptom. They associate a specific 'meaning' or reason to the somatic complaint.
- Behavioral change related to the symptom – The symptom causing distress is associated with an identifiable change in the patient's behavior.

Hypervigilance, or excessive preoccupation about one or more symptoms, is another clue. A phenomenon termed somatosensory amplification, the experience of otherwise normal bodily sensations as intense, harmful, or disturbing, could be another clue. Usually, the patient selects out the weaker and relatively minor symptom of the multitude of symptoms and gives it undue importance or reacts in an exaggerated way that further worsens the impact of the symptom. The illness behavior amplifies the illness, thereby blurring disease definitions.

The psychiatrist may need to obtain additional tests to understand the etiology better. It is also pertinent to ask about the impact of the symptoms on family, social situations, career, and interpersonal relationships.

Specific commonly encountered somatoform symptoms are listed below -

- *Pain* - In the head, abdomen, back, joints, extremities, chest, and rectum, and pain during menstruation, sexual intercourse, and urination.
- *GI symptoms* - Nausea, bloating, vomiting, diarrhea, intolerance to different foods, vomiting throughout pregnancy.
- *Sexual and gynecological symptoms* - Sexual indifference, erectile dysfunction, ejaculatory dysfunction, irregular menses, excessive menstrual flow.
- *Neurological symptoms* - Amnesia, seizures, loss of consciousness, impaired coordination or balance, paralysis, localized weakness, involuntary movements, difficulties in swallowing, lump in the throat, aphonia, loss of touch or pain sensation, deafness, double vision, hallucinations, urinary retention.

Clinical Interview

Interviewing a patient with somatoform disorder could be a challenging task. I shall break the interview process into simpler parts –

How did the referral happen?

Before seeing the patient, analyze how the referral was brought to you. Did the referral mention a specific reason for which a psychiatrist referral was sought, or did it simply say, 'need a psychiatric opinion'? Read between the lines here. Getting to know the referring physician and talking to them directly or in person is essential and recommended. A 'difficult to handle' patient, a patient with recalcitrant symptoms, profound physician bias, patients dissatisfied with the current medical provider, pending litigation, unpleasant physician-patient relationships, or an intention to transfer or 'dump' the patient's care to another physician or specialty may be a reason for psychiatrist referral too.

Preparing for the interview

Read all the physician and referring documents before seeing the patient. Some psychiatrists may prefer to see and interview the patient before reading the prior notes to keep an open mind and a fresh look at the patient's problems without pre-existing bias. I find this an acceptable approach, too. However, I prefer to thoroughly review the documents and look for hidden 'clues' that may be valuable in making the first interview fruitful. The advantages of going through the documents first are -

- It gives an idea about the extent of the problem and the treatment undertaken until the current time.
- The patient develops confidence in the psychiatrist after knowing that an effort has been made to review their medical records in detail.
- Medical records give clues to psychosocial stressors and precipitating factors for the onset and exacerbation of somatic complaints.
- Aspects of the patient's personality and interpersonal dynamics that may explain the symptom pattern better.
- Aspects of the patient's personality might have caused disturbances in the prior doctor-patient relationships.

Explaining the rationale for psychiatric referral ——————

In the patient's mind, the symptoms are all related to bodily dysfunction and 'not in their head'. The patient might perceive the psychiatric referral as a way to dismiss their real complaints and 'dump it on a shrink'. These patients are looking for one diagnosis to explain all their symptoms and are expecting a cure. They believe that if the diagnosis is made correctly, the treatment for cure could be easily inferred. So, explain to the patient that the referring doctor has legitimate reasons to consider the referral and that, as a psychiatrist, you will stay relevant to the patient's ongoing care from the standpoint of the presenting somatic complaints. Explain that the mind is also a part of the physical body, and its ailments may require treatments or medications, which are part of the psychiatrist's expertise. Articulate explicitly that their complaints and suffering are real. Also, explain to them that our current knowledge of medicine, despite being vast, has limitations and that doctors cannot diagnose or treat all ailments. Recognizing the patient's suffering, good listening, and diligent thinking are necessary.

Differentiating between the major types of somatoform conditions

- **Acting** – is a conscious act. The patient is not suffering. The intention for the act is not related to psychological factors. Both the performer and the observer are aware of the act.

- **Malingering** – is also a conscious act. The performer has psychological disturbances that lead to the act. Usually, the performer knows it is an act, but the observer presumes it is not.

- **Factitious disorder** – partly conscious and partly subconscious. The patient does make up complaints or tamper with the results of tests to validate their complaints consciously. Still, their intentions to do so and the psychological distress driving them to perform in such a manner are unconsciously driven. These patients do suffer and need psychiatric help.

- **Somatoform disorder** – an entirely subconscious phenomenon where the patient's psychological distress is manifested through somatic complaints. The observer and the patient both trust that the complaints are bodily in origin. The symptoms may be related to voluntary or autonomic nervous dysfunction.

- **Conversion disorder** – an entirely subconscious phenomenon where the patient's psychological distress manifests through a burst of deviant or abnormal behavior, where the patient is unaware that their behavior is falsely driven. A clinching feature for diagnosis is that the manifestation is purely related to the voluntary motor system or sensory dysfunction.

- **Psychosomatic disorder** – an entirely subconscious phenomenon where the patient's psychological distress is manifest primarily through symptoms related to the autonomic nervous system.

General Principles in the Management of Somatic Symptom Disorders

- Approach the patient with empathy and acceptance.

- Recognize the patient's symptoms are causing suffering.
- Reassure the patient that their complaints are taken seriously.
- Avoid using medical jargon or overlapping medical terminologies while talking to the patient.
- Obtain a psychosocial history.
- Evaluate the presence and level of insight.
- Search for anxiety or depression symptoms.
- Evaluate for the presence of secondary gain.
- Focus on symptom management rather than 'cure'.
- Discourage doctor shopping.
- Schedule repeat appointments based on time needed or not based on symptoms.

General Principles in the Management of Factitious Disorders

- **Clues –** Observe if the patient uses medical jargon or gives a classic textbook description of the disease. Are there frequent visitors to the patient's home, and is there a temporal relationship between patients' symptoms and the visitors?

- **Do's –** Anticipate and accept resistance from the patient for psychiatric care. Set aside ample time for the interview. Address the patient's reluctance and objections directly. Review the patient's history and medical records thoroughly ahead of time. Start with their symptoms and listen to them in detail. 'Medicalize' your questioning. Keep your questions short and objective. Emphasize your medical credentials without coming across as condescending.

- **Don't's –** Do not assume that the patient is thrilled or pleased to see you. Do not try to act nice or smooth things over. Do not emphasize your psychiatric credentials. Avoid concluding your assessment after a single interview. Do not walk straight to the psychological aspects before addressing the somatic complaints at the patient's pace. Finally, do not doubt your skills.

- **General tips –** Focus on the patient's symptoms and the evolution of the symptoms over time. Attempting to bring in emotions, thoughts, and other psychological aspects to explain the somatic symptoms backfires in these patients. First, get a detailed history of the physical symptoms and establish a chronology. With an unbiased mind, exclude other medical causes for these undiagnosed symptoms. For this reason, the psychiatrist must be familiar with medical and psychiatric diagnoses. Ask the patient to narrate a 'typical day' or an hour-by-hour review of the symptoms. Establish the impact of these symptoms on daily life and activities of daily living such as self-care, hygiene, toilet habits, kitchen work, worship, housekeeping, work, and interpersonal relationships. Can they perform adequately as a parent, spouse, or colleague? Build a healthy rapport with the patient, and slowly forge a deeper investigatory questioning as the rapport builds.

Conversion Disorder

When abnormal behavior is understood through the presence of a specific psychological motivation, it used to be called 'hysterical' behavior, now referred to as 'conversion'. Typically, this understanding is along the lines of the Freudian understanding of the mind. There is a subconscious mind and a conscious mind, and the subconscious mind is undergoing a 'conflict' (please refer to an earlier chapter on the basics of the mind). The conscious mind is unable to resolve or cope with the conflict, resulting in a psychological condition where the person 'bursts out' in an episode of abnormal behavior or complaints, the result of which is understood to benefit the conflicted subconscious mind. In other words, these hysterical conditions are psychogenic in nature – i.e., precipitated (brought about by) a psychological stimulus that has assumed importance in the patient's mind. In other words, the motivations of the unconscious mind effect a 'conversion' of a psychological problem into a physical complaint (which may be a sensory, motor, or behavioral disruption).

An important clue to the clinical diagnosis of conversion is the role of voluntary muscle activity in the presentation of the complaints. The presence of involuntary or autonomic complaints does not solicit the same level of attention from the clinician – for example, if a psychological problem manifests as anxiety, insomnia, or dyspepsia, it is not called conversion disorder or hysteria. If a person faints at the sight of blood or on hearing devastating news, it is not called conversion or hysteria. The label is quite exclusively and specifically used when a disruption of muscles of volition is observed. Volition (or 'will') is the conscious capability of an individual to exert control (to act or not to act) in a certain way. For example, musculoskeletal movements of the body are the result of volition. Volitional complaints include positive complaints, such as twisting of the limbs or torso, or negative complaints, such as paralysis of a limb.

Another clue for conversion disorders is the dramatic (sudden or rapid) onset and disappearance of the complaints. They are often related to a specific psychological stimulus, person(s), event, circumstance, or stressor. Hysterical complaints often possess the qualities of dramatization, exaggeration, and lack of genuineness.

A third clue is the absence of the expected emotional reaction to these complaints, called *'la belle indifférence'* (meaning 'so beautifully indifferent'). Patients tend to dissociate themselves from their symptoms and regard themselves as separate from what is happening to them.

The most common complaints related to hysterical complaints are disturbances of sensations, motility, consciousness, complete loss of memory, amnesias, fugue, hysterical trances, and splitting of personality.

Although the patient's personality type is a risk factor for conversion disorder, it is the precipitating factor that is more consistently seen across the outbursts of hysterical activity.

Conversion vs Dissociation: These are two conceptually similar phenomena, except that the term 'conversion' is preferred when the symptoms are primarily related to bodily complaints or motor behavior, while 'dissociation' is the preferred term when symptoms or complaints are primarily psychological in nature. In general, dissociation could occur in 2 forms (as per the Holmes and Brown model) – compartmentalization or detachment. It has been suggested that the prefrontal cortices could play a vital role in controlling actions that are noted to be involved in conversion disorder. It may be possible in the future that functional brain imaging may be utilized to diagnose conversion disorders.

Social historians believe that the 'hysteria' as a clinical condition shall and is disappearing from clinical practice. What was previously considered hysteria is now understood to be various other disorders. Nevertheless, the burden of chronic hysteria is far more impactful and higher than we were led to believe from what is now described in standard psychiatry and clinical neurology textbooks.

Key components during the interview of a patient with conversion disorder include age at onset, mode of onset, recent life events or difficulties, prior history of unexplained symptoms, psychiatric co-morbidity, history of neurological complaints or diagnoses, secondary gain or litigation history, and corroborative history from family or informants.

Clinical features of conversion disorder may be motor or sensory in nature. Motor symptoms include paralysis, functional weakness, gait disturbances, seizure-like activity, or abnormal movement patterns. Sensory symptoms include visual, auditory, and tactile abnormalities. They involve a distribution that is not explained readily through known neuroanatomy, such as sensory loss involving a particular part of half of the entire body, a 'top-to-toe' of a specific half, or sometimes a glove-stocking type of distribution. The distribution may sometimes demarcate precisely at the midline of the body.

Keep in mind that the prognosis is poor! Disability produced by conversion disorders could be extraordinary. Often, these patients are ignored and not treated adequately, and iatrogenic injury from unnecessary investigations and treatments could be further damaging. I have known patients who have spent years in a wheelchair due to these disorders.

Hypochondriasis

I decided to discuss hypochondriasis as a separate section here due to the common myths and misunderstandings associated with using this term. The term 'hypochondria' has been used for several centuries but has been used to imply different conditions during different ages. The term has been used since the times of Hippocrates and Galen. Strictly speaking, 'hypochondria' refers to 'below the ribs', as it used to be believed that 'bile' (which is in the gallbladder and liver beneath the ribs) was the cause of illness or sickness. If the pathophysiology could not be witnessed, the cause of suffering was squarely blamed on the bile – what else could it be if not for the bile going bad?... was the prevalent logic at that time. Hence, later in the 18th and 19th centuries, the term 'hypochondriasis' became used to refer to a condition where the person reported a sickness or sadness about a bodily illness, where a cause could not be found. In other words, it was 'melancholia without cause'. A review of historical writing related to hypochondriasis demonstrates that the primary problem was psychological – a profound sadness (melancholy), depression, or anxiety about a bodily illness. Freud called it an 'actual neurosis', not amenable to psychoanalytic therapy. The term has been used in the last century to imply a condition characterized by significant mental preoccupation about a physical or mental illness (Gillespie, 1928). There are also concerns within the psychiatric community if hypochondriasis deserves to be recognized as a clinical diagnosis in and of itself or if it is merely a type of manifestation of a known psychiatric illness such as depression or anxiety. The DSM-5 has replaced the term with 'somatoform symptom disorder' and 'illness anxiety disorder'. In this section, I shall discuss hypochondriasis as a psychiatric condition characterized by pathological preoccupation arising from the perception of being afflicted by an illness.

Hypochondriasis is not uncommon, both in general medical and psychiatric clinical practice. A minor level of hypochondriasis is prevalent in a bigger portion of the general population, which in turn becomes a market for several over-the-counter treatments for 'upset stomach', constipation, dyspepsia, heartburn, body aches, joint pain, headaches, sleeplessness, urinary complaints, sexual dysfunction, 'heart health', 'memory problems', fatigue, etc. Social media-based advertisements and promotion of 'tips for health' target these audiences. A flurry of medications, 'oils', herbal remedies, unique plant or animal extracts, etc., are also sold to these audiences.

The hallmark clinical sign of hypochondriasis is the elicitation of a belief that they are suffering from a severe illness, accompanied by fear and preoccupation about the seriousness of the disease. Fear is a mood, a manifestation of anxiety. Preoccupation refers to thoughts of the illness. These fears and preoccupations typically arise from misinterpreting normal bodily processes, such as heart rate, breathing, sweating, peristalsis, flatulence, or minor skin changes such as pimples or furuncles. Cognitive interpretations of these otherwise normal bodily processes are erroneous and dysfunctional. Constipation and irregularities of bowel function are particularly common targets.

Risk factors – Age is a crucial factor. Older adults are common among those who present with somatoform complaints and illness anxiety. A more significant proportion of men present during middle age. Athletes and medical students are also a common demographic. Certain personality types predispose to hypochondriacal preoccupations.

Symptoms - The symptoms frequently pertain to the 'heart', such as palpitations, chest pressure, chest pain, or abdominal complaints such as pain, soreness, or bloating. Other symptoms include urinary, menstrual, pelvic, or genital discomfort, muscular weakness, pain, and strange sensations in the head or spine. There is a constitutional basis; by the latter, I mean that the condition is associated with specific personality traits. I have also noticed families with many hypochondriacal members.

It is essential for the clinician to keep in mind that sensations of tingling, warmth or coldness in the limbs, mild aches, and pains of a dull or sharp quality, feelings of fullness in the stomach, distension of the bladder or rectum, headaches, sensation of tightness, pressure on the head, etc. are felt by all human beings, are left to pass unheeded and do not form the subject of complaint in the usual state of being. In the hypochondriacal state, these sensations bring forth conscious appreciation and heightened awareness of such bodily processes. They are perceived to be the cause of discomfort or malaise. They are so preoccupied that they begin to interfere with routine life activities. They constantly check their body for signs of severe disease, check their pulse, look for lumps, and examine themselves in the mirror, using oximeters, thermometers, etc. Conversations and activities are dominated by medical concerns, which lead to self-absorption, and consequently, their interest in others and pursuits become withdrawn. They comb through dubious medical resources, such as those on social media, for the meaning of their symptoms and keep asking friends, family, and medical professionals for reassurance. Their search may lead to excessive utilization of health care services. They become preoccupied with eating natural foods, achieving physical fitness, and living a healthy lifestyle with activities that reflect an idealized conception of good health. Due to their low self-esteem, they develop negative expectations from others, including medical professionals. They feel unworthy and unlovable. Personality type, developmental factors, life events, cognitive and perceptual factors, interpersonal factors, and social and cultural factors must be considered to be possible contributing factors to hypochondriasis. These patients also fear severe disability, death, or dying, with specific imageries.

Hypochondriasis is associated with depressive, anxious, and hysterical symptoms as well. The majority of persistently hypochondriacal men present initially with anxiety and features of obsessive personality. Conversely, women are associated with a relatively bland and complacent affect, with elements of hysterical personality. Symptoms may overlap, too. Personality traits with obsessional and perfectionist tendencies drive these individuals to strive for bodily fitness. These traits are commonly found along with cognitive inflexibility and low agreeableness, which renders physician reassurances useless in relieving their anxiety about the illness. Such reassurances are countered by doubts of a compulsive nature.

The presentation may initially focus on one symptom (i.e., monosymp-tomatic hypochondriasis), but with time and increased exposure to medical terms and knowledge and association with similar patients, the patient may pick up specific symptoms along the course of the illness through imitation. They may even compile evidence of their illness to contradict physician reassurances. They seek to secure vicariously, through illness and invalidation, the sympathy, affection, and concern they feel deprived of in their personal relationships - deprivation results from their own emotional shallowness and unrealistic excessive demands in their relationships with loved ones.

Reassurance seeking is a prominent feature. Despite their tendency to argue with physicians and combat their reassurances, they may go to lengths to assert invalidation or disability to seek reassurance.

In summary, essential features of hypochondriasis are a fear of severe disease, disease conviction, preoccupation about bodily function and processes, and reassurance seeking.

Iatrogenic aggravation – Much of the damage in hypochondriasis is iatrogenic. Physicians contribute to or precipitate hypochondriasis in at-risk individuals. Social media and unauthorized health information also contribute to the problem. Physicians tend to take a patient's word for the validity of the complaint and go with it. For example, if a patient complains of abdominal pain, the physician reflexively resorts to investigations such as abdominal ultrasound, CT scan, or endoscopy. The practice of rigorous history-taking about the qualities of the complaint and thorough physical examination is becoming extinct. With the latter approach, patients with somatoform complaints or hypochondriasis are subject to many investigations and procedures. Multiple specialty consultations are often sought, and regular follow-up visits or tests are scheduled. Thus, substantial time spent with various physician visits and investigations prevents the patient from forgetting its existence. Physician's failure to consider hypochondriasis and somatoform disorders in the differential diagnosis disallows self-limitation of hypochondriacal tendencies, reinforces their dysfunctional perceptions, promotes chronicity of complaints, and eventually worsens the outcomes. Before the use of advanced imaging studies, these patients would have undergone multiple unnecessary laparotomies or gynecological or orthopedic surgery. This is referred to as iatrogenic aggravation (Mananalam Clinic Experience).

The key message is that physicians play an important role in aggravating hypochondriasis. Some physicians tend to make alarming statements to patients without the necessary reassurances. They order unnecessary investigations, picking up clinically unimpactful incidental findings that may now gain importance in the patient's mind. Physicians are reluctant to address these complaints as psychiatric or hypochondriacal and keep uttering statements like 'everything is normal', 'nothing is wrong', 'nothing to worry', or *'nothing serious'.* By doing so, they challenge and reject these patients and inadvertently contribute to their suffering and alienation from the healthcare system.

Cultural factors - The importance of cultural factors in the course and evolution of hypochondriacal patients cannot be overemphasized. Throughout history, humans have used symptoms of illness as vehicles of communication of mental distress. In everyday language, mental stressors are often called 'headaches', 'pains', and 'pain in the rear'. Communication of signs of physical illness, such as these utterances, is a type of signaling of the individual to others - a signal to other members of society to adjust the behavior of others towards the individual. It allows the individual to assume the *'sick role',* which incites others to adopt a caretaking role and behave in a comforting way towards the individual. The sick role grants certain privileges and reduces expectations of obligations from the individual, enabling the affected individual to return to health and optimal functioning. This social programming is 'hijacked' in somatoform and hypochondriacal diseases. I use the word 'hijack' because the unconscious mind employs this strategy, and the individual does not consciously decide to report physical complaints to secure these privileges. People who are socially isolated or perceive needing more social support are more likely to manifest such care-eliciting behavior seen in hypochondriasis. Some cultures emphasize specific physical attributes, which may be predisposing factors in at-risk individuals.

Clinical course and outcome – Hypochondriasis may begin at any age. Onset is usually associated with a stressful life event. In some patients, it may be transient; in others, it may become chronic and fluctuate in severity throughout life. After the initial clinical visit, most patients will improve. In about four years, two-thirds of the patients will get labeled with a diagnosis, while one-third will have persistent symptoms. Despite their improvement, they may continue to be more hypochondriacal, impaired, and symptomatic. In a few instances, severe medical illness may relieve hypochondriacal concerns by legitimizing the symptoms. Failure to remission during the early course of therapy predicts higher severity, more psychiatric co-morbidity, poorer perception of health, and greater neuroticism.

Take Home Points

Symptoms are real – it is the cognition about the symptoms that is dysfunctional. Don't argue. Reassure but do not get pulled into the lead taken by the patient. Do not say 'everything is normal' or 'it is all just in the mind'. Polypharmacy must be recognized, and medications must be reconciled to the minimum required. Cardiac and GI symptoms are the most common symptom categories. Physicians play an extraordinarily impactful role in the course and outcome of these disorders by being conscious of the phenomenon of iatrogenic aggravation. Words should be chosen carefully during conversations with the patients. It is an actual disease, and suffering must be recognized. Avoid misusing the diagnosis of somatoform disorders to protect the inability to make a non-psychiatric diagnosis, and refrain from using 'normal reports' of labs and imaging studies as proof to argue with patients that 'everything is normal'. Do not hesitate to reach out to a senior psychiatrist with expertise in somatoform disorders.

Despite being a challenging clinical condition, it is gratifying for the treating psychiatrist when managed appropriately.

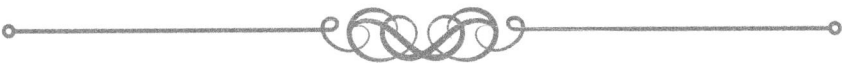

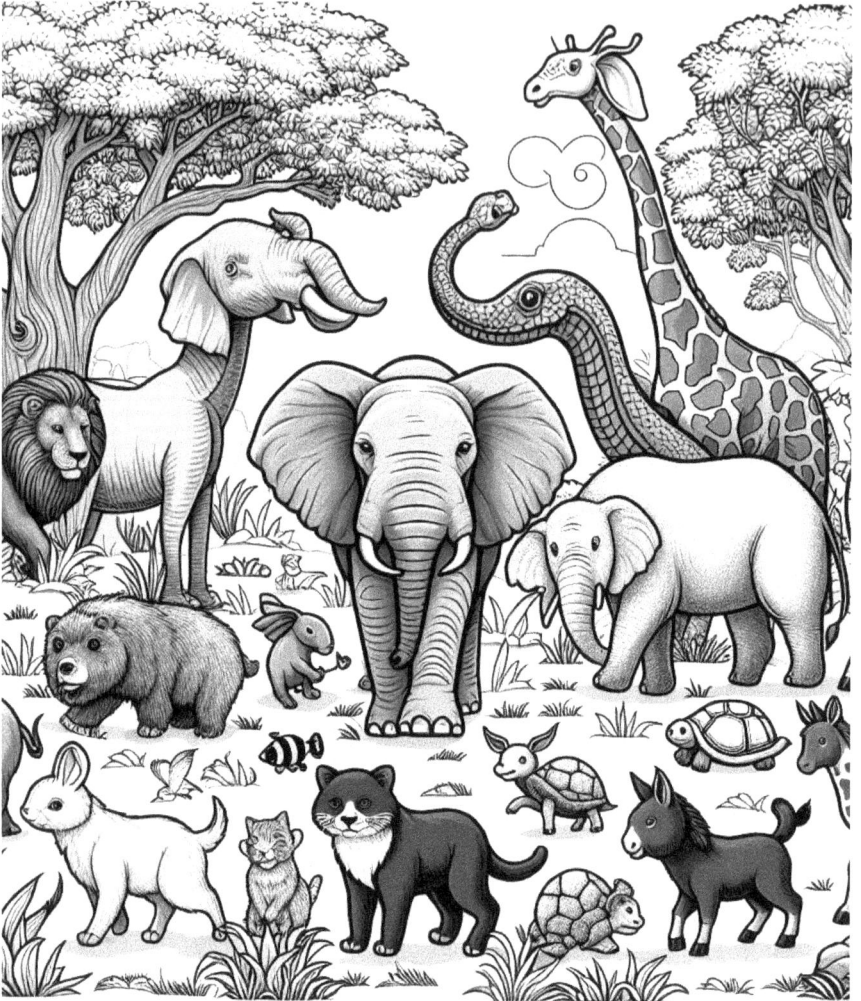

CHAPTER 17

Personality and Personality Disorders

What is Personality?

The word 'personality' in English means 'type of person'. The term 'personality' is used loosely to describe a person, especially the characteristics of the person that make them distinguishable. For example, 'nice personality', 'irritating personality', 'generous personality' etc., are some of the usages of the word 'personality' in everyday language, as is used interchangeably in the context of a person's character, demeanor, and behavior.

In academic medicine, the word 'personality' has stricter usage, and healthcare professionals must use this word carefully and accurately. In this regard, let us consider the relevant terminologies: trait, temperament, and personality.

Trait refers to a single quality of a person's nature. For example, 'generous', 'stingy', 'suspicious', 'faithful', 'loyal', 'social', 'antisocial', 'adjustable', 'impulsive', 'organized', 'superstitious', etc., are all examples of traits. Hundreds, if not thousands, of traits, are described in the literature. Around 300 BC, Greek philosopher Theophrastus described 32 such 'characters'. The founder of psychometrics, Sir Francis Galton (1822-1911 AD), reported that he counted the number of words in the dictionary that described prominent character descriptions and noted that at least 1000 words conveyed a 'separate shade of meaning'. Building on the latter, in 1926, Perkins presented his review of 400,000 words from Webster's New International Dictionary and honed it down to 3,000 trait-related words. An entire field of study called psycho-lexicology deals with analyzing words to describe personality traits. Allport and Odbert came up with a list of 17,953 words instead. Although there may be thousands of trait descriptions, most are not independent and random – by that, I mean most of the traits often occur together in the same person. In the same vein, certain traits are often not found to occur together. For example, optimistic individuals are often more outgoing, open to new experiences, risk-taking, social, etc., while pessimistic people are more reserved and cautious about new experiences. This approach to finding broad groups in which traits appear together or separate from each other is called the 'lumping-splitting' approach. In 1947, German-British psychologist Hans Eysenck (1916-1997) at the Institute of Psychiatry at King's College in London lumped and split descriptions into two broad dimensions of understanding personality traits, namely 'introversion-extroversion', and 'neuroticism-stability'. Further studies have panned out more such dimensions of understanding personality patterns.

For clinical practice, the clinician must be familiar with the following five major personality trait dimensions (often dubbed as the *'Big Five'*) –

1. **Extroversion** – A dimension where one end of the spectrum is being outgoing and social, while the other is being solitary and reserved. Extroversion is a trait pattern focusing more on external experiences, primarily through interaction with others. Unlike introverted individuals, extroverted individuals feel charged or energized by social interaction. They tend to be less self-critical, readily seek new experiences, look for excitement, and tend to 'live in the moment'. They tend to be more impulsive, quickly bored and have a lower tolerance for boredom and frustration, which may lead to difficulties in their life. Being low on extroversion is referred to as introversion. Introversion is a trait pattern that focuses more on the inner self, being more self-critical and slower to warm up to newer situations and relationships. These individuals feel quickly exhausted by social interaction but tend to be more creative and thoughtful about the future. They are bothered more by uncertainty and are prone to anxiety, avoidance behavior, and depression during periods of transition or uncertainty. They have difficulty relaxing, worry more (especially about minor matters), and are excessively self-critical.

2. **Openness** – A trait dimension of being welcoming to new situations, experiences, and, most importantly, ideas and ways of executing tasks. High openness scores are associated with being more liberal about diversity, curious about new ways, culturally inquisitive, imaginative, and creative. High openness levels could be associated with being positive, increased job performance, and overall well-being, and may lead to being non-conformists, agents of change, or independent

thinkers. Extremely high openness could be associated with impulsivity, decreased pragmatism, or even being perceived as 'unusual'. Openness may have a negative influence on intimate relationships. On the other hand, low openness scores are associated with trust in established wisdom, such as traditions, customs, and rituals, being consistent and cautious, data-driven, realistic, and pragmatic. Extremely low openness may be perceived as being 'close-minded' or 'rigid'.

3. **Agreeableness** – A trait dimension dealing with the nature of an individual to relate to others. In essence, it is a measure of the level of disagreement an individual can tolerate, i.e., high agreeableness implies low tolerance to being in a situation of disagreeability with another individual(s). In contrast, low agreeableness implies high tolerance or even being dismissive of disagreement with another individual(s). High agreeableness is associated with being cooperative, polite, friendly, trusting, and a good team player. They prefer harmony, tolerate others' opinions and ideas to prevail over theirs, and are respectful and empathetic. Overall, agreeable people forgive, are more satisfied, are less likely to complain, are unlikely to cause trouble or 'rock the boat' and are more peace-loving. Agreeability also increases the likelihood of experiencing a placebo effect with medical treatments. Life through hardship and increasing age generally make people more agreeable. However, high agreeableness may negatively impact outcomes in material/financial negotiations. Nevertheless, once they get their foot in the door in professional circles, agreeable individuals have more opportunities for growth and promotions.

4. **Conscientiousness** – A trait dimension of regulating oneself. The higher end of the spectrum in this dimension involves being methodical, well-planned, systematic, and organized in approaching problems or executing tasks and consequently is perceived as persevering and enduring. Such individuals constantly focus on self-improvement. Very high levels of conscientiousness could be associated with menial perfectionism, inflexibility, and stubbornness. Lower levels of conscientiousness are associated with more 'gut-driven' approaches and 'going with the flow'. Such people do not persist in non-yielding undertakings and are more spontaneous.

5. **Neuroticism** – A trait dimension measuring the stability of emotions

in the context of external stimuli. Neuroticism, as a trait dimension, must not be confused with 'neuroticism' or 'neuroses' described in Freudian literature. High scores on this trait dimension imply ready emotional reactivity to surrounding situations, i.e., being more sensitive to incoming signals. They are happier under favorable circumstances, sadder with adverse circumstances, and transitioning from one emotion to another quicker. They tend to experience life in all aspects and can express them more clearly in art forms relatable to others. Very high neuroticism scores could be perceived as being more 'dramatic', emotionally labile, or having 'mood swings'. Lower levels of neuroticism tend to react more evenly and similarly to a diverse range of stimuli and are preferred in more professional situations where emotional reactivity could be counter-productive and less preferred in interpersonal relationships where they may be considered 'boring'.

Apart from the above five trait dimensions, there are multiple others. The resultant sum of the intensity and combination of all traits in an individual is called 'personality'. There are innumerable combinations of traits, each being expressed at varying amounts, resulting in the uniqueness of everyone in humankind. The key concept here is that there is no such thing as a good vs lousy trait, good vs bad personality, or good vs bad score on any trait dimension. Each trait has its importance in human life and human evolution. No judgment (moral or ethical) must be levied on any trait or personality.

What is a Personality Disorder?

When one or a cluster of traits predominate a personality in a pervasive manner, the personality becomes a source of problems for the individual, causing distress to oneself and others. At that point, the individual is said to have a 'personality disorder'. However, such an objective, verifiable definition is needed for clinical purposes. Several definitions and criteria exist, but I use the following set of 5 criteria to clinch the diagnosis of personality disorder –

Diagnosis of Personality Disorder
- Mananalam Clinic Experience

MCE

- **Pervasiveness** – An identifiable single or cluster of traits must pervade all aspects of the individual's life. For example, suspiciousness is a trait, and some individuals are more suspicious overall than others. However, there are certain spheres of life where the suspicious trait needs to be curtailed, such as friendships, family, and intimate relationships. If the suspiciousness also pervades uncontrollably into the latter areas, it results in conflicts and issues. Pervasiveness can be identified as the impact of the trait on both cognitive and affective processes, i.e., affecting how the trait impacts the understanding and perception of self, society, and the universe (i.e., cognitive processes), and the impact on emotional type, lability, impulse control, and interpersonal functioning
(affective processes).

- **Extremeness** – There must be an 'extreme' level of one or more traits, resulting in scores of the trait outside the 'normal' variation seen in the general population. Extremes of the trait, even if non-pervasive, could cause distress to the individual.

- **Rigidity** – The trait(s) must be uncontrollably expressed, unable to be modified by the individual even while brought to their attention. (Refer to Ulan concept – the mood, thought, and intellect always act in union and congruently. So, the inflexible and rigid trait is associated with congruent alterations in thought and intellect. Consequently, individuals with a rigid trait tend to harbor thoughts and ideologies that support their extremeness and rigidity in that trait. Some could be argumentative about it, causing more distress in interpersonal relationships). Rigidity can lead to loss of employment, disability, marital discord, irreversible damage to relationships, and economic loss.

- **Lack of insight –** The individual does not have insight into the depth and magnitude of the personality-related issues. They may be aware that they think or behave differently or possess a different nature, but not aware of the extent to which it is different or the impact on one's or others' lives.

  - **Clinically identifiable distress –** The personality may be causative of distress to the patient or others (refer to the Ulan concept's third mental health criterion).

The DSM approach to the diagnosis of PD is a bit different – it understands PD to be a 'characteristic pattern of difficulties' (which the DSM later then elaborates on), affecting multiple areas of functioning, including cognition, affectivity, interpersonal functioning, and impulse control. The latter describes the 'pervasiveness' mentioned in the Mananalam clinic criteria as above. The DSM also adds that such difficulties are inflexible, associated with significant distress, and evident as an enduring pattern throughout life, with onset in early childhood. It also cautions the clinician to ensure that such difficulties are not a manifestation of other primary psychiatric illnesses and substance abuse.

Why is it Important to Know About Personality Disorders?

Knowledge of personality types and disorders transforms one's outlook on people and life. It makes the physician more compassionate, empathetic, and diligent about psychiatry and healthcare-related issues. Approximately 12% of the population is reported to be affected by personality disorders, and approximately 50% of those seeking mental health services could be affected by personality disorders. Furthermore, PD is an adverse prognostic indicator for psychiatric outcomes in general. PD is also associated with poor compliance and unhealthy doctor-patient relationships in general medical and surgical practice. Overall, PD could affect the quality of life – the rigidity of the traits could cause failures in professional progress, prolonged dysphoria and unhappiness, low frustration tolerance, coping issues, and interpersonal conflicts. In essence, it leads to activities with self-destructive tendencies, resulting in overall decreased enjoyment of the lifetime.

Classification of Personality Disorders

Since traits are numerous, and personalities could be innumerable due to varying compositions of traits in varying proportions, the interrater reliability in scoring or diagnosing PD tends to be relatively low. Hence, the clinical classification of PDs is approached by identifying three broad 'baskets' where each PD could be put. The rationale for this approach is that, as mentioned earlier in the chapter, traits tend to 'cluster'; hence, disorders related to personalities also tend to be in clusters. The clusters can be understood through the Ulan concept of mind and mental health as below –

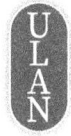

U L A N

Understanding the Clusters of PD through the Ulan concept of mind and mental health

Cluster A - Characterized by atypia in the 'thought' component of the Ulan. Essentially, patients in this cluster have 'odd' thoughts and ideas. They are perceived as 'eccentric'. This thought pattern pervasively affects their cognition (how they perceive themselves and the world) and affective processes (mood, emotion, reaction pattern, etc.). How they perceive themselves affects the first criteria of the Ulan concept of mental health (i.e., knowledge of oneself) and thus disturbs the mental health equilibrium.

The subtypes include paranoid, schizoid, and schizotypal personality disorders.

Cluster B - Characterized by deficits in the second criterion of the Ulan concept of mental health (ability to relate well with others). Essentially, patients in this cluster are more focused on the self and lack sensitivity to others' emotions, which then causes a characteristic pattern of difficulties relating to others.

The subtypes include antisocial, borderline, histrionic, and narcissistic personality disorders.

Cluster C – Characterized by instability in the 'mood' component of the Ulan. Essentially, patients in this cluster tend to have unstable or labile mood patterns, which pervasively affect their cognitive process, leading to disturbances in the third criterion of the Ulan concept of mental health (actions not being beneficial to self).

The subtypes include anxious, dependent, and obsessive-compulsive personality disorders.

Understanding the Types of Personality Disorders

I will not discuss each type or subtype of PD in detail, as it is outside the scope of this book. However, I would like to drill down into certain clinically relevant aspects of the most common PDs, the most clinically relevant PDs, and the aspects that cause clinical ambiguity. Many PDs are misunderstood, often misdiagnosed, and underdiagnosed. Often, other psychiatric conditions are misdiagnosed as PD.

In general, Cluster A PDs are the more disabling and damaging PDs and are associated with profound compromise in the individual's functioning across many domains and could cause the individual to lead an isolated life. Cluster A PDs are the most difficult to summon the patient to treatment. They maintain limited contact with other people in general. They usually manage to keep a job, albeit with difficulty. Under stress, they may exhibit psychotic features transiently, which in turn may require treatment. Typically, it isn't easy to establish a solid doctor-patient relationship with these individuals.

Schizoid PD

The patients are perceived as cold, reserved, distant, unsociable, aloof, and indifferent. They are inhibited in social situations and feel little need for relationships. They have difficulty initiating relationships and come across as being 'closed off' in relationships. They struggle to express emotions, rarely tolerate eye contact, and respond to questions in short sentences. They also get uneasy when asked to discuss their emotions. They may engage in fantasy relationships. They are preoccupied and overly conscious about their self and self-image or with abstract philosophical ideas or odd scientific topics of mathematics, physics, or chemistry. They might seem absorbed in their own world and otherwise insignificant matters. They do not appear concerned about others and are usually indifferent to praise or criticism. Their facial expressions are childlike when trying to be humorous or engage in comical discussion. They face threats (real or imagined) with a sense of fantasized omnipotence or resignation. They are attracted to and perform well in solitary jobs where social interaction is minimally required and would remain original and creative in ideas. Sexuality is predominantly fantasy-related, and they rarely engage in mature sexual relationships. Typically, they lack insight into their condition, have a poor sense of identity, and have a poor capacity to evaluate interpersonal events. Clinicians find it difficult to engage the patient in a therapeutic relationship, but these individuals depend highly on the relationship with the clinician once engaged.

Schizotypal PD

These patients do not have a definitive thought disorder, but they are almost there! The ICD 10 labels this PD as 'latent schizophrenia' and is more common in first-degree relatives of patients with schizophrenia. Their primarily dysfunctional trait pattern is unusual cognition – with odd beliefs (outside the social norm), ideas of reference, magical thinking, peculiar thought patterns, linguistic peculiarities, and bizarre ideologies. The onset of this thought pattern is apparent in childhood or early adolescence, which invites peer teasing and bullying. In school, there may be academic underachievement. Affective processes are also congruently impacted – they are emotionally constricted, often aloof and solitary, avoid social interaction, avoid eye contact, are hypersensitive to criticism, have poor peer friendships, and may indulge in self-talk. Speech may be circumstantial, overinclusive, and challenging to follow. They dress poorly, appear disheveled, and have an unusual choice of colors or costumes. Due to perceptional unusualness (such as experiencing a 'sixth sense' or an odd belief pattern) or distorted perceptions (such as the experience of sounds or visions), interpersonal relationships get affected adversely, and they rarely have friends or intimate partners. People who know them or have had unpleasant experiences with them may want to damage their reputation, and hence, these patients increasingly avoid relationships and social interactions. Dysphoria, anxiety, and depression may ensue due to these life stressors arising from their PD. Stressful situations may result in psychosis lasting for minutes or hours and occasionally long enough to warrant treatment. Major depressive disorder is a common comorbid condition, making diagnosis difficult.

Paranoid PD

The hallmark traits of this PD are suspiciousness and irritability. There is a pervasive, persistent, and inappropriate 'angry mistrust'. Typically, these patients interpret others' motives as malevolent, exploitative, or deceptive. They question the loyalty and trustworthiness of friends, spouses, family, colleagues, and intimate partners. They are exquisitely sensitive to comments and criticisms and may turn otherwise innocent remarks or jokes into arguments and brawls. They tend to overread or misinterpret otherwise routine or benign remarks. They may misinterpret unintended errors as planned threats or sabotage. Providing evidence to disprove their assumptions is useless, as they also mistrust objective evidence; they may collect trivial information and data to prove their point. Due to their internal solid conviction and being at odds with others, they tend to withhold valuable information from dear ones or may fail to reach out for help even while in trouble, causing interpersonal relationship problems. Pathological jealousy also destroys relationships. Acutely stressful conditions may exacerbate the suspiciousness, which may become overly pervasive. Paranoid PD is prevalent in about 2.5 to 5% of the population and is more common in men. Paranoid PD is distinguished from schizophrenia by the absence of hallucinations or delusions. Paranoid PD differs from schizotypal PD by the absence of bizarre or magical thought patterns seen in the latter. Caution should be exercised in differentiating paranoid PD from hostile social attitudes towards minority groups, immigrants, and ethnic and political groups.

Antisocial PD

The hallmark feature of this PD is a pervasive lack of concern for other individuals. Over the centuries, this PD has been recognized and described in varying forms. In 1935, British physician James Prichard coined the term 'moral insanity' to describe the traits of the loss of 'feelings' and all ethical sense. Intellectual abilities are unimpaired in this condition, but moral principles are defective or non-existent. It was like they did not even have a conscience. In 1891, German physician Julius Koch described conditions of 'psychopathic', 'psychopathic inferior', or 'constitutionally inferior' deviants in personality. In 1900, it was described as the 'morbid variety of normal' personality. Eventually, the DSM I recognized 'sociopathic disorder' when an individual's behavior was non-conforming to the prevailing cultural milieu, including subtypes such as antisocial reaction, dissocial reaction, sexual deviation, and addiction. The DSM II combined antisocial and dissocial reactions as an antisocial personality disorder. With no significant changes in the DSM-III and the DSM-IV, changes ushered in the DSM-5 where the diagnosis of antisocial PD required at least 3 of 7 pathological traits – deceitfulness, impulsivity, irritability, aggressiveness, irresponsibility, lack of remorse, and hostility. In essence, these individuals are not necessarily criminals but are indifferent to others' emotions and well-being to an extreme and inflexible extent. They do not seek pleasure or gain happiness from being antisocial; they are simply indifferent and have no remorse for the adverse consequences that their actions may bring upon others. Often, these individuals are encountered by the judicial system, from where they may be referred for psychiatric evaluation or treatment. Their criminal behavior is linked to their mental infrastructure; this condition has fueled the age-old debate of 'mad vs bad' being the cause of criminal behavior.

In my opinion, antisocial PD is a mental health condition based on the 2nd and 3rd criteria of the Utilitarian model of mental health, which identifies the ability to relate well with others and the actions of the individual not being detrimental to others as criteria for mental health. Usually, red flags for this disorder are seen in early adolescence or high school and may fit the diagnosis of a conduct disorder. Essentially, these individuals engage in facile, superficial displays of affection when it benefits them and may indulge in repeated acts of lying, stealing, arrests, recklessness, conning, cheating, or vandalism. A clinching diagnostic clue is the presence of impulsiveness and erratic unplanned acts. They come across on first interaction as charming, seductive, and clever, but long-term acquaintances may perceive them as unreliable, selfish, or manipulative. Presenting complaints include a history of disturbed functioning in the domains of self, love, sexuality, interpersonal relations, and the general cognitive outlook of the world. Internalized moral values are absent and are manifested as lying, truancy, delinquency, running away from home, thefts, vandalism, brawls, substance abuse, and illegal activities, all of which may be seen as early as childhood or adolescence. They are exploitative, demanding, egocentric, incapable of feeling guilt, intense and persistent anger, and have no capacity for reflective mourning or sadness. Frequent suicide threats or attempts may be present in their history. Sexual perversions, pedophilia, and abuse are frequent, too. Deficient parenting abilities are also present. Impulsiveness and aggression decline with age, although the trait pattern remains lifelong. Nevertheless, despite all these features, they are generally successful in life.

Borderline PD

   The hallmark feature of this PD is what its name indicates – 'borderline'. These individuals are borderline between normal and psychotic, borderline between normal and neurotic, borderline between psychotic and neurotic, and borderline between functional and impaired. Essentially, their affect is unstable and labile, and the thought pattern also fluctuates between being in touch with reality but with a disturbed variant of perception. Their pattern of unstable behavior is pervasive, affecting interpersonal relationships, workplace functioning, self-image, and overall functioning. They frantically fear real or imagined abandonment, frequently complain of having no sense of direction in life, and are depressed but overwhelmed with feelings of anger, emptiness, and boredom (rather than sadness). Acutely stressful situations may provoke psychotic features and impulsive actions such as spending frenzy, substance abuse, long-distance driving, binge eating, and self-harm. Occasionally, they may be severe enough to manifest as regression, paranoia, dissociation, and hallucination. Primitive defense mechanisms such as rejection, denial, splitting, projective identi-fication, derealization, depersonalization, etc., are manifested at times of stress. Although the latter results in genuine suffering of the individual, they are perceived by others as being self-serving.

   As mentioned above, there is a profound fear of being left alone, and they go to great lengths to seek out company – such as indiscriminate sexual affairs, making phone calls at odd times, unwarranted frequent visits to acquaintances, etc. They oscillate between overvaluing and undervalu-ing/devaluing their partner but remain dependent on them. Despite the stability, they remain susceptible to the threat of rejection or abandonment. Recognizing and assuaging their internal state is extremely difficult. They project their unwanted affective states onto their partners and act in such a way as to coerce the partner to respond to the projected emotions, which then strains intimacy in the relationship.

A ' diffuse sense of identity ' is another distinguishing clinical marker for borderline PD. Difficulties with self-identity may manifest as difficulties with gender identity or marital/family roles. They lack cognitive flexibility and view world matters in distinct buckets of white or black. Patients with borderline PD have extreme difficulty engaging in therapy. They also oscillate in their relationship with the clinician, ranging from complete dependence and admiration to suspicion and hostility. The primary differential diagnosis of BPD is Type II Bipolar disorder. Comorbid conditions associated with borderline PD are affective disorders, anxiety disorders, PTSD, somatization disorders, and alcohol abuse. BPD patients report profound dysfunction in many vital aspects of life, including education, work, marriage, and intimate relationships. Psychosexual and alcohol problems are frequent. Repeated deliberate self-harm and premature death from suicide are consequences of BPD. Reportedly, there is an overall 8-10% risk of suicide associated with borderline PD, and hence suicidal gestures must be taken seriously.

Narcissistic PD

The hallmark trait pattern in this PD is the desire to be loved, praised, and admired. The desire to be the object of admiration becomes the motivation for the individual's behavior, pervasively in all aspects of life. They are energetic, work arduously, and are socially successful, too, but the primary motivation behind their work is the need to be admired. They believe that they alone should be admired, no one else. They come across as boastful and pretentious, exaggerating their accomplishments and feeling offended when others do not praise them. Their cognition is also congruently affected, as they believe that only 'special' people can recognize their talents and that usual rules do not apply to them. They have low empathy towards others, harbor a fragile self-image, and yet view themselves in high regard and others in low regard. Minor criticisms may overwhelm them, pushing them to depression and self-loathing as complete failures or manifest as anger with resentment and vengeance.

Chronic envy may exist, and defenses against such envy, such as devaluation, a sense of omnipotence, control, and narcissistic withdrawal, may be present. Despite success in their work lives, they may feel it is 'not enough' and feel emptiness and frustration. They may have frequent mood swings, hypomanic exaltation, and bipolar-like affect changes. Regarding others, they are incapable of genuine feelings for others, sadness or longing, lack emotional depth, are unable to 'fall in love', and may harbor fantasies of 'ideal love'. Sexuality is trivialized, and sexual intercourse is viewed as for physical pleasure alone. Boredom is common, and resultantly, perverse fantasies, devaluation of objects, and promiscuous behavior may be seen. Interpersonal tendencies are dominated by idealizing people. They expect to feed them with admiration and contempt by disparaging those who do not praise them, thereby appearing exploitative and manipulative. They cherry-pick only the positive comments towards them and consider praise a sign of success.

The primary differential diagnosis for narcissistic PD includes borderline PD, antisocial PD, passive-aggressive PD, and schizotypal PD. Comorbid conditions associated with narcissistic PD include major depression, dysthymia, substance abuse, and anorexia nervosa. Typical distinguishing clues for clinical differentiation from other PDs are that narcissistic PD is associated with relatively better impulse control, more significant social adjustment, better anxiety tolerance, less self-harm/suicidal attempts, and lesser psychosis or fragmentation. A severe form of this PD, called malignant narcissism, is also associated with antisocial tendencies. Typically, individuals with narcissistic PD display depression or defensively become hypomanic sometime in their middle age due to a vicious cycle of disappointments and frustrations and an expected lack of praise.

Histrionic PD

The word 'histrionic' is derived from the word 'hysteric'; the hallmark trait pattern in this PD is the strong desire to love and be loved. The ramification of the latter desire leads to behavior patterns and defense mechanisms that characterize this PD, including emotionality, dramatization, exhibitionism, and impulsivity. They are inappropriately seductive, demanding, emotionally enthusiastic, novelty craving, and tend to throw temper tantrums, all in some way motivated by the need for attention, love, and emotional reassurance.

In more severe forms, they may display accusative, guilt-inducing, and infantile indifference. They may indiscriminately scandalize non-sexual relations in various spheres of life. Pseudo-sexuality is present and is perceived as frigidity. A romantic outlook or a superficially adoring attitude disguises the need for dependency and emotional attachment. Individuals with a more severe form of this PD may be promiscuous and engage in multiple deviant and perversive activities. The cognitive outlook on life and the world is non-specific, impressionistic, diffuse, and lacks sharpness of details. Speech is inhibited and has malapropisms. Education is superficial, and they are better at communicating nonverbally. They are excited when they are the center of attention and highly disappointed and uncomfortable when ignored. They draw attention by acting and speaking in a charming, flirtatious manner. They are quick to respond to others intimately, treating superficial acquittances as if they were long-term friends. The trajectory of their trait pattern is that others need to be impressed or shown attention to receive attention, and the strategy to achieve it is through dramatization.

Obsessive Compulsive PD

The hallmark trait pattern in this PD is 'controlling', which pervades all aspects of life, and is called 'anankastic personality' (anankastic meaning 'force' in Greek). They are typically fearful, insecure, and compulsive. They try to control those around them, especially those who are close to them, and are controlling thoughts, emotions, and events. They hate uncertainty, increasing their insecurity, fear, and anxiety. They wish to make the world a predictable place. Their affect, cognition, and thoughts become accordingly impacted – they avoid internal aggressive drives or motivations, avoid free emotional expression, and organize even trivial things to the last detail. Eventually, this mental nature leads to extreme and inflexible stubbornness for order and organization and intolerance to change. They emphasize rules, regulations, protocols, schedules, and punctuality. They pay attention to trivial details, which get perceived as 'perfectionist'. However, they become a problem to themselves and others in their drive for perfectionism, eventually derailing the outcome of the task they are perfectionists about.

They do not relax or enjoy leisurely activities and consider such activities a waste of time. They insist on the perfect performance of casual activities and sports, which interferes with parenting and intimate relationships.

Typically, they expect things to be done their way, are intolerant and indifferent to reasonable changes, resistant to reasonable explanations, and want others to surrender to their ways. They render elaborate explanations to justify their actions and get irritated with alternative suggestions. Due to this inflexibility, they cannot delegate tasks to others and end up drowning themselves in work, which causes stress. Their stubbornness is founded on suspicion, doubt, and indecisiveness (all of which pertain to thought-related abnormalities of this PD). There is a fear of making mistakes, which underlies their stubbornness.

In the arena of morality and ethics, they are even more inflexible and tend to be judgmental. They respect authority and react with anger to criticism. They are usually stingy or miserly, live below their means, and believe in saving money for the future. They do not discard things that may end up in hoarding. They are humorless, lack spontaneity, and may be passive-aggressive. Their affect is controlled, stilted, and constricted – medical students tend to describe these patients as having a 'flat affect'. They may not readily laugh or cry. In a nutshell, they love order, neatness, sameness, spontaneity, and avoid novelty or change.

Usually, this PD presents in early adulthood and may be associated with multiple psychiatric comorbidities. However, there is no certainty that this PD would lead to OCD. If they end up with a submissive spouse, I have seen these individuals enjoy marital harmony and have a fulfilling domestic life.

Dependent PD

The hallmark trait pattern of this PD is dependency and the fear of rejection or abandonment. German psychiatrist Emil Kraepelin used an accurate term, 'abulic' to describe this trait pattern. Abulia means lack of willpower or indecisiveness, which underlies this trait pattern. Schneider called it 'immature'. There is a pervasive and persistent behavior pattern to avoid the loss of relationships, especially the close and intimate ones. Essentially, these individuals view themselves as weak or helpless (unrealistically) and perceive others as powerful and protective (unwarrantedly). Hence, they allow others to control a significant portion of their lives, expecting them to be safeguarded by them. They are passive, rarely express needs, less sexual, not aggressive, and avoid significant responsibilities. They shun making decisions concerning the significant areas in their life. They want others to decide for them and want continuous guidance. They may depend on others even for simple, day-to-day activities. They display self-doubt, lack confidence, low self-esteem, and are pessimistic. They yearn for affection, seek constant company, and do not tolerate being alone. They like jobs that do not require independent decision-making and function very well in jobs that involve what is clearly instructed to them. They may also accept unpleasant tasks that require sacrifices and tolerate verbal, physical, or sexual abuse to maintain their subordinate position. They will tolerate an abusive relationship if attachment and contact are preserved. Once an existing relationship ends due to separation or death, they would rapidly, and sometimes even indiscriminately, attach themselves to someone else, even if it means belittling their position by depicting themselves as inept.

This PD is apparent in adolescence and evolves further during adulthood. It may appear after separation anxiety in childhood or chronic physical illnesses that require long-term dependency from caretakers. There is an increased risk of depression, anxiety, and adjustment disorders with this PD. They may function adequately in a closed and protected environment but will struggle or even find it difficult to survive when left alone. They do well in jobs that require regular protocols and would enjoy marital harmony with a dominant spouse.

Avoidant PD

The hallmark trait pattern in this PD is avoiding social interaction pervasively in all spheres of life. The ICD 10 uses the label 'anxious PD' based on the assumption that the avoidant nature is due to anxiety that arises from social interaction. However, in the clinical setting, I have seen that the primary problem is fear of rejection, criticism, and mockery, to which they react strongly. Feelings of inferiority, low self-esteem, shyness, self-doubt, insecurity, and emotional lability drive their concept of self and worldview. They proactively isolate themselves from socially busy situations, avoid public speaking entirely, and prefer jobs that require no social interaction. They long for intimate partnerships and friendships but avoid making such relationships due to the fear of rejection. They misinterpret the slightest and most innocent remarks as criticism and approach others as harmful and antagonistic. They tend to use self-defeating expressions while talking, which may invite further ridicule from others, thereby reaffirming their hesitations for social interaction. They assume themselves to be unattractive, disproportionately weigh the negatives of a situation, and exaggerate the risk of action. Typically, they lack intimate relationships and are low on sexual desires. They may have fantasy ideas as an escape from reality. On clinical examination, they come across as being ashamed of their life.

Other PDs

Certain other PDs may be helpful for the reader to seek more information on but are outside the scope of this book. They are passive-aggressive (negativistic) PD, self-defeating (masochistic) PD, sadistic PD, and depressive PD.

Clinical Examination

In general, interviewing a PD patient is quite challenging. The most helpful tool is the history elicited from patients or caregivers and those who have closely observed the patient. Eliciting a trait is simple, but establishing the presence of a maladaptive trait across several domains of living over a long period is difficult. Establishing that the maladaptive trait is not an expression of other psychiatric disorders is an arduous task that requires time. The patient does not 'complain' of anything, but there are presenting problems brought to attention by family (or sometimes by the patient). The problems that result in clinical presentation are usually a result of the behaviors influenced by the maladaptive trait(s).

I suggest a three-step process for detecting the presence of and establishing the diagnosis of PDs. First, establish the source of the information. There are three major sources of information for PD – the patient interview, self-reported questionnaires, and information from a third party (caregiver, employer, school faculty, etc.). During patient interviews, the most helpful information is asking them to describe their nature or 'type' in their words. Observing the cardinal features of PD (listed below) during this self-description gives the most yielding information. The questionnaires useful in PDs include the Personality Diagnostic Questionnaire, Million Clinical Multiaxial Inventory, etc. These questionnaires have the possibility of false and misleading responses but may help narrow the vast diagnostic possibilities to a few more probable ones. An interview with a third party is beneficial, as PD patients often lack insight into the severity of the impact of their maladaptive or disruptive behavior. Second, look for clues for personality trait(s) being the primary factor behind the presenting problem. Third, determine if there is pervasiveness of the trait(s) that makes it eligible for diagnosis of a personality disorder. Finally, with the above information, construct a 'narrative'. You must reconstruct a mental image of how the patient might lead their life. Then, use closed-ended, specific, and directed lines of questioning to further refine the accuracy of the narrative. Essentially, you are constructing a 'model' of the patient's behavioral infrastructure, which you can use for further treatment strategizing.

Cardinal features observable during the interview of PD patient- Mananalam Clinic Experience — MCE

Note – 'Cardinal feature' here implies that the absence of it during the clinical interview makes the diagnosis of the PD improbable, compelling the clinician to re-consider the diagnosis of the respective PD. The cardinal feature is the first single-word attribute (italicized) mentioned for each of the PDs below.

- Paranoid PD – *Guarded.* Essentially, the patient refuses to provide information readily. Responses to questions are unrevealing, and the patient may be hostile.
- Schizotypal PD – *Circumstantial.* The patient and the history are challenging to follow. Responses are circumstantial and digressive.
- Schizoid PD – *Incoherent.* The history would lack coherence, and the clinician would find it challenging to construct a narrative.
- Antisocial PD - *Manipulative.* The clinician can sense that responses are engineered with a specific agenda or to make the clinician conclude in a certain way. Bullying and glib are commonly encountered during the interview.

- Narcissistic PD – ***Demanding.*** The patient constantly attempts to devalue the interview process, making it difficult to get a realistic impression of the patient's past and current life experiences.
- Borderline PD – ***Labile (affect).*** The patient usually appears visibly angered and is unable to provide a clear history.
- Avoidant PD – ***Self-denigrating.*** The patient speaks themselves down yet is reluctant to reveal their vulnerabilities.
- Dependent PD – ***Clingy.*** The patient comes across as needy and overly ingratiating.
- Obsessional PD – ***Emotionless.*** The patient comes across as controlling, stripped of emotions, and could be subtly critical of the examiner or the clinical interview.

The next step would be to assess if a personality disorder exists in the patient, independent of other diagnoses. This is a particularly challenging task since, as described in a previous chapter ('What is normal?'), the demarcating line to differentiate an individual's personality from a personality disorder becomes blurred in clinical practice. I use the following clues to detect if the personality is the underlying primary factor behind the patient's presenting complaints.

Clinical Clues to the presence of a personality disorder - Mananalam Clinic Experience   MCE

Note – The following leads are simply clues and pointers for the clinician to consider the diagnosis of a personality disorder as the primary factor behind the presenting complaints. If the answer to any of the following questions is a 'no', then the clinician must seriously reconsider the diagnosis of a personality disorder and seek more senior help or guidance from a psychiatrist with expertise in personality disorders.

- Has the patient been chronically unhappy or adversely affected by their behavior? (a reverse way of inquiry is – is the patient someone who has enjoyed life for significant periods, and if the answer is a 'yes', then the diagnosis of a personality must be reconsidered. Also, inquire about any behavior or conduct disturbances in childhood and adolescence).
- Is there a history of impulsivity? Or poorly planned acts that have resulted in destructive, non-profitable, or detrimental effects on oneself?
- Is the patient's assessment or judgment of others unusual, extreme, or improbable? (Usually overly critical, suspicious, untrusting of others or the examiner).
- Does the patient's concept of oneself markedly at odds with reality? (Usually overly self-critical, putting down oneself more than necessary, or a general attitude of inferiority or superiority).
- Is there a consistent pattern or theme of a particular trait(s) that keeps repeating when the patient is asked to give their narrative of the self or events?

Key point – Anytime the diagnosis of whether a mental health disorder exists, go back to the basics! The basics of mental health have been discussed in the earlier chapters of this book. Ask yourself - Does the patient know about himself well? (i.e., is there a realistic perspective of the self?) Is the patient able to relate well with others? (i.e., maintain relationships with family members, friends, colleagues, etc.) Is the patient's actions and behavior beneficial to themselves and not palpably detrimental to others?

Challenges

There are some specific challenges while dealing with a PD patient, such as

- **Disturbing impact on the clinician -** The doctor is also human, with a personality (or personality disorder). Interaction with another strong personality (as in the patient's case) can provoke strong emotional reactions and defense mechanisms within the clinician. Try hard not to be judgmental and acknowledge the problems and distress of the patient with an empathetic and professional approach. Take enough time to decide. Seek the help of experienced clinicians.

- **Dysfunctional family or caregiver relationships** – Patients with PD rarely seek help independently. They are usually referred by a therapist or brought to the doctor by a caregiver, typically a family member such as a parent or spouse. The caregiver is concerned if the patient has a psychiatric illness and may have preconceived notions, for which they may seek affirmation from the doctor. The doctor's opinion may make the situation hostile. In such situations, it is better to interview the patient alone or with another caregiver or friend, depending on who is seeking such affirmation. The doctor must not lose focus and be determined to get through the interview.

- **Cultural challenges** – This is more common in affluent families in the West and among middle-class and affluent families in India and Southeast Asian countries, where deviant, unusual, or extreme traits and behaviors are swept under the carpet by the family for a long time to save the 'honor of the family'. The latter culture makes even the most obvious personality disorder challenging to diagnose. In Asian countries, school counselors, documentation, and legal records that could support school dysfunction, delinquency, and conduct disorders are maintained poorly, easily manipulated, unreliable, or unavailable. Parents and spouses also tend to downplay these problems to protect their family's 'honor', reputation, and social prestige. Breaking across this barrier could be burdensome for the clinicians in these nations.

Take home points

There is no such thing as a good or bad trait or a good or bad personality. All traits and variations of these traits, and the innumerable flavors of personalities, make human society vibrant, diversely competent, wholesome, and functional. Personality disorder is a mental health condition caused by a pervasive expression of a rigid and inflexible trait cluster. Personality disorders, like personalities, come in innumerable flavors, and each PD may not fit snuggly into one of the known diagnostic labels (although most will). The critical aspect of management is educating the patient and making them introspective about their condition and how it adversely affects themselves and others. The clinician needs remarkable patience, clinical acumen, and determination to manage personality disorders successfully.

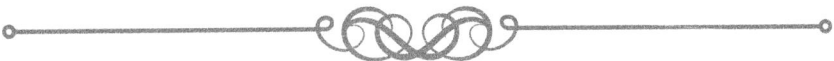

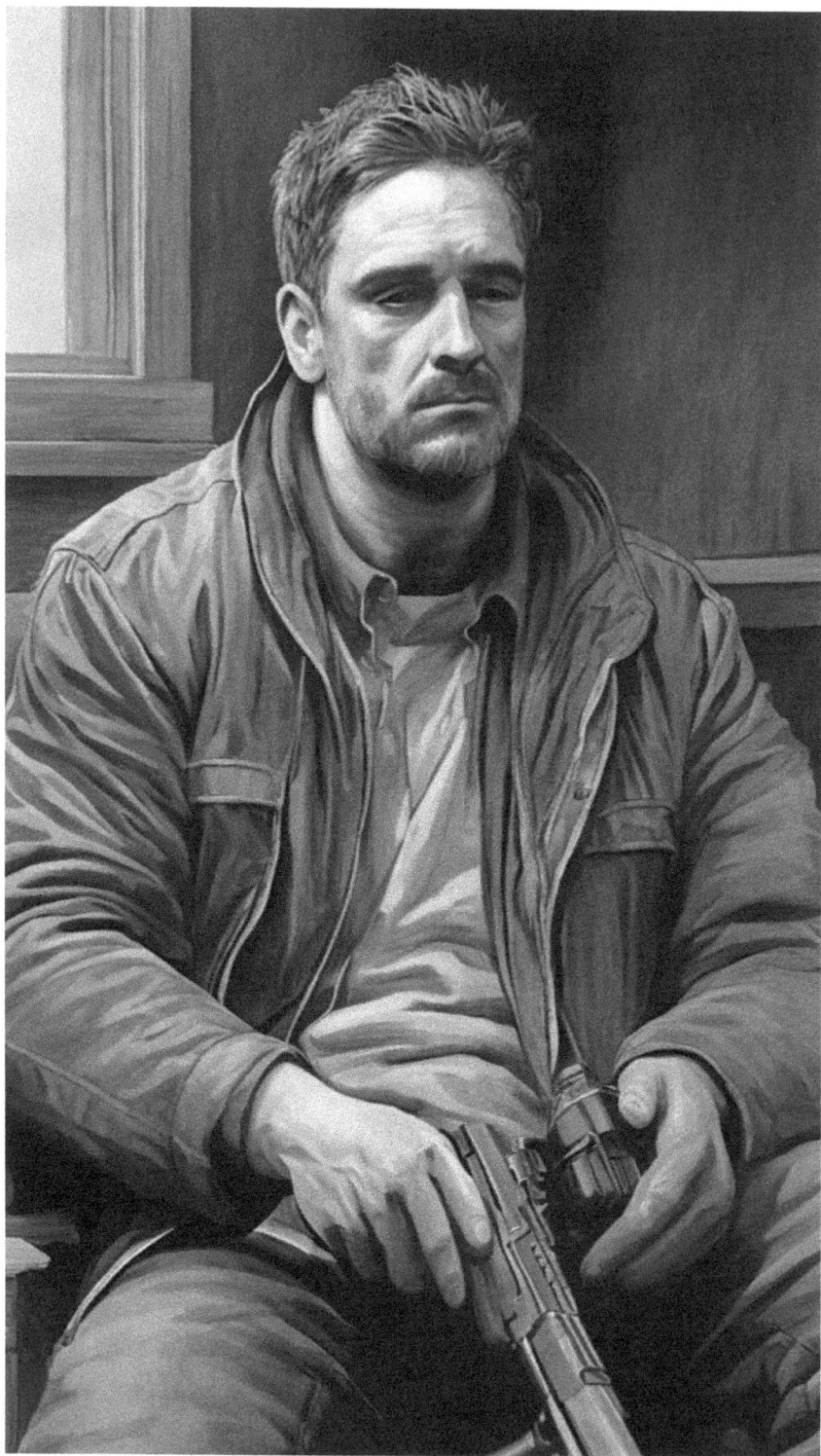

CHAPTER 18

Suicidal Behavior

Suicide is a vast topic. It intersects various psychiatric diagnoses and non-psychiatric medical conditions. It is influenced by personal, social, political, legal, religious, cultural, ethnic, and economic factors. The stigma associated with suicide is powerful and universal. It is easier to understand suicide in the context of any individual diagnosis, but the psychiatrist does not have that luxury – typically, a patient is brought to psychiatric consultation for suicidal attempts or tendencies. The psychiatrist must start from scratch to explore and dissect various aspects of the patient's mental and physical health and then come to a reasonable assessment of the causative factors. The psychiatrist then assesses the risk of imminent and long-term risk of suicide, drafts a practical management strategy, and develops a rapport strong enough to summon the cooperation of the patient and the family to the management strategy.

For this purpose, I shall approach the topic of suicide through an approach different from what is conventionally used in academic textbooks. I aim to introduce the reader to a broad bird's eye view of the scope of the topic of suicide and educate on the relevant fundamental clinical concepts. At some point, most, if not every, physician would come across patients who have either attempted suicide in the past or have a patient who would die by suicide while under the physician's care. It happens more commonly to primary care physicians than to psychiatrists, which makes education on suicide mandatory for general practitioners. Most of the suicides in patients under the care of non-psychiatrists become included in the statistics of suicide in patients with medical illnesses.

Definition

The etymology of suicide is 'su-' or 'sui-', meaning 'self', and '-cide', meaning 'to kill' or 'to slay'. Thus, suicide is the act of killing oneself. In clinical medicine, suicide refers to the conscious, deliberate, and planned act that ends in the instantaneous death of oneself. Typically, suicide occurs because the individual concludes that ending one's own life is the only and most suitable option for their problems. Suicide is usually premeditated, but sometimes the unintended or accidental consequence of an impulsive act.

Fundamental Concepts

Certain key principles are indispensable to the management of suicidal patients, or while approaching a patient at risk for suicide.

Suicide is not a disease

Suicide is neither a medical nor psychiatric condition. Instead, suicide is a behavior. The behavior could result from many reasons, and hence cannot be explained through a generalization. It is a common misconception that suicide is due to depression, which has resulted in most of the discussion about suicide revolving around depression.

Suicidal behavior is not a trait

Suicidal behavior is not an enduring trait. By that, I mean that no patient must be approached with the notion that suicide or suicidal behavior could be an inherent characteristic of their personality.

Parasuicide

Suicide must be differentiated from parasuicide. Parasuicide refers to a behavior of inflicting harm on the self, where the intended consequence is not necessarily death. Suicidal behavior, on the other hand, is an act of inflicting harm on the self where the intended consequence is death. Parasuicidal acts may result in death and thus may end up being labelled 'suicide'. Conversely, all suicides are not the result of parasuicides either. Parasuicidal behavior is far more common than suicidal behavior, and a small proportion of parasuicidal attempts (~10%) accidentally result in death. However, due to the relatively higher prevalence of parasuicidal behavior, that 10% of deaths is still more than the proportion of successful/completed suicides resulting from suicidal behavior. Conversely, a proportion of well-planned attempts at death through suicidal behavior could fail, resulting in survivors. These survivors may be clinically misdiagnosed as having parasuicidal behavior, failing to protect them against ongoing suicidal behavior that may eventually result in suicide. Enormous decreases in mortality through self-harm could be brought about even by addressing parasuicidal behavior with the same attention given to suicidal behavior. Impulsivity is a risk factor for suicidal and parasuicidal behavior.

Suicide is predetermined

Suicide, unlike parasuicidal behavior, is not a sudden event. Typically, a pre-existing psychopathology evolves over a period, resulting in suicides. The psychopathology begins with sporadic thoughts of ending life, a stage of 'suicidal thoughts'. While thoughts of ending life may occur widely in many individuals, occasionally without any recurrence, individuals who eventually commit suicide have had recurring thoughts of suicide. With time, these thoughts become organized and consolidated – i.e., the thought has now become an 'idea'. This is the stage of 'suicidal ideation'. In essence, it is through repeated occurrences of suicidal thoughts that suicidal ideation develops. This is why, traditionally, there has been extraordinary reluctance and taboo related to any public mention or discussion of suicide, as it is feared that such discussion may promote repeated suicidal thoughts. It is believed that discussing suicide openly in public may 'seed the idea' in a vulnerable person's mind. This is also why there are now mandatory warnings for viewers of movies if there is any picturization of suicide. These warnings have become more severe, extending to any reference to suicide in dialogues. Most suicidal ideations, however, do not persist.

In some individuals, suicidal ideas persist and become unremovable from the person's thought process. At this point, the reader must refer to earlier chapters on the definition of normal vs abnormal thought. A thought is considered abnormal when it cannot be dismissed by the person at will. When suicidal thoughts become persistent and unable to be dispensed by will, the individual becomes preoccupied with recurring suicidal ideas, a stage referred to as *'suicidal rumination'*.

Over time, the individual sees suicide as an eventual possibility and starts changing their life accordingly. For example, the individual may write a will, close bank accounts, clear debts, etc., which may be motivated by the perception that suicide is an eventuality. These acts are called *'suicidal gestures'*.

Finally, the person plans the exact way to end life, a stage called 'suicidal planning'. The individual executes the plan, sometimes through trial and error, which may or may not end in death. Failed attempts result in survivors who are brought to medical attention and considered '**suicide attempters**', while others result in death. Thus, suicide results from a long-drawn process characterized by predictable stage-wise evolution of psychopathology over a long period, typically months and sometimes even years. The latter statement brings two meaningful inferences –

- Firstly, suicide arising from suicidal behavior marks a failure on the part of the family, society, and sometimes the physician to recognize the long-drawn process that could have been interrupted multiple times. Suicide implies repeated failures to rescue and not one, but multiple failed opportunities.

- Secondly, survivors of suicide attempts through suicidal behavior, having already passed through all the proximal stages, are at the highest risk for mortality from suicide. Some survivors of suicide attempts regret a failed attempt and may die in future attempts, while some survivors are glad they survived.

Suicide attempts and suicides are multifactorial, even in severe mental illnesses; hence, accurate risk prediction is difficult. There are suicides where such a clear delineation of stages is not identifiable. Parasuicides may not have such a clear distinction of stages as well.

Special Terminology

Let us now discuss specific terms that you must be familiar with for discussions about suicide. Do not use these words casually or interchangeably.

Psychache

The word literally means 'a hurting mind'. American psychologist and pioneer in suicidology, Dr. Edwin Shneidman, introduced the concept of psychache. Through his extensive work researching suicidal notes, he concluded that although there is a multitude of affective states, such as anger, humiliation, depression, anguish, frustration, desperation, hopelessness, etc., there was one thing that was common to all patients – and that is, the affective state (whatever it may be) rises to the level of causing intense 'mental pain'. For example, it is not just anger; it is anger that is so intense it causes mental pain; it is not just humiliation; it is humiliation to the point of causing mental pain. In other words, the predominant affective state is not the cause, but merely the flavor of the psychache. This unbearable mental pain called psychache becomes suffering, and death appears as the only solution to that unbearable cognizable by the individual. Psychache may sound like depression, but it is not. Multiple studies have validated the presence of psychache as an accurate, independent predictor of the risk of death by suicide.

Perturbation

It refers to the level to which an individual is affected by the psychache or suicidal psychopathology. This was also a term introduced by Dr. Shneidman, who used it to describe the risk of suicidality, as in, the more perturbed an individual is, the higher the suicidal risk. He also asserted that psychotherapy is less effective if the individual is highly perturbed. He advocated that the therapist must put 'a hook' on the perturbation and do whatever is necessary to bring the level of perturbation down to de-escalate the acuteness of suicidality and *then* resume psychotherapy once the risk of lethality is much lower.

Constriction

This is another term used by Dr. Shneidman to refer to a perceptive state of seeing no solution other than killing oneself. Constriction is a cognitive state of aberrant thought, where the individual's mind is unable to perceive any other solution that may be readily apparent otherwise. In essence, constriction refers to the patient's perception that suicide is the only logical solution to their current predicament. Sometimes, constriction is too severe to be specific enough to detail the time and method of suicide. Dr. Shneidman reported a case of a young pregnant woman who was intensely perturbed - her psychache was characterized by the shame of unwed pregnancy, where she sees shooting herself as the only solution. Dr. Shneidman observed that not only did the patient see killing herself as the only solution to her psychache of shame, but also shooting was the only way to kill herself. The individual is 'thinking inside a box' and appears shut off to any other solution. He accounts that the patient was offered several ways to escape her shame of pregnancy. Still, she rationalized each of the other solutions as not the solution and somehow honed in on shooting herself to death as the ***only*** solution to her situation. This cognitive state of seeing suicide as the only 'way out' of the problem is called 'constriction'. Note that psychache is an affective state, and constriction is a cognitive state.

Impulsivity

Impulsivity, as a term in the context of suicide, is used differently than in the rest of academic psychiatry. We know that impulsiveness is discussed as a trait and symptom or consequence of irritability in depression. In the context of suicide, it is used as a surrogate marker for the risk of lethality from suicide. The risk of a suicidal patient setting into action a process that results in death is called impulsivity. Essentially, it is the risk of the patient 'flying off the handle'. Impulsivity causes the person to choose the mode of harm closest at hand, which could be more deadly than initially intended by the patient. Impulsivity is amenable to clinical therapeutic intervention and is considered a dynamic risk factor for suicide (discussed below). Antipsychotic medications have been proven effective in reducing impulsivity, challenging the notion that serotonin is the only neurotransmitter involved in impulse control. Alcohol dependence and substance abuse aggravate impulsivity.

Lethality

It refers to the risk of death of a suicidal person. Lethality is directly proportional to all the risk factors mentioned above, such as psychache, constriction, perturbation, and impulsivity. However, it is impractical to quantify the actual risk in terms of numbers. Lethality also depends on the patient's knowledge base, skill, and intelligence. For example, an individual with less knowledge but less perturbed may erroneously choose a method with more lethality risk than intended.

Hopelessness

This term is also used with a slightly different connotation in the context of suicide than with depression. In the case of depression, hopelessness implies an affective state of despair and gloom and a sense that the despair would not improve. In suicidology, hopelessness is a cognitive state of seeing cessation of life as the only solution to the psychache. In my practice, a subjective sense of hopelessness is the most useful clinical predictor of the risk of suicide. It may not predict lethality, however. Hopelessness may be so severe that the individual may not even find the completion of suicide possible. The psychiatrist must be vigilant during the first few weeks of antidepressant therapy, as suicides could be more common in this period – a possible reason is the persistent presence of hopelessness about life, but just enough decreased hopelessness about completing the suicidal act, along with the return of psychomotor energy to execute the act.

Deceptive calm

It refers to a period of apparent reduced/resolved suicidality in an individual who then surprises everyone by silently taking their life. It is an arduous clinical task to identify this psychological attribute, which implies a 'quality' of suicidality – the person's acceptance of suicidal eventuality. It is impractical to be able to remove all opportunities for a person to be able to commit suicide when they appear clinically non-suicidal.

Risk Factors for Suicide

Risk factors are different from predictive factors. ***'Risk factors'*** refers to factors associated with increased prevalence of (i.e., predisposes to) suicidal behavior and, hence, suicide. ***'Predictive factors'*** are those factors (signs or symptoms) among suicidal patients associated with a higher probability of suicide. Psychache, high level of perturbance, constriction, and lethality are not risk factors, but predictive factors associated with a higher risk of suicide.

The risk factors of suicidality could be understood as static or dynamic factors. Static factors are not subject to change, i.e., non-modifiable variables, and include demographics, prior established psychiatric diagnoses, previous history of suicide attempts, comorbid medical illnesses, and enduring traits such as intellectual disability or personality disorder. Dynamic factors are potentially amenable to change, i.e., modifiable variables, categorized into clinical and situational variables. Clinical variables include specific clinical symptoms (discussed below) amenable to psychotherapy or clinical intervention and the presence/absence of therapeutic alliance. Situational variables include social support, interpersonal conflict, employment status, and access to lethal objects. These risk factors do not necessarily predict suicidal events in suicidal patients, but they are instrumental in understanding the patient's situation and drafting management strategies. We shall now discuss certain important risk factors in more detail –

- **Major Depressive Disorder –** Approximately 90% of people who commit suicide have an Axis I diagnosis at the time of death; in 10% of suicides, no underlying psychiatric diagnosis is discovered. Furthermore, 5% of suicides occur in people with terminal illnesses. About 10% of individuals with depression have a family history of suicide. Suicides are more common in either the initial stages of depression or in the most advanced stages. It is for this reason that it is advisable not to begin antidepressant therapy with high initial doses.

- **Prior history of suicide –** Nearly 40% of suicides in patients who are being clinically followed for a prior suicide attempt occur during the first year since the prior attempt (called 'short-term suicides'), and the remaining 60% occur after a year ('long term suicides'). In general, nine clinical symptoms are prospectively associated with suicides. Six of them, namely panic attacks, anxiety, decreased concentration, insomnia, alcohol abuse, and anhedonia, are associated with short-term suicides. The other three, namely hopelessness, suicidal ideation, and a history of suicide attempts are associated with long-term suicides. All these associations are derived through statistical analyses. Clinically, a subjective sense of hopelessness is the most useful predictive factor. Remember, 60% to 90% of persons who commit suicide have not previously attempted suicide. Thus, even if every person who had attempted suicide in the past were somehow prevented from doing so in the future, most suicides would still occur.

- **Alcohol dependence and substance abuse –** Approximately 20% of those who commit suicide have been diagnosed with alcohol dependence, and 3% of individuals with alcoholism die of suicide. Suicide is more common in those who have undergone inpatient treatment for alcohol dependence than outpatient treatment alone, suggesting a higher risk of suicide with more severe forms of alcohol dependence.

In this context, up to 40% of those who underwent hospitalization could be at risk for suicide within a year of the hospitalization, and 40% of them have a history of a previous suicide attempt. Polysubstance abuse is also strongly associated with suicide, and overdose could be the reason. Cocaine withdrawal is also associated with a higher risk of suicide. Often, suicide in the background of polysubstance abuse is associated with losing an interpersonal relationship as a precipitating factor.

- **The 'depressed alcoholic'** – Depression and alcohol are an explosive combination, so much so that it is worth mentioning this combination as a separate risk factor. Many patients with alcohol dependence who commit suicide were noted to be depressed during inpatient stays. However, it is difficult to ascertain whether the depression is secondary to alcohol dependence or due to medical complications of alcohol dependence. In many cases, the depression was either not treated adequately or not treated at all. Since alcohol intoxication is associated with a depressed mood and loss of inhibitions, many individuals commit suicide while intoxicated. Depression in alcohol dependence is exacerbated by social isolation resulting from strained relationships with family and friends. Nearly 50% of suicides with alcohol dependence have been associated with losing a close relationship during the previous year. Depressed persons with alcoholism are at greater risk for suicide after successful detoxification, and this risk is particularly high in the absence of adequate social support. Depressive episodes could precipitate a recurrence of alcoholism, and alcohol intake could precipitate a depressive episode. As a rule, patients with depression must not touch alcohol at all, forever!

- **Schizophrenia** – Approximately 30% of people with schizophrenia attempt suicide, and ultimately 10% results in death. Many commit suicide during the first year of the illness. Single unmarried status, social isolation, and feelings of inadequacy point toward higher risk. Greater severity of negative symptoms of schizophrenia does not correlate with a higher risk of suicide. Instead, later onset, better premorbid functioning, greater capacity for abstract thinking, and better insight are associated with a higher risk of suicide. Suicide is common in the post-psychotic depressive phase. Other higher-risk periods include personal or interpersonal loss and periods when the patient gains greater insight into a chronic and morbid illness. Physicians tend to be less aggressive in recognizing and treating post-psychotic depression.

- **Medical illness** – Retrospective studies suggest that 25% to 75% of suicides are associated with medical illnesses, including terminal illnesses. In the Indian setting, peptic ulcer-related chronic abdominal pain and gynecological disorders related to painful menstruation are commonly cited in this regard. Gleaning the data further, it appears that medical illness and age may not be independent risk factors – rather, medical illnesses acting as psychological stressors may be a more appropriate understanding of the association with medical illnesses. Interpersonal conflicts, separations, and rejections are primary contributory life stressors in adolescents and young adults. In the 40–60-year age group, economic problems appear to be the most significant stressors. Over the age 60, medical illness plays a more prominent contributory role; over age 80, medical illness is the most significant factor.

- **Other static risk factors** – Eating disorders, panic disorders, delirious disorders, and epilepsy are also associated with suicide lethality.

- **Therapeutic alliance** – A dynamic risk factor that can impact the occurrence of suicide. A solid therapeutic alliance, sometimes established solidly through a no-self-harm contract, could help deter or distract suicidal attempts. A request for such a contract elicits a response from the patient, which could be used to gauge the patient's mental position toward suicide. Some patients may readily sign the contract, only to violate it later. Some clinicians assign too much importance to the contract – it must be noted that these contracts do not assure the patient will not commit suicide.

- **Access to lethal methods** – Availability and access to lethal methods are crucial as situational variable type dynamic risk factors. For example, purchasing a handgun could be related to a 50 times higher likelihood of committing suicide the week following the purchase, with increased risk persisting up to 6 years after the purchase. The MSE should focus on this variable – questions related to the procurement plan of the tools needed to execute the suicide must be asked. This is especially relevant in a country like India, where overdose is a prevalent method of suicide. Pesticide ingestion is also common in rural and agricultural communities in India, as leftover pesticides are commonly found in many households. Hanging is a prevalent method of suicide in correctional facilities. Suicide does happen in psychiatric units, too. No place is entirely suicide-proof.

- **Other dynamic risk factors** - The presence or absence of social support, interpersonal conflicts, financial stressors, employment instability (and unemployment), and residential instability are other situational-type dynamic risk factors.

The clinician must identify all the relevant risk factors and act on them. The clinician must document the risk factors (absence or presence of each) and the action taken to mitigate the risk, keeping in mind that 'if it is not documented, it did not happen'. Some clinicians believe that not touching on the topic of suicide and avoiding probing-type questions could help protect them from liability – it is quite the contrary. Failure to look for suicidal risk could be viewed as deviance from the standard of care, amounting to negligence. In my experience, in the area of suicide, clinicians are more prone to liability for errors of omission than errors of judgment.

Protective Factors for Suicide

Certain clinically identifiable factors may be associated with a decreased risk of suicide or lethality. Some of them are listed below –

Stoicism – Stoicism is essentially the ability to bear misfortune. Typically, stoic individuals rely more on logic and less on emotions. They prefer to do things because it is the right way to do. These individuals tend to resist and deter suicidal thoughts and intentions.

- **Adaptability** - Refers to the ability of oneself to change their attitudes, perceptions, and approach to a problem or situation to suit the needs of survival or success. These individuals are practical and less conformist.

- **Alternate seeking** - Refers to a behavior of seeking or searching for alternative solutions to a problem. It is the antithesis of the cognitive state of constriction seen in suicidal patients.

- **Abhorrence** - Refers to a personal disgust towards suicide. It may be intrinsic to their personality or be taught through religious or cultural norms. Abhorrence is a significant deterrent to suicide and is commonly seen in Islamic communities.

- **Anchorage -** Refers to a strong commitment or obligation (personal or social) that makes suicide a bad choice. For example, the presence of young children to be reared is associated with less suicide.

- **Compliance -** Cooperation to treatment, willingness to present for psychiatric visits, and communicative patients are protective factors, too.

The 'Suicider Profile' (Mananalam Clinic Experience)

The medical literature identifies a list of risk factors and protective factors. How would you use this expanding and increasingly complex list of factors in your clinic? It would be best if you had a mental schema that is readily applicable and easy to use in the clinic. In essence, you must envision the typical profile of a 'suicider', i.e., an imaginary person who has committed suicide in the future, but is alive today and in your clinic now. You must develop this profile in your mind through evidence from academic literature, learnings from colleagues, and ongoing personal clinical experience. I shall share the suicider profile I have built through my clinical experience over the years -

- Age – Elderly or middle-aged.
- Gender – Male.
- Education level – uneducated or low education level.
- Social status – low.
- Economic status – weak (no savings).
- Employment status – unemployment (may have a 'job', not a career), insecure employment status.
- Marital status – not happily married (i.e., single, chronically unmarried, separated, divorced, or widowed).
- Living situation – alone or living with pets.
- Anchorage – none (i.e., no children).
- Professional type – farmer, student, military .
- Special subpopulations – refugees, female doctor/health

professionals, affiliations to unique or minor religious or spiritual groups, immigrants, prisoners, chronic facility inhabitants (in hospitals, nursing homes).

- Geography – lowly populated areas, especially rural communities, living in the outskirts, or urban areas with secluded living.
- Timing of the year (for eventual suicide) – spring, autumn, weekend, evenings, anniversary.
- Life experiences – personal history of death of a loved one/ family member, separations, estrangements, abandonments, absence of long-term relationships, criminal charges.
- Social support system – low.
- Social integration – absent or minimal (no consistent long-term relationships or friendships), having only one or two friends.
- Medical history – severe or chronic medical conditions.
- Psychiatric history – psychosis, substance abuse.

The suicider profile is not meant to be a sensitive test to identify every potential case of suicide, but is meant to prevent you from failing to recognize a high-risk patient. The suicider profile may be individualized to the area and scope of your practice and is specific to the geographical area catered by your practice.

The Suicide-Attempters

Suicide, being a lethal event, is not a clinical presentation. In practice, the clinician faces two types of patients – patients at risk for suicide (i.e., suicidal patients) or those who have attempted suicide (i.e., 'suicide attempters'). Suicide attempts must be differentiated from those who commit self-harm – the difference being that a suicide attempt is associated with an awareness that the attempt could result in death. However, the intent of the suicide attempt must not be viewed as a binary (i.e., all-or-none type) variable. Suicide attempters may wish to ultimately survive their attempt, although they are aware that death could occur – and for this reason, it must not be considered as parasuicide. Suicide attempts could be acute or chronic, planned or impulsive, single or repetitive, with the seriousness of intentionality or ambivalence, with weak or absolute resolve. Suicide attempters are typically deficient in problem-solving skills due to cognitive distortion ('constriction'). Most suicide attempts are impulsive. Two-thirds of suicide attempters have their first thought about doing so less than an hour before the attempt.

Weisman and Worden assessed the lethality (defined as the probability of inflicting irreversible damage) in a quantitate way through a 'risk-rescue rating' method where the actual risk of death by the method used for the suicide attempt and the ability to be able to rescue the victim was determined. Simply put, the clinician must assess the following - how dangerous was the suicide method? Did the person genuinely believe that they would die? Was the victim surprised to have survived? Was it impulsive or premeditated? Was there a suicidal note? Did the victim take steps to increase or decrease the likelihood of being rescued? Based on these factors, the risk-rescue types are four-fold: high risk - high rescue, low risk – high rescue, high risk -low rescue, and low risk – low rescue. Assessing the risk-rescue type helps understand the situation better. The clinician should consider all these types equally important and approach them with the same seriousness regardless of the type.

Neil Kessel and Ed Shneidman also used another type of classification of suicide attempts to understand the victim better. They postulated four types - intended cessation, sub-intended cessation, intended interruption, and intended continuation. Intended cessation is when the victim intends for the suicide attempt to cease; hence, they are absolute failed suicide attempts unless an accident results in death. Sub-intended cessation is when there is ambivalence - predominantly favoring cessation of the suicidal process and about 15% ambivalent hoping for death. Intended interruption is also associated with ambivalence, but 40% hope things will improve once they become conscious. Intended continuation is associated with interpersonal gains.

In my personal experience, there is ambivalence even in the most seriously suicidal person – in almost everyone, there seems to be an instinct to want to live. The clinician must search for this window of opportunity and exploit it to deter suicidality.

Risk factors for committing suicide after a prior suicide attempt include older age, male gender, unemployed or retired employment status, separated/divorced or widowed marital status, living alone, poor physical health, psychiatric disorder (particularly depression, alcoholism, schizophrenia, and sociopathic personality disorder), high suicidal intent in the current episode, violent method involved in current attempt (such as attempted hanging, shooting, jumping, immolation), and leaving a suicide note.

Self-Harm and Self-Mutilation

As mentioned above, self-harm and self-mutilation are different from suicide attempts. Here, there is no actual intention to die. Occasionally, they may end in death and end up being labeled as parasuicides. Acts of self-harm are deliberate attempts to injure one's physical body, and the motivation behind these acts is to alter the life situation or course of events to make it feel better. Unfortunately, these cases are often misdiagnosed as suicide attempts. Self-harm could be due to various psychiatric diagnoses; hence, the term 'deliberate self-harm' (DSH) is preferred for a presenting complaint. Self-mutilation is a specific form of deliberate self-harm. It begins in adolescence and is common in young females. The reasons given for such self-mutilation is the subjective feeling of relief from anger, tension, or dissociative numbness that happens while cutting an arm, thigh, breast, or torso with a sharp object. Some patients burn themselves with cigarettes or a hot iron or may bang their heads against a wall. The physical pain or the sight of their blood is reported to bring emotional relief and a sense of 'feeling real again'. The skin of such people may demonstrate a complex grid of vertical and horizontal scars in various stages of healing. Persons with schizophrenia or psychotic depression also mutilate themselves, but the self-mutilation in the latter conditions is much more severe, such as piercing the abdomen with a knife, amputating the genitals, or cutting off the tongue. I have encountered a case of self-enucleation of the eyeball.

'Understanding the Predicament'

Establishing a friendly, non-distractive atmosphere, maintaining privacy, and empathetic language are some fundamental requisites for the interview of the suicidal patient, as they would with any other psychiatric interview. The distinguishing feature in the case of a suicidal patient is the need for a semi-structured interview style, with the aim of ***understanding the predicament*** – and by that, I mean that the interviewer must follow a set structure of obtaining information but with the flexibility needed to establish the nature of the troubled situation entrapping the patient. Typically, the narrative goes like this - the suicidal patient has a long history of problems that have led to the perspective of being 'trapped' in a hopeless situation, the solution to which is suicide and suicide alone. That particular 'trapped situation' for which suicide is the only way out is the predicament. Information must be gathered in a way that enables the psychiatrist to reconstruct the predicament, as perceived by the patient reliably.

In essence, how did the patient find themselves in this situation? How did the patient's parents, siblings, friends, spouse, employer, or children contribute to (or deter) the current predicament? Begin with childhood history and the patient's perception of the parents and other members of the family. Reconstruct details about the person as if your understanding flows like reading through a rich, detailed, critical biography. Details about the formative influences of family, culture, educational environment, and psychosexual development, including peer and sexual relationships, must be gathered. The physician must elicit the person's life experiences, dreams, needs, wants and desires, and reactions to situations to understand how they might arrive at suicide as the solution to their predicament. Delve into depression, degree of despair, hopelessness, helplessness, anxiety, degree of obsessions, perceptual and cognitive distortions, internal guilt, and self-blame, if any.

Remember that the suicidal patient has cognitive disruptions (such as constriction), which means suicide is rationalized as the only solution to their suffering. Being the examiner is devoid of such cognitive disruptions, and the thinking process in the patient might be silly, trivial, or unlikely to you, making you unable to reconstruct the predicament in the patient's mind. You have to resist this pitfall constantly. This pitfall is the reason for missing a potentially suicidal patient. When a patient under the care of a psychiatrist commits suicide, the psychiatrist may say post-hoc, 'I didn't think the patient was this troubled' – Well, it means you didn't understand the predicament correctly. Be agreeable and empathetic to the patient. The interview process should proceed in a manner reminiscent of one confiding in the other, like a confession.

The interview must establish the predicament leading to suicidality *and* how sinister it could be. At this point, the psychiatrist must be able to gauge the level of intent (or ambivalence) and the changes necessary in the patient's life to keep them alive. Then, the physician needs to discover what changes in the person's life are necessary to take to keep the person alive. This might help in treatment and assist in prognosis. The degree of seriousness (i.e., level of intent) of suicidality is inversely related to the level of ambivalence about dying. Questions should never be asked in a hurry.

The 'Breakthrough Moment' (Mananalam Clinic Experience)

The suicidal patient is often embarrassed and ashamed of their predicament. Avoiding eye contact, trembling lashes, or flushing on the cheek might indicate an effort to conceal suicidal intent. The psychiatrist must study facial mannerisms and bodily language constantly. The psychiatrist must calmly, empathetically, and non-judgmentally approach the patient with a firmness that 'breaks the mantle', typically resulting in crying or emotional outpouring. In the Mananalam clinic, this is called the 'breakthrough moment'. The occurrence of the breakthrough moment implies that you are on the right track and progress is being made. After the breakthrough moment, the patient readily opens up to the psychiatrist, providing information in a forthcoming fashion. Cooperation, compliance, and therapeutic alliance are much more reliable after the breakthrough moment. Some breakthrough moments are less dramatic or obvious than others, but if you have no clue of a breakthrough moment, you must seriously re-evaluate your interview process.

Let me summarize certain important 'do's' during the assessment of a person in the context of suicide evaluation

- *Do* form a positive therapeutic alliance
- *Do* wait until the alliance is formed before making recommendations.
- *Do* gather corroborative information from family, work, and friends.
- *Do* a thorough MSE always.

- ***Do*** a biopsychosocial assessment.
- ***Do*** document all your findings diligently.
- ***Do*** remain objective and stay away from personal bias and judgmental approaches.
- ***Do*** conclude based on facts (and not on intuition).
- ***Do*** keep the patient always in the vision of family or staff.
- ***Do*** ask for help and supervision from colleagues, primarily from senior and experienced psychiatrists.

Assessing the 'Dangerousness' of a Suicidal Patient

What is meant by the term 'dangerousness' or 'risk of dangerousness' of a suicidal patient? Dangerousness is neither a clinical symptom nor sign nor diagnosis. Instead, it is a legal term equivalent to the clinical term of lethality. Dangerousness is commonly misunderstood and erroneously treated like a trait, a quantifiable non-modifiable risk factor. The psychiatrist is expected to know the risk, and the psychiatrist's competence is assessed retrospectively based on what happens to the patient in the coming weeks or months following the initial assessment. Dangerousness is not an accurately quantifiable variable. Dangerousness is a modifiable variable that may change with time and environmental situations. The public and the legal system believe that a clinician must be able to assess which patient is 'dangerous' to oneself. Popular media such as journals, social media discussions, and movies seem to pedal this notion. They see every suicide of a patient under a psychiatrist's care as a failure in assessing dangerousness. Furthermore, the legal system summons expert opinions from mental health professionals to arbitrate on matters where an individual's dangerousness needs to be ascertained. Sometimes, school counselors and employers ask for such assessments. Clinicians are ***not*** trained to assess the dangerousness of a suicidal patient, like how the public or law expects the clinician to have assessed it. I don't think it is even possible to quantify dangerousness.

In medicine, clinicians assess risk using statistical methods to the study population. The assessment of risk depends on the population studied and the control group used to compare the effect of the risk on the study population. These risk valuations are ***meant for the physician, not the patient or***

the legal system. These risks are statistically expressed as 'odds ratios' – i.e., the odds (or chances) of associating a specific diagnosis with the risk of suicide. These numbers are not directly translatable to a person seen in the clinical setting. Even if the psychiatrist assigns a specific risk estimate based on a detailed assessment of risk factors, many other variables cannot be accounted for in the practical setting.

The psychiatrist usually has reliable information on the severity of the chosen method of harm (i.e., a single cut vs a hanging attempt or the use of a poison vs knife) and the likelihood of such behavior (no prior attempts vs multiple attempts in the past). Using these factors, the psychiatrist could make a sensible decision on the immediate threat to life and decide whether to commit the patient to admission or release the patient to their habitat. That is the most a psychiatrist can do – a psychiatrist cannot entirely prevent suicide for the foreseeable future. Also, several other downstream factors after this decision may affect the eventual outcome – for example, what if the patient declines admission? What if the family is not cooperative with inpatient management? How compliant and diligent is the family in following the psychiatrist's instructions for outpatient management?

Psychiatrists often have difficulty deciding how to proceed when a person declines a voluntary admission. In a country like India, admitting a patient for suicidality is more of a social issue than a clinical one. In a country like the USA, the decision becomes a question of legality, i.e., restricting the scope of constitutionally guaranteed liberties rather than a clinical or social issue. For a psychiatrist like me who encounters Indian patients living in the USA, the problem is doubly more complex.

In these situations, there are two competing ethical interests – the principle of beneficence (to protect the patients from their illness) and the principle of autonomy (to protect a person's right to make medical decisions independently). Doctors and lawyers would find themselves at a crossroads here.

Doctors are trained to 'do no harm' (the ethical principle of non-maleficence). So, they err on the side of caution – 'when in doubt, admit'. On the other hand, lawyers prioritize individual liberty as the cornerstone of the constitution, and a person can be committed against their will only under extraordinary circumstances that could be proven beyond doubt. Thus, they err on the side of liberty – 'when in doubt, acquit'. Despite these inherent contradictions, clinicians are called upon to use their skills to determine who is potentially suicidal and who is not accurately. Releasing a patient who proceeds to commit suicide will be viewed as medical error or negligence, and admitting a patient who may not be considered to commit suicide is viewed as a crime. Thus, the psychiatrist would find themselves stuck between a rock and a hard place.

The judicial system might call upon the psychiatrist to provide clinical input in determining the treatment needs in the context of suicide and other situations, including domestic violence, parole petitioners, persons on probation, sexual offenders, and transfers from prison to hospital and hospital to prison. In all these situations, clinicians should ***restrict the scope of their opinions to the clinical issues only and avoid making predictions about future dangerousness.*** Clinicians should also avoid making absolute statements and speak in terms of the relative probability of the person committing suicide. The clinician must clearly articulate the difference between their clinical and legal duties. The clinician's clinical duty is to assess suicidal risk based on clinical factors to draft an effective management strategy. The clinician's legal duty is to identify and document the reason for involuntary confinement without ambiguity. For the latter, the clinician must persuade the patient of the need for hospitalization. The patient may exercise the legal right to refuse admission, in which case the judicial system may be approached to override the patient's will. The psychiatrist must think ten steps ahead of the patient to get what is intended successfully. The criteria for involuntary confinement and the procedure to approach the judiciary depend on local laws, and the psychiatrist must be familiar with these procedures. The psychiatrist must prepare for such situations ahead of time rather than scrambling to figure out what to do when faced with a defiant patient.

There are certain documents that the patient can sign, such as 'suicide contracts' or 'safety contracts. Essentially, these documents spell out that the patient has been educated on the risk of suicide and given adequate information to identify times of increased risk and the methods to seek help and prevent suicide. These contracts are controversial and are believed to be useless, if not detrimental to the patient. In my view, these contracts do not prevent suicide. They may, however, serve as documents to protect the physician against severe forms of liability. It becomes an instrument to prove that the physician has recognized suicide as a risk and has acted on it in some form. Remember - the contract is between the patient and the doctor – the hospital or institution is not involved in this contract.

The Decision to Admit

The decision to admit a suicidal patient is one of the most daunting situations for a psychiatrist, especially for a patient who has been under their established care for a while. The psychiatrist is often seen as unreasonable by the patient and family and as an overreaction to the situation. In the ideal world, the psychiatrist would want to admit any patient, even with the smallest suicidal ideation, and discharge the patient only after the ideation has disappeared. However, admitting a patient has profound personal, social, and legal implications, and such a decision is often antagonized or criticized. The patient usually resists admission, and the family and friends of the patient often want to be on the agreeable side of the patient and join the chorus of resistance. The psychiatrist must consciously seek and destroy any desire to be friendly and agreeable. The patient being alive is more important than maintaining niceties. The psychiatrist must not hesitate to involve the family or the legal system to commit the patient involuntarily if the situation demands it. Psychiatrists in private practice or solo practice are the ones who find it challenging to deal with this situation.

There are many guidelines and recommendations from various sources on the indications and selection criteria for admission. It is impractical to follow them to the dot in the clinical setting.

At our Mananalam clinic, I use a simple rule of thumb – the ***presence of active suicidal ideation*** is a strong indicator of benefit from inpatient admission and management. Active suicidal ideation means the individual is actively contemplating or entertaining the idea of suicide as a foreseeable solution to their problems – they are thinking about it, planning it, assessing its risks and benefits, working out the possible obstacles to executing the plan, working on backup plans to successfully overcome obstacles, purchasing or accessing a lethal weapon or method, etc. Patients with an acute psychotic episode, a major depressive episode, severe psychache, and suicidal ideation are at even higher risk. Also, I will likely admit patients with suicidal ideation ***and*** no anchorage, regardless of other factors. On the other hand, the presence of a psychiatric diagnosis with a published high risk of suicide is not an indicator of benefit from inpatient admission. I am less likely to admit patients with no suicidal ideation if a willing and cooperative family can be safely observed. In general, it is safer to lean towards admission in the case of psychosis with suicidal ideation. Also, patients who are not compliant with admission are the ones who are at high risk of committing suicide if not admitted. The psychiatrist must double down on the efforts to admit the more it is resisted.

Another situation where I prefer to admit is when a patient is brought for a recent suicide attempt where there is evidence of high suicidal intent. Examples of high suicidal intent include a suicide attempt carried out in isolation, a suicide attempt timed to make rescue unlikely, precautions are taken to avoid discovery, preparatory suicidal gestures (such as enacting a will, organizing life insurance), accessing lethal methods (buying or saving up tablets, poisons, guns), communicating to close contacts about intent, extensive premedication, leaving a note, and alerting potential helpers after a failed attempt.

Whenever a patient is admitted for suicidal ideation, the nearest of kin or family must be contacted. In countries like the USA, privacy of health information is a concern. In countries like India, not divulging such information to the family (even in the absence of informed consent to inform the family) would be considered unethical. When contacting the family, clearly articulate your decision's logical reasoning and medical rationale. Document the same in simple language. If the family declines admission, simply have them sign documents that they wish to remove the patient from the doctor's care despite education on the risk of suicide.

Predicting Suicide

The million-dollar question in psychiatry is if it is possible to predict ***who*** will commit suicide. The billion-dollar question is predicting when it will happen. The risk factors for suicide are well-identified in the literature but are more applicable in research papers than in the clinic. Risk factors are reliable and statistically valid when applied to groups of people but are not so useful for the person interviewed in the clinical setting. Suicides are indeed rare events in the general population – so any method with enough sensitivity would be over-predicting suicides (i.e., a high number of false positives).

The *'suicide paradox' (a Mananalam Clinic Experience)* is where those judged to be at the highest risk of suicide by any research method and subject to appropriate, effective suicide mitigation interventions would be the least likely to commit suicide. It would thus be impossible to determine if the decreased incidence of suicide is a result of inaccurate prediction modeling or effective treatment strategies. This is why psychiatrists must approach all suicidal cases with equal importance. There are multiple reasons to explain the paradox.

- Persons who seriously wish and contemplate dying take actions to nullify obstacles to their suicide. Thus, they are careful to conceal the depth of their intentions and are more likely to lie or misrepresent their situation in tests or interviews. Observing the patient's general attitude towards psychiatric care is the best way to identify if the patient is genuinely non-suicidal or is willfully misrepresenting. Actively suicidal patients do not view psychiatrists, medical help, and resources as allies but as obstacles. They are likely to be passively non-cooperative. Eliciting the breakthrough moment (see above) is a reliable marker that the patient was indeed actively suicidal. Still, the psychiatrist has successfully 'broken into' the mantle that protects their desire to perish. Patients in this group tend to be older, male, and have medical comorbidities, substance abuse, and psychosis.

- Persons who are not seriously contemplating suicide and do not wish to die but indulge in self-harmful behavior to gain attention or for other secondary gains may willfully misrepresent their intentions as serious, thereby being scored as high risk for suicide. DSH, parasuicides, adjustment disorders, and personality disorders are differential diagnoses in this context. Patients in this group tend to be younger, female and have Cluster B-type personality traits.

- Intrinsic risk of failure due to human error – Any human endeavor has a risk of failure due to poor planning, ineffective execution, or unforeseen circumstances. I would say roughly 10% falls into this category. So, 10% of those attempting suicide with intentions to die may fail and thus show up as suicide attempts or misdiagnosed as DSH, parasuicides, or sometimes as malingering. Similarly, 10% of those who enact a DSH or suicidal attempt expecting not to die may die. These individuals do end up being included in the statistics on suicide. Retrospectively, both these groups of people fudge the post hoc estimation of the validity of the prediction models.

- Prediction models used to identify the high-risk person might have been inaccurate (i.e., false positives or using a prediction score that has low positive predictive value).

- The treatment strategy employed was successful, thereby preventing suicides.

- Due to this paradox, suicide prediction models cannot be solely relied upon. The psychiatrist must use diligence, acumen, and the accumulated wisdom of senior and experienced colleagues.

The usual question from a psychiatry student is - when one can't accurately predict, why this exhaustive study and search for the risk factors of suicide? The answer is – that the aim is not to predict suicide as a yes/no occurrence in the future but to position the patient in the continuum of risk based on known factors, to more effectively inform the psychiatrist of treatment options, and then track the movement of the patient along the continuum in the direction of safety.

Predicting suicide is like a weather forecast – the accuracy of any prediction is higher for the shorter term. The most the psychiatrist can do is be able to identify acute suicidality (i.e., death by suicide within the next 24 to 48 hours) and 'defuse' the situation by inpatient admission, removing access to lethal methods, disrupting the constrictive thought process, and exploiting the ambivalence of the patient to restore pro-survival intentions. Sometimes, experienced psychiatric nurses or ward staff could sense acute suicidality and may alert psychiatrists.

Losing a Patient to Suicide

Being in the medical profession, you would encounter a patient who commits suicide at some point. Consider yourself blessed if you don't. It is a destabilizing moment for any physician, especially for a psychiatrist, who would feel responsible for not preventing it. It is a difficult moment, even for a veteran psychiatrist. The physician may feel guilt, shame, or aversion to their career and may be tempted to dismiss traditional clinical wisdom as inaccurate. Facing the patient's grieving family is another daunting task. Nuances in dealing with the situation at the personal, professional, and public levels can only be learned by tutelage and apprenticeship under an experienced psychiatrist. For this reason, I recommend novice psychiatrists actively seek help from seniors when dealing with suicidal patients. Here are some tips –

- **At the personal level –** do not punish or blame yourself. We all make mistakes, and our mind and mental health knowledge is not exhaustive. Remember that losing a patient to suicide is akin to the death of a patient to any other doctor of another specialty. Fortunately, we psychiatrists do not lose our patients to death from the illness we treat as much as other medical specialties do. But that is also why we may not be stress-inoculated enough to deal with the loss. Losing a patient is part of the practice of medicine. Get up and start working again.

- **At the professional level –** you must take the death very seriously. You must present the case at mortality conferences to other psychiatrists and discuss what might have been done differently to prevent the suicide. Was the diagnostic assessment correct and comprehensive? Was the MSE thorough? Was the risk modeling accurate? Was anything missed? You must do everything possible to reassess your thought process and how it needs to be modified to prevent this from happening to the next patient. You must verbalize, write down, and implement changes in your clinical practice.

- **At the public level –** Do not condone suicide. Do not justify any personal, social, or political reasons assigned by the patient's family or public to the cause of suicide. Do not glorify any death from suicide, and do not glorify any person who died by suicide. Do not perform post-hoc analysis or psychological autopsy on a dead patient to the public. Suicide can be discussed at a professional level to the lay public as a health problem – a doctor must avoid commenting on any individual death by suicide to the public or media.

Population-Based Strategies

As I have discussed above, the scope of a psychiatrist in preventing suicide is indeed limited. Many extra-clinical factors strongly influence the occurrence of suicide. As mentioned above, the best a psychiatrist can do is recognize acute suicidality and prevent suicide in the short term. However, there are population-based strategies that could help us in the long run. Some of them are:

- **Education –** of medical students and primary care physicians – There is a wealth of medical literature, research, and studies on suicide. Except in well-developed countries like the USA, this literature is neither applied in everyday clinical practice nor taught to medical students with the needed emphasis in their syllabus. Testing on suicide-related knowledge and skills is low, even in psychiatry residency programs.

- **Media influence –** There is data to show that the incidence of suicides rises after media coverage of suicides of celebrities. Movies now have mandatory warnings that caution audiences about scenes related to suicide (like warnings related to smoking, violence, foul language, nudity, etc.). The latter reinforces my first point – suicide is a behavior subject to positive reinforcement by others' behaviors. Suicide behavior is modeled in society. Thus, there is a strong case to take a hardline stance against condoning, glorifying, or justifying suicide in any form. It is to reinforce this strong point, that this chapter is titled 'suicidal behavior'.

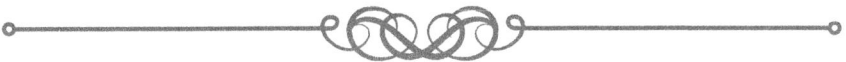

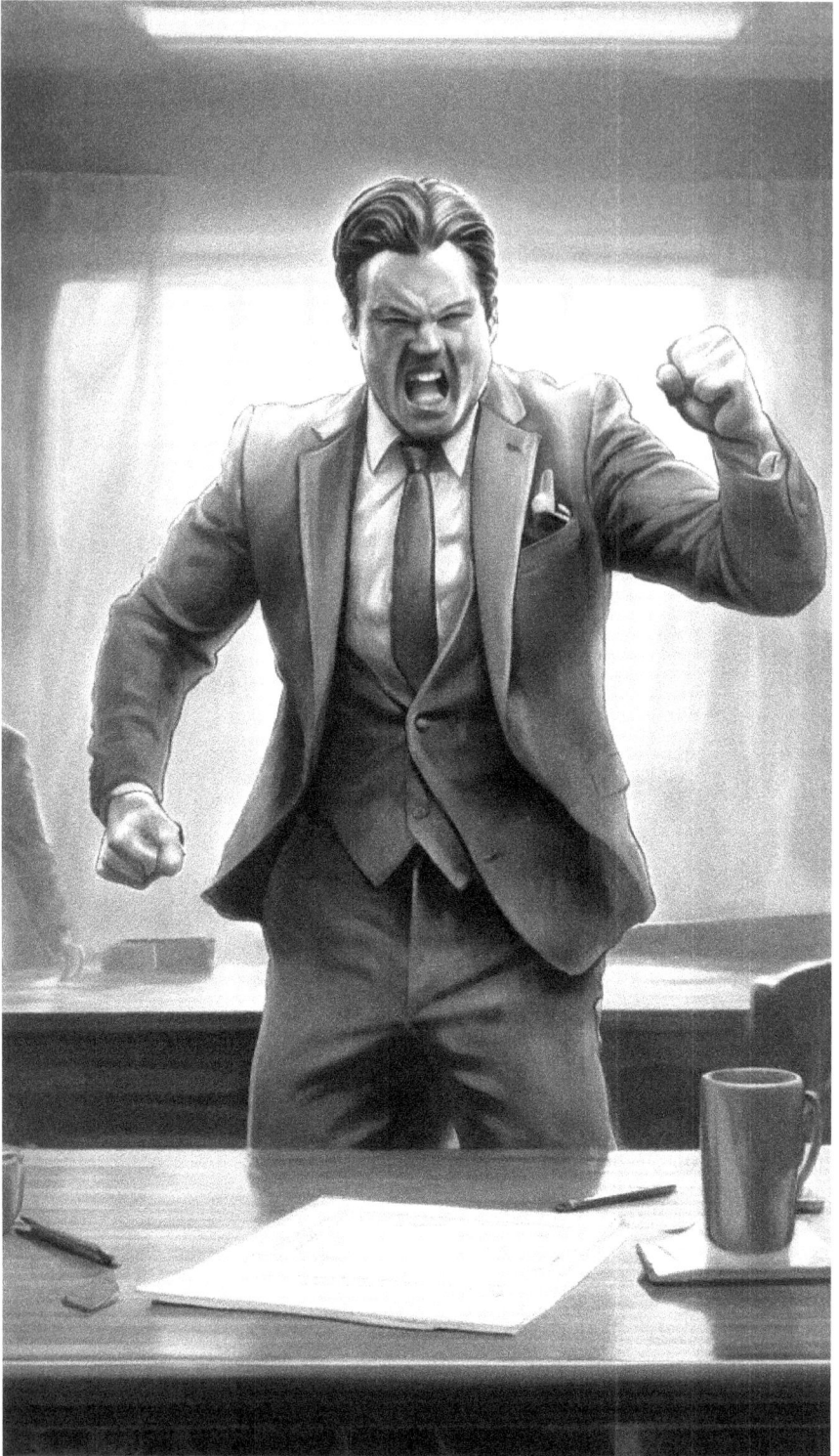

CHAPTER 19

Violent Behavior

What is violence?

In the context of violence, clarifying the meanings of specific terms is crucial to avoid misleading interchangeable use.

- **Aggression –** the root word '-gress' refers to 'moving' or 'stepping'. 'Progress' means moving forward, 'regress' means moving backward, and 'aggress' means moving towards. The most common reaction of an organism facing danger is to flee. Instead, if an organism intentionally moves towards potential conflict or danger, it is called 'aggression'. Aggression is not necessarily a bad or good thing and implies a phenomenon of moving towards a target or situation despite the possibility of difficulty or conflict. Aggressiveness is a trait. In certain professions, such as sales, sports, and marketing, aggressiveness would be a desirable trait.

- **Anger –**an affective state characterized by feelings of antagonism (i.e., being against) towards a person, target, or situation. In other words, anger is an affective state characterized by hostility towards another object, person, or situation. It is an unpleasant affective state, which means that the individual experiencing this state feels compelled to act in a way to get rid of the unpleasantness – i.e., to destroy the target, object, person, or situation perceived to be the cause of the unpleasantness.

- **Agitation –** a psychomotor state associated with the affective state of anger. Psychomotor activity that results from anger (loud voice, angry expression, fisting, clenching, slamming, or throwing) is called agitation.

- **Violence –** a behavior that physically damages a person, object, target, or situation. Violence may happen due to anger or in the absence of anger.

To summarize, aggressiveness is a trait or nature of a person. Aggressiveness does not necessarily imply an angry mood or violent behavior. Anger is an unpleasant emotional or affective state that may drive a person to act in a way that causes physical damage. Violence is a behavior that directly or indirectly causes physical damage but may not be necessarily driven by anger or aggressiveness.

Understanding the Types of Violence

All violence is not the same. Certain types of violence are needed for self-defense or disciplinary action. Violence can also be differentiated as 'instrumental' vs 'reactive'. The instrumental type is goal-directed, premeditated, unprovoked, and less amenable to modification through clinical intervention. The reactive type of violence often follows some form of provocation and calms down after the disappearance of the provocative stimulus. Reactive-type violence is more amenable to pharmacotherapy and behavioral intervention. I find this type of classification less useful, as provocation is hard to objectify – nearly all violent individuals perceive some form of provocation or justification for their violent behavior.

Instead, it is helpful to classify violence into two forms: maleficent and ***non-maleficent (Mananalam Clinic Experience)***. Maleficence implies ill intent. Maleficent violence is often premeditated, motivated by intentions to cause harm, to derive pleasure from others' loss or suffering. Usually, it is accompanied by a lack of remorse or concern for consequences. Non-maleficent violence is non-premeditated, not motivated by ill will or intention to cause harm and follows impulsive reaction to anger or perceived hostility. The differential diagnoses of maleficent violence include antisocial personality disorder, substance abuse disorder, and schizophrenia. In contrast, those related to non-maleficent violence include dementia, bipolar disorder, personality disorders other than antisocial PD, traumatic brain injury, mental retardation, autism, impulse control disorders, and seizure disorders.

Is violence a Mental Health Problem?

There is a general perception among the public that violent behavior is rooted in mental disorders. One could see that in everyday parlay – if a person displays extreme rage or violent behavior, they are called a 'psycho'. The general public believes that to be extraordinarily violent, one must have lost one's mind. The inverse of this line of perception also exists among the public – if a person has mental health problems, they may be violent or potentially dangerous to be around. Most of these perceptions are introduced and reinforced by popular media. This has led to public stigma and reluctance to treat psychiatric illnesses in the community setting. The highly protective and securitized imagery of psychiatric wards in movies and novels has also contributed to this perception.

The truth is contrary to this perception – most mental health patients are harmless and not violent. They are more likely to be victims rather than perpetrators of violence. The exceptions to this generalization are antisocial personality disorders and substance abuse disorders, often associated with maleficent violence. Antisocial personality disorders carry a higher risk of violence – but this type of personality disorder constitutes only a minor fraction of the overall population, so violence due to this diagnosis does not constitute a significant burden. The other and more prevalent mental health-related cause of violent behavior is substance abuse. The base rate of violence in the substance abuse population is significantly higher than in the general population. Contrary to popular belief, substance abuse with marijuana also carries a higher risk of violence.

Education of the public that mental health patients are not necessarily dangerous people is essential. Violence is more of a public health problem, but this aspect of violence is not relevant to clinical practice and is outside the scope of this textbook.

However, psychiatrists and non-psychiatrists will have to deal with patients with violent behavior at some point in their careers. The most common situations related to violence faced by the psychiatrist in clinical practice are -

- **Defiant behavior –** When a patient resists treatment or instructions, the situation escalates into conflict and often precipitates anger and rage in the patient. A psychiatrist is then consulted to evaluate the patient for 'violent behavior' or 'aggressive behavior'. Often, this is not violence at all and does not happen if the patient is not put in a position to act against their wishes. Examples include patients with dementia who yell or topple objects when trying to be fed or bathed.

- **Requests to evaluate future risk of violence –** Psychiatrists are often asked to evaluate individuals considered at risk for acting out in violence. One typical example is when schoolchildren make verbal or behavioral threats. They are brought to the psychiatrist by the school counselor to evaluate the potential for actual violence in the future. In these situations, the psychiatrist must refrain from quantifying or certifying risk and stick to clinical evaluation of the person and treatment of associated psychiatric diagnoses alone.

- **Objectively verifiable acts of physical damage** – These are patients with a history of violent episodes, verifiable and witnessed, resulting in measurable physical damage to a person or property.

Risk Factors for Violent Behavior

Risk factors may be categorized as static or dynamic based on the fluidity of the risk factor in the patient's life.

Static risk factors include demographic variables such as age, sex, race, family history, psychiatric diagnosis, mental retardation, or enduring personality traits. Dynamic risk factors include clinical variables such as psychotic symptoms, alcohol/substance abuse, and strength of the therapeutic alliance, and situational variables such as social support, interpersonal conflict, occupational status, access to weapons, and the availability of potential victims.

Psychiatric diagnoses and violence

The base rate of violence in the general population is low, in the range of 2%. In the presence of one psychiatric diagnosis other than substance abuse, the risk ranges from 2-8%. In substance abuse disorders, the risk increases to ~21%. In the presence of substance abuse and another psychiatric diagnosis, the risk varies between 20% to 30%. Within substance abuse disorders, the risk of violence is ~19% with marijuana use, ~25% with alcohol use, and ~35% with other substances. These are rough estimates and may vary across different societies. Nevertheless, the take-home message is that the risk of violence increases only marginally with the presence of psychiatric diagnoses other than substance abuse, and this increase could also be due to the reporting of defiant and non-cooperative responses to treatment as violence. The absolute risk of violence by individuals with mental illness, particularly the more severe violence, remains minimal. Substance abuse is associated with a marked increase in propensity for violence.

Dementia deserves special mention in this regard. According to some data sources, working in nursing homes (or homes for older adults) could be more dangerous than working in mines or construction! This is due to violence perpetrated by old individuals with dementia on their caretakers. It usually takes the form of 'catastrophic reactions' during attempts to redirect or assist them with bathing, toileting, or dressing. These events tend to happen in the evening, a phenomenon called 'sundowning'.

Patients with closed head injuries typically display a combination of apathy, impulsiveness, irritability, and occasional outbursts of violence. Violent behavior may be related to injury to specific neuroanatomical regions – injury to a particular region in the brain's amygdala may lead to rage responses. In contrast, injury to another amygdala region may cause inhibited expression of anger. There have been studies that have demonstrated a higher rate of EEG abnormalities among impulsive and aggressive individuals. However, these findings are non-specific, and it is clinically impossible (at least with the knowledge and methods available) to associate violent behavior in a patient with a neuroanatomical anomaly or injury.

Patients with seizure disorders become violent during the ictal state or the state of postictal confusion. Violence during the postictal phase is disorganized and not goal-directed. Some with seizure disorder exhibit violent outbursts out of proportion to provocative stimuli. Such individuals may have underlying neuropsychological impairments, lower IQ, or a comorbid psychiatric illness.

There is a strong independent negative correlation between IQ and the risk of violence (i.e., the lower the IQ, the higher the risk of violence). When studied in the UK general adult population, the risk of violence perpetration fell linearly from 16% for IQ 70-79 to a low of 2% for IQ 120 and above, and this correlation was independent of demographic variables, behavioral factors, childhood adversity, and psychiatric comorbidity.

Personality traits are enduring factors and may increase the risk of violence in a durable fashion. Those who display easy ability to get frustrated or have difficulty controlling their expression of anger or displeasure, instability of affective states and impulsiveness are at higher risk for perpetrating violence. Some of these traits may cluster consistently, allowing for the diagnosis of specific personality disorders, especially borderline PD and antisocial PD.

Sex Differences in Violence

There are distinct differences in the characteristics of violence between men and women. Men are three times more likely to engage in violent behavior than women. The difference gets blunted in the setting of psychiatric illnesses. Targets (or victims) of women's acts of violence are more likely to be family members, while those of men are more likely to be either acquaintances or strangers. Violent acts by women are more likely to occur at home, whereas those by men are more likely to occur outdoors, on the streets. Violence by men is more likely to be associated with alcohol or substance use intoxication. Violence by men is more likely to be more severe in intensity, associated with grievous injury, and more likely to invite legal trouble. Psychiatrists are likely to be more accurate in predicting the risk of violence in men than women. Despite these differences, caution must be exercised in assigning the sex of an individual as a causative factor or predominant predictive factor for violence.

Children and Violence

Being a victim or witness of violence is a risk factor for violence in adulthood. Children can often be perpetrators or victims of violence. Childhood abuse and neglect are often associated with a lack of adequate supervision during the phase of moral sense development, which also correlates with the risk of violence, especially of the maleficent type. The availability of lethal weapons is a significant factor in child homicides. High-end firearms and lethal weapons are commonly present in some homogeneous ethnic and rural areas, especially in certain parts of Northern India. Still, the rates are far below compared to urban areas with a lower density of firearms.

Childhood learning disorders and ADHD are also associated with an increased risk of violence. Children with ADHD receive little reward from academics and soon find the entire educative environment unrewarding. Eventually, they become disruptive and ultimately drop out of school. Enjoying no support from their family or the school system, their impulsiveness is more likely to become linked to socially disruptive behavior. While taking the patient's social history during the psychiatric assessment, developmental history must be explored in detail for this reason.

Domestic Violence

Most domestic violence incidents are not reported to legal authorities, which necessitates detailed awareness on the part of the clinicians. The battering of females is more prevalent, and the perpetrator may not necessarily be male. Perpetrators could be spouses, intimate partners, family members, or frequent acquaintances. Some studies suggest that roughly one-third of emergency room visits by women result from domestic violence, and more severe forms of such violence may end in homicide. About 22% of the homicides are committed by a stranger, 44% by an acquaintance, and 20% by a family member. Battered women suffer from depression, substance use disorder, and PTSD. Children in these households are at greater risk of being abused themselves. Abuse may not necessarily be by the male partner. When spousal abuse occurs in a household, it can be associated with anxiety, depression, emotional disturbances, low esteem, and school problems in children. Children growing up in these households may exhibit violent behavior during childhood and adulthood.

Workplace Violence

Workplace violence, which includes violence (verbal and physical) related and not related to the work environment but happening in the workplace, is a cause of lost work time, productivity, employee burnout, occupational injury, or death. Data points to the most common attacker being a customer, stranger, co-worker, employer, or former employee, in that order. Commonly cited reasons include revenge, jealousy, and financial gain. Non-fatal assault is much more common in the healthcare sector. In some instances of workplace violence, the background job stress in the work environment may be so high that the victim and the co-workers experience pervasive fear, stress, or depression.

Interviewing Patients with Violent Behavior

An exhaustive interview is typically impossible if the patient is violent or agitated. The psychiatrist must have an agenda first to establish certain critical information and then to proceed to more detailed interviews in another setting. In this context, first, try to understand the nature of the violent behavior by establishing the following aspects –

- **Magnitude –** refers to the scope of the violent behavior. It spans from verbal outbursts to pushing, slapping, hitting, battering, or severe enough to cause grievous injury or death.

- **Likelihood –** refers to the probability of the violent behavior happening, given the likelihood of the situations that precipitate it. For example, if violence happens when the patient is intoxicated, gather information on how frequently they visit the bar or drink.

- **Imminence –** refers to the possibility of violence happening anytime soon. Violence may be imminent under certain circumstances and not under certain circumstances. Clinicians must be able to identify this aspect accurately and are most often good at doing it.

- **Frequency –** refers to the number of times the violent behavior has occurred within a certain period. Is it rare or a common occurrence? Sometimes, even infrequent or one-time occurrences could have been severe enough to invite legal consequences (e.g., child abuse).

Next, establish the stage or phase of violent behavior the patient is in and then take the appropriate measures to mitigate it and protect yourself. The phases are as follows –

- **Safety phase –** This is a phase where the patient could be imminently dangerous. Such patients are often impulsive and seem to be in turbulent emotional crisis. They are labile, volatile, and may act at any time. This situation is indeed a clinical challenge. Physicians cannot conduct a fruitful psychiatric assessment if they feel threatened or intimidated. If patients are in this phase, first secure them in a safe and quiet location with no hazardous objects, preferably in the presence of other personnel trained in the physical restraint of patients. If the family or attendees of the patient are found to be valuable and protective, keep them around. If they may precipitate or aggravate the violence, ask them to leave.

- **Calm phase –** This phase is where the patient is reliably calm, cooperative, relaxed, and willing to undergo the interview. A more detailed assessment is possible in this phase.

- **Agitated phase –** This phase is where the patient exhibits psychomotor activity that suggests impulsiveness or imminence of violence. For example, pacing the room, foot tapping, fisting, clenching, etc. Such patients experience intense anxiety, pervasive uneasiness, and sometimes confusion. They may also exhibit approach-avoidance type psychomotor activity – for example, they may walk to another person or an object invitingly, stare or analyze it, feel disgusted or uneasy, and then walk away. These patients may be able to provide valuable and reliable information but need some catharsis or ventilation for their anxiety and uneasiness. Facial expressions reveal their internal mental state reliably in this phase. The psychiatrist must engage these patients through constant questioning and chatting but with unassuming, non-judgmental, and empathetic questions. Appear relaxed and confident and maintain good eye contact with the patient. Let the patient vent.

- **Verbally aggressive phase - This is a phase where the patient is verbally aggressive –** yelling, cussing, cursing, and threatening. They become defensive, question authority (asking to speak to someone higher in authority or report a complaint against the psychiatrist), and may become increasingly demanding and insistent – this usually means that physical violence is imminent. In this phase, a detailed interview is not possible. Summon security or nursing staff. However, do it in such a way that the patient does not feel 'trapped' in the room, as it may precipitate violence. A detailed assessment is not possible in this phase, so use the time to focus on exploring the cause of the patient's rage and loss of control. Stay at least one meter or an arm/leg distance away from the patient, seated at a 45-degree angle to the patient's face, and closer to the door to leave anytime. Appear calm and relaxed and converse with the patient in a gentle but firm tone. Use short, firm, closed-ended , and non-threatening sentences. If they are confused or agitated, use firm verbal cues to redirect them. Questions must be directed towards allowing the patient to discuss their reasons for rage, allowing them to vent and feel empowered. Allow the patient to employ coping strategies that may decrease their anger. Unnecessary delay in de-escalating the verbal aggressiveness could result in physical violence. If verbal aggression escalates, terminate the interview before physical violence happens. Patients may be offered drugs to help them calm, if appropriate. Parental medications may be administered if the patient is willing and permits.

- **Physically aggressive phase** – Patients are intimidating in this phase. They commit or attempt an assault, throw or fling objects, damage property, and grab or attack people. If verbal commands fail to affect the behavior immediately, a 'show of force' through physical restraint or involuntary pharmacological therapy is necessary to prevent injury to the patient, physician, and others. Placing the patient in seclusion or restraints is possible and sometimes the safest option, but it is unpleasant for the patient. When patients regain control, they feel guilty and ashamed of their actions. Assure them that the mental health personnel will continue to help maintain their control. Patients may resent the use of restraints - remind them it is for their safety and those of others. Staff trained in physical restraint and the use of medications in this situation are beneficial to the psychiatrist.

In general, violent patients feel justified in their violence. They try to explain, sometimes quite convincingly, the provocations that justify their acts of violence. Do not argue, explain, or lecture. Allow and encourage them to talk more – usually, it helps de-escalate their anger. Sometimes, the physician may feel convinced of their explanation, sympathetic towards the patient's situation, and behave over-protectively. The latter should also be avoided. Sometimes, novice clinicians or trainees focus more on their performance in this situation and may miss obvious clinical cues necessary for mitigating the situation. Avoid appearing intimidated by the patient as well. In this short interim, focus on gathering information on precipitating factors, cues to de-escalate the anger, and a psychosocial support system available for the patient. Try to understand if the patient's social network is precipitating or failing to mitigate the violent tendencies of the patient. Suppose it appears that the patient will return to a social situation or a network that is hostile, unsympathetic, or toxic to the patient's situation. In that case, the patient must be excluded from those networks.

Focus on substance abuse history and interpersonal conflicts usually prevalent in this patient population.

If time permits, look for repetitive dysfunctional patterns currently being relived. Elicit past stressors and traumas. Prior incidents, prior hospitalizations related to violent incidents, prior history of psychiatric diagnosis, and other seminal events from past psychosocial, family, occupational, and medical histories should be inquired. If possible, the physician should also explore the past circumstances of all violent episodes, including the patient's state of mind, environment, and target of the violence during the episode.

Certain dimensional variables obtained through history taking reflect 'core' aspects of a personality dimension that increases the propensity of violence, especially of the maleficent type (Mananalam Clinic Experience). They include a history of being charged with reckless driving offenses causing grievous injury, multiple job transitions without spending long in any one (likely due to being fired for truant behavior), public intoxication, childhood fire setting, fights and brawls, shoplifting, cruelty to animals, school truancy, suspensions, drug use, sexual promiscuity, coercive sexual activities, destruction of property, deceitfulness and lack of remorse.

Managing Violence in Psychiatric Inpatient Units

Although most psychiatric inpatients are not violent, violence in psychiatric inpatient units is not uncommon. Such incidents commonly go undocumented and are accompanied by some level of injury to the staff. Most assaults and injuries occur during seclusion or restraint of a patient (i.e., non-maleficent, unplanned, and defiant behavior). Violent behavior is more prevalent in acute admission wards and locked units because it houses the most unstable patients. Assaults occur during periods of 'increased activity' such as visiting days or during periods of 'relative inactivity' in chronically admitted patients.

The psychiatric diagnoses commonly associated with inpatient violence include mania, schizophrenia, dementia, personality disorders, and alcoholism. The violence associated with mania often results from increased irritability and behavioral disinhibition and is not associated with prior threats or premeditation.

The violence associated with schizophrenia is associated with prior threats and executed after prior planning. The persecutory deluded patient formulates a plan, procures a weapon, predetermines the victim, and executes the plan at a determined time. The disorganized schizophrenic is more likely to engage in unplanned violence during a long-term admission.

Typically, the staff members who appear or are described as strict, intolerant, rigid, authoritarian, and adversarial are at greater risk of being assaulted.

Predicting Violent Behavior

The psychiatrist is sometimes, and increasingly commonly, called upon to provide an 'opinion' on a person's dangerousness. In essence, the psychiatrist is asked to predict the risk of violence perpetrated by the person in question. Sometimes, it may be necessary for psychiatrists to divulge patient information to protect third parties from unforeseen violence that the patient could perpetrate. In these situations, the psychiatrist may find themselves conflicted between societal and ethical obligations towards the patient.

Dangerousness is not a trait, a symptom, a risk factor, or a clinical diagnosis. It is a measure of the propensity of a particular event across a specific time interval – it is assessed for legal purposes to document the patient's qualification to be subject to inpatient admission or involuntary detention. It is impossible to quantify this propensity precisely; therefore, psychiatrists must refrain from making categorical statements or quantifying risk calculations. Instead, it is more appropriate to state the risk in relative terms – such as 'higher than usual probability of...' or 'higher than prior risk of...'. Risk calculations comparing a patient's risk of future violence to their prior risk are more reliable and clinically useful than comparing the patient's risk to historically published data based on MSE variables.

The determination of the risk is not the same as the decision to commit the patient to involuntary confinement. The determination of the risk of violent behavior is to enable the goal of treatment, which is not to eliminate all the risk (it is not possible anyway), but to intervene on modifiable risk factors to reduce the risk of violent behavior to a lower level than it was initially or before intervention. The decision to commit a patient to involuntary commitment is based on the imminence and magnitude of the violence – which in turn depends on patient-specific dimensional variables (as discussed above). Generally, the psychiatrist must estimate the raw risk of violence by considering the demographic variables and published data, then adjust the risk based on patient-specific individual dimensional variables (such as impulsivity, enduring personality traits, psychosocial history, and social support). The latter could vary based on cultural, ethnic, and local factors. Eventually, the psychiatrist could develop their personal algorithm based on local factors and personal experience. I say this because the risk associated with specific types of delusions or command-type hallucinations and the patient's tendency to respond to those stimuli vary significantly.

The factors that best help make this nuanced adjustment are derived from specific personality dimensions that are not apparent during brief interviews or from impersonal study of the medical records alone. Core antisocial personality traits such as lack of empathy, absence of remorse, disdain for societal rules and obligations, disregard for others' rights, presence of violent fantasies, impulsiveness, and irritability are best assessed only through comprehensive, time-consuming examination. Sometimes, such comprehensive assessment needs multiple sessions. Corroborating history from witnesses of the violence is also valuable for assessing the core traits mentioned above. Listening to the patient's own description of the conduct of the violence throws light on the state of mind, perception of reality, presence of remorse or empathy, and the regard of the patient for the victims of violence.

A prior history of violence is the best standalone predictor of violent behavior. The legal system understands this pattern better, which is why the 'history of priors' (i.e., history of prior offenses or convictions) plays a vital role in the judge's decision to pardon or convict a defendant and allow bail. According to a statistic, the probability of committing an offense is 80% if there is a history of 4 priors and nearly 100% if there is a history of 5 priors.

This chapter's crucial take-home message is that it is best to approach violence as a 'behavior' rather than a clinical condition.

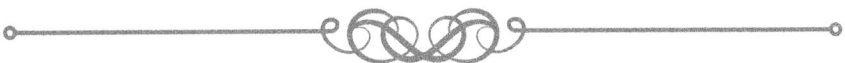

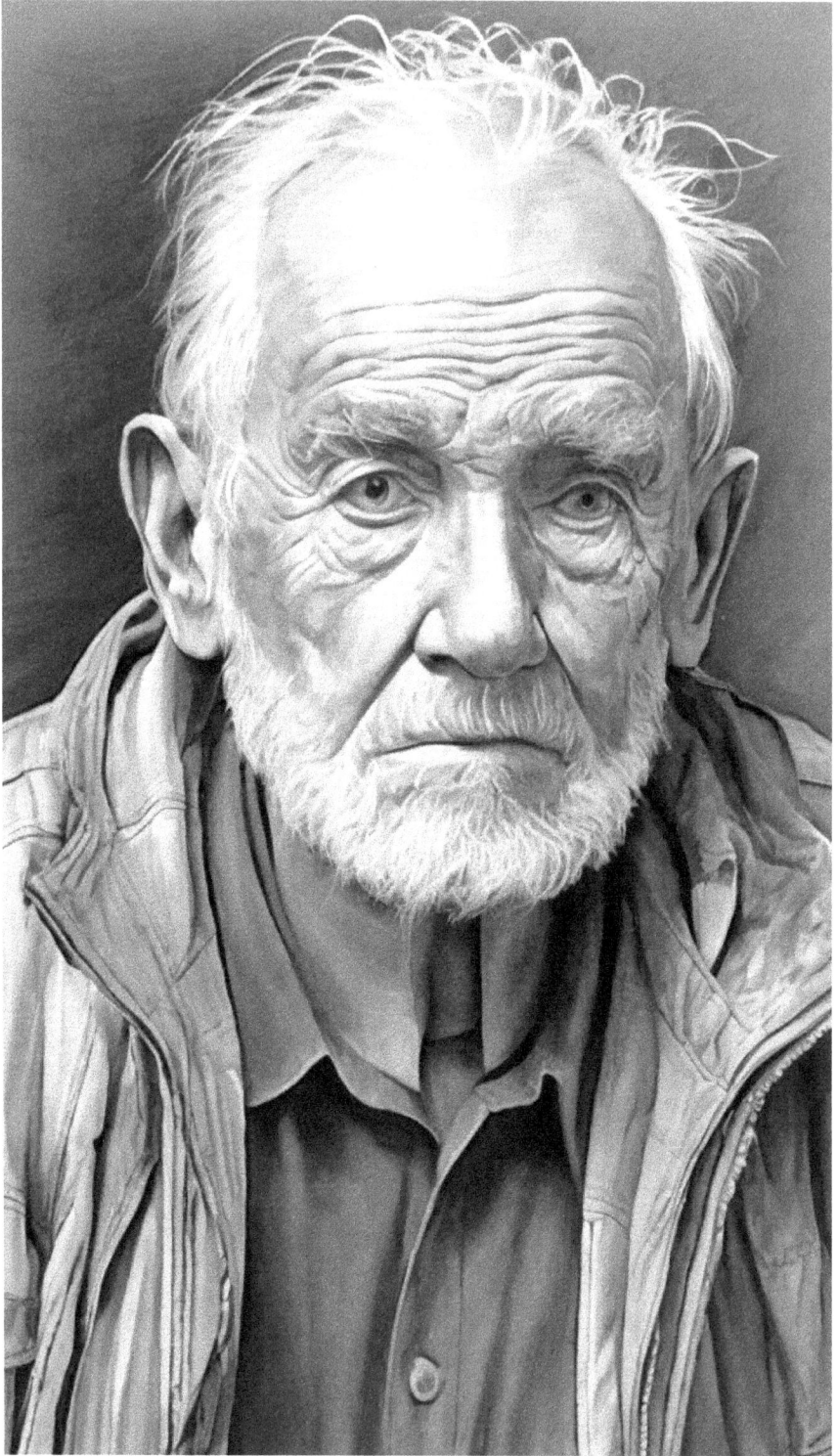

CHAPTER 20

Geriatric Psychiatry

The world is growing older. In all known history, the last century has been the most liveable, prosperous, and stable for humankind. Most people over 80 would remember that world geopolitics was almost always unstable and unpredictable during their early life. Every person of the older generation has seen some version of war and foreign armies in their land. Borders were fluid, and migrations and displacements were common. Most of the world, regardless of nationality, lived in abject poverty. Early death was routine – infections, sickness, childbirth, trauma, and war took plenty of lives. Maternal and infant mortality were not uncommon. To have lived another year was a success, which is why celebrating birthdays was meaningful. Those who survived to adulthood were considered blessed, and those who survived to old age were considered extraordinarily gifted and lucky. Amongst most societies, especially in the Eastern hemisphere, respecting, revere, and honoring older individuals is a virtue. It is still common practice in South Asia to celebrate 60th and 70th birthdays with extra fanfare and re-enact the marital rituals on these birthdays. Generally, if women survived childbirth, they ended up living longer than men, who were subject to riskier livelihoods outdoors. Due to a lack of medical advances, only those who were inherently physically healthy and mentally resilient survived to old age. Thus, a common observational bias was that older individuals were generally wise, strong, and resourceful.

However, after World War II, the world's geopolitics has been relatively stable until now. The advent of nuclear weapons and the emergence of extraordinarily militarily strong nation-states has deterred the tendency for conflict. In many countries, generations of people are about to enter the geriatric age without having ever seen a foreign army in their homelands in their lifetime. Globalization of the economy has shifted and distributed the labor burden to much poorer nations that now have developed more stable government systems with reasonable health care and education. This has allowed for growth in science and technology, which has positively impacted health care, resulting in longer life spans in several underdeveloped countries. Vaccinations, antibiotics, surgeries, medications, emergency resuscitation, and intensive care facilities have deterred death on a massive scale. Consequently, the world population has grown significantly in the last century, with a growing elderly population. While this may be good news, the flip side is that the assumption that the older population was generally healthier and wiser is no longer valid. The older population is increasingly unhealthy, both physically and mentally. They are considered a nuisance in lower socioeconomic societies, and elder abuse has become increasingly reported. Older people are segregated into facilities and institutions such as old-age homes, nursing homes, etc.

Geriatric medicine has become a well-established specialty during the last few decades. The mental health field has only been recently warming up to this development. During my training in Tamil Nadu in the 1970s, one of my senior professors mentioned that he had 'never' come across a patient with dementia, and it was only found through descriptions found in Western medical textbooks. Even during the busiest times of my practice in Tamil Nadu before the year 2000, older patients (in their 60s or 70s) were rare. Today, I see at least 2-3 new patients above 60 years, per week in my practice. Psychiatric disorders in the geriatric population may be new onset psychiatric illnesses, the discovery of chronic conditions that have existed before, or complications of medical comorbidities.

The flagship psychiatric disorder in the geriatric population is dementia. Dementia, as the word indicates, is 'de-mentation'. It is an organic brain syndrome, where structural deterioration results in the deterioration of the brain's functioning, affecting mental processes. I ask the reader to refer to the initial chapter on the Ulan. The Ulan is a functional concept, an amalgamation of mood, thought, and intellect. The seat of the Ulan is the body, specifically the brain. The aging process of the brain thus affects the functioning of the Ulan. Intellect is the primary component of the Ulan that is affected by dementia. Medical textbooks describe various 'types' of dementia – the psychiatrist needs to be familiar with the types, but these are of academic importance only. In clinical practice, recognition of early dementia is a challenging task. Very little can be done to improve the condition. Educating the caregiver and honing the cognition of the caregiver is the mainstay of treatment.

As mentioned above, the component of the Ulan primarily affected by dementia is the intellect. The mood (i.e., affect) is relatively well preserved.

Intellectual deficits, however, result in thought and mood disturbances as a downstream effect. In the disease's most subtle and early stages, dementia manifests as behavioral abnormalities. It is only in later stages that memory deficits begin to manifest more clearly. Furthermore, it is uncommon for patients to present with memory deficits as the chief complaint. Usually, it is some behavioral abnormality that results in psychiatric referral. Some of the typical early manifestations encountered in my clinical practice *(Mananalam Clinic Experience)* are as follows –

- **Grammatical mistakes** – early dementia is manifested by linguistic slips, especially in grammar, syntax, or choice of words. Those who have been fluent and proficient in language may be seen to have glaring slips in grammar, and when prompted to their mistake, would adamantly argue and justify it (unlike their usual self). Those around may concede to their arguments out of respect and courtesy. They may forget the right choice of a word, may use a poorly chosen substitute word, and persist on its use as being accurate. Even after the incident, they are preoccupied with proving their mistakes as accurate, which leads to the breakdown of interpersonal relationships.

- **Searching** – They may search for lost things, and sometimes things that are not lost. They search for missing things in places where they are unlikely to find them. They may blame others for misplacing them or suspect they stole them.

- **Argumentative and Quarreling** – Patients engage in arguments beneath their position. A highly positioned officer or judge would end by picking up an argument with an unseemly bystander, a doorman, or the waitress at a restaurant. These arguments are impulsive and often for silly issues. They 'make a scene' for no good reason and do not regret it. They tend to 'pick up' quarrels or fight over silly disagreements.

- **Strange behavior** – Patient may engage in behavior outside their usual nature. They may make traffic stops in unlikely places and buy unneeded items. Friends and families notice this as surprising behavior. They may either praise or criticize someone, like a bystander on the street or someone in a room, for no real reason and may continue with that line of thought for an unusually long time.

- **Verbal looseness** – They may utter silly comments, foul words, obscene phrases, or engage in disgraceful gestures they have never indulged in before. They may smile or giggle inappropriately, such as giggling at a funeral. They don't regret these actions.

- **Unexplained friendliness** – They may have lost a long-held hatred for an enemy or adversary and speak to them with sudden friendliness. These unexpected changes in social patterns may disrupt existing social relationships.

- **Childish behavior** – Their taste in choices or demeanor generally becomes childish. They may ask for an extra serving during dinner like a child would, may get excited when they see a new object or a toy, or may childishly engage with teenagers, all of which may stir unnecessary gossip or ill will among family members, who may conclude that the patient is perverted or mean.

- **Financial failings** – They exhibit major flaws in spending, accounting, cash handling, or bills. These are manifestations of intellectual deficits and may lead to compensatory behaviors such as shunning responsibilities, delinquencies, and withdrawal-type behavior.

- **Abrupt change in long-held routines** – One who has always gone for a morning walk or run with friends for years would drop this routine. In India, those who have been going to temples on a specific day for years may stop doing so.

- **Loss of long-held beliefs** – These usually pertain to religious rituals. Those who have long held strong beliefs about ideologies or religious concepts would be seen to have 'let go' of such ideologies and beliefs.

- **Loss of patience** – They tend to have a lower threshold for losing patience than usual. This is not to be confused with irritability or emotional lability.

- **Getting lost** – They may lose their way, even from well-known routes from work or home. They may lose the concept of time in social situations or public places and may be seen wandering away from the group for a long time. In India, it usually happens during pilgrimages to crowded temple sites, where they might get lost. The families, usually due to pre-existing animosity from disruptive behavior by them, tend to let them be lost and abandon them. These individuals may forget to clean themselves, search for food, and may appear like homeless individuals. They get mistaken for conmen or liars by the public and are considered a nuisance.

- **Violent behavior** - According to one statistic from the Western world, the nursing home for the elderly is one of the most dangerous places to work due to unforeseen acts of violence perpetrated by inhabitants on the nursing aids and caregivers. Demented individuals may unexpectedly strike, slap, or throw objects at others, especially the caregivers. They may strike away the feeding hand of the caregiver or splash them with food. These acts are unplanned, not malicious, arising from altered perceptions or cognitive deficits. They neither remember these acts nor express regret.

- **Sexual misbehavior** - This is a common complaint. However, these sexual advances are not actually sexual in nature, and are not done for sexual gratification. They are due to cognitive deficits or perceptual abnormalities. Sometimes, they may hold on to a person and be unable to let go of their posture, which may be misunderstood as a sexual grab.

- **Deliberate self-harm** - During the early stages of dementia, the patient regrets their repeated untoward and bizarre mistakes and becomes ashamed of their behavior. Their affect is still preserved, so they deeply regret their mistakes, resulting in deliberate self-harm and punishment. This is quite typical in early dementia; hence, any deliberate self-harm in the geriatric population must raise the suspicion of early dementia.

- **Other symptoms** - Unexplained loss of appetite, unintentional weight loss, forgetting to flush the toilet, urinating or soiling the bed, urgency in urination (especially in women), exiting the restroom or their room without putting on the clothes back on, sleep disturbances, unable to handover messages to others, wandering, forgetting meal times, forgetting names, etc are some of the other features in early dementia.

It is commonly taught that the predominant manifestation of dementia is memory loss. However, I have yet to see any dementia patient being brought by their family for memory loss. In other words, in day-to-day clinical practice, memory loss is not the presenting complaint that results in an eventual diagnosis of dementia. Instead, the most common presenting complaint is some behavioral issue – some form of behavior alteration that results in interpersonal, social, or relationship problems. This is because the commoner believes memory loss is an expected 'normal' consequence of advancing age. Furthermore, the commoner believes that the strength of the memory is directly proportional to the time it is held. For example, the memory of events that happened years or decades ago is believed to be stronger than the memory of events that happened the day before. As we know, dementia typically begins with short-term memory loss with relative sparing of long-term memory. Patients with early dementia tend to recount their memories accurately from childhood or early adulthood. So, their caregivers tend to disregard dementia as a possible diagnosis for their short-term memory loss. Instead, they attribute it to transient illnesses, stress, recent travel, etc.

Early dementia, through its behavioral disturbances, produces significant conflict within the family and may lead to elder neglect or abuse. The immediate family and friends become significantly stressed and distressed. Educating the caregivers and the family about the disease of dementia and how it affects their behavior allows them to be forgiving, compassionate, and caring of their loved ones. This is where I find the education of the Ulan concept (as mentioned in the earlier chapter on Ulan) very useful. When caregivers understand how the Ulan operates, their dislike flips to sympathy and compassion. Education should emphasize that this is an organic brain syndrome, and no one is 'immune' to it. Family must be educated to avoid hiding these individuals from social situations to prevent their embarrassment.

The onset of dementia is notoriously insidious and gets more apparent in the setting of an unrelated medical illness. Dementia could get acutely exacerbated during infections, such as urinary tract infections common in the geriatric population. Falls, fractures, and head injuries are also common. Lack of self-care and poor personal hygiene must be looked for and cared for by the caregivers. Segregating them in institutions is not a good idea and must be avoided whenever possible.

There is a lot of research on dementia and how to avoid or slow down the process. The data is unclear for the most part. Still, from my experience, there are two ways that could reliably prevent accelerated dementation

– the first is regular aerobic exercise enhances cerebral blood flow and neuronal oxygen delivery. The other is avoidance of alcohol (earlier in life), which is known to have cumulative subclinical metabolic encephalopathic effects even with minor use.

Another observation noted in the Mananalam Clinic is the difficulty working individuals and couples face in caring for their elderly parents. This difficulty creates significant inconveniences, losses, and disruptions that unconsciously leads to resentment, neglect, and abuse, leading to clinical deterioration in the presence of dementia or other psychiatric diagnoses. Moving them to an old-age or nursing home often increases resentment and clinical deterioration. Instead, I suggest a daycare model for older adults, where working men and women can drop off their elderly folk and pick them up on their way back from work. The latter allows them social interaction and physical activity during the day and while having family time in the evenings. That, I think, would be a happy medium.

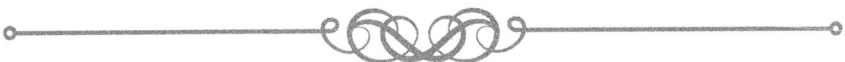

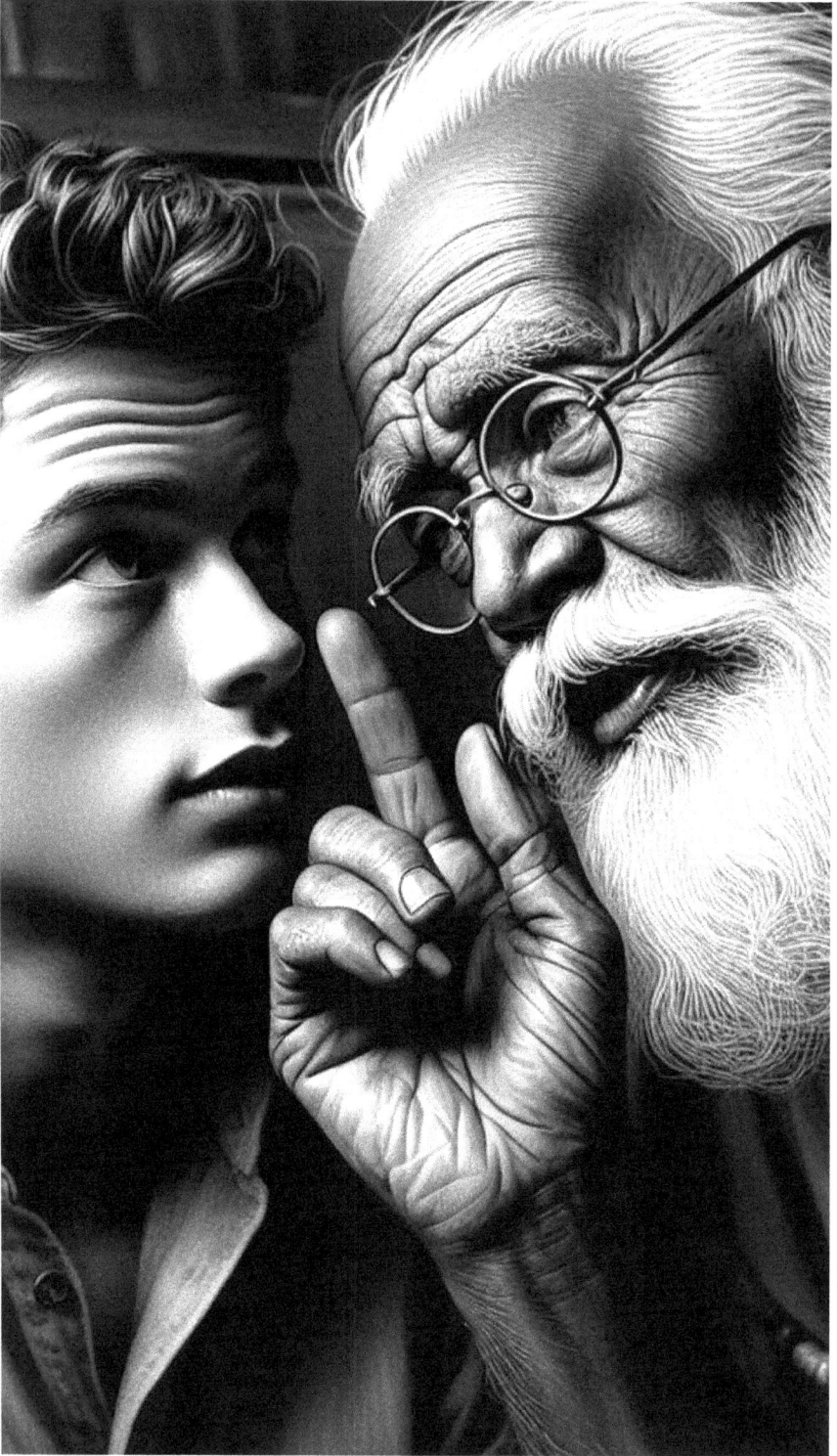

CHAPTER 21

Points of Wisdom for the Practicing Psychiatrist

#1 Know the Tongue.

Language is the ether of psychiatry. Mood is expressed in language. Thoughts are processed and expressed through words. The ability to handle language reflects intelligence. Regardless of your native tongue or medium of instruction during school and college, you must master the language of the people you cater to. You may have mastered psychiatric knowledge and skills and may be the most intelligent person in the room. Still, you are only as good a psychiatrist as your proficiency in your patient's language.

Patients express themselves in imperfect language. They do not choose words accurately, may use words interchangeably, and may not be not adept in grammar. Most of the time, their vocabulary and grammar are incorrect. You must know the common inaccuracies and imperfections of their language so you can interpret their words correctly. In other words, *you must be correct about their wrongs.* When you speak, use simple and short sentences. Avoid overly medical terms.

The best way to go about mastering any language is to use the dictionary while you study. If you use the dictionary while reading the textbook, you would be surprised how often you have misunderstood the meanings of words you were so confident about.

You must also be familiar with the local dialect or vocabulary of the language specific to the county or zip code. This would also improve the rapport with the patient.

#2 Watch Your Step.

Have you noticed a disproportionately acute displeasure and anger towards someone who might have stepped on your foot? The stomper might have been a stranger. It might have been a total accident or the result of your fault. The stomper might have profusely apologized to you as well. Still, you might develop an instant aversion to the person. Why? Because you were hurt, and it happened off guard. Any unpleasant experience, regardless of how it happened, reflexively polarizes you to the person associated with the experience.

The same principle holds in a doctor-patient relationship. If you induced hurt psychologically, however unknowingly and innocently as it may be, it would be counterproductive to your rapport with the patient. So, be careful about your choice of words. Make every effort to understand your patient's lifestyle, worldview, and habits. Learn what is essential for them and what their sensitivities are. Make every conscious effort to not hurt their sensibilities, ego, sentiments, or pride. Don't talk down their priorities. For example, if they adore their dog, ask about their dog every time.

Simply put, don't hurt their feelings. And I mean this not as an ethical principle but as a clinical strategy. Every adverse comment, argument (passive or active), and judgmental remark (good or bad) will irreversibly move you away from the patient. The psychiatrist does not mean to hurt the patient intentionally. It is essential to make intentional efforts to limit unintentional mistakes.

#3 Respect the Disease.

No disease happens overnight. Every disease has established its roots over months, if not years, before it becomes clinically apparent. Our physiology is incredibly effective at mounting several layers of defense against any disruptive process. The very existence of disease implies a process that has successfully overcome several layers of the body's defense mechanisms. The disease process knows how to hide itself from its cure. It knows how to camouflage and mislead the physician. It knows how to exploit the host to prevent it from seeking or undergoing correction. The disease has done its work! You cannot win it over with ease. So, learn to respect the disease process. You must put in as much effort and work as the disease has put in to nullify it.

When I first started practicing psychiatry, I would conclude with a diagnosis within the first 24 hours of presentation. After 40 years of practice, I make it a point to repeatedly examine the patient, usually at least three visits, before finalizing a diagnosis. With experience, I have learned to take more time, even if the diagnosis appears obvious. I take even more time before recommending treatments and management strategies. One must resist the temptation of being able to make a snap diagnosis or treatment plan.

Have a low threshold when it comes to asking for help from a more experienced or senior colleague or for a second opinion to review your diagnosis and treatment. Yes, you may have seen more patients than your senior colleague, yet they may know something by their experience, which you may lack. Haughtiness and pride can blind your eye to even the simplest of clinical challenges.

#4 Don't Underestimate Your Patients.

Yes, you went to medical school, and the patient may not have. Yes, you may be smarter than the patient. Yes, you may be right and the patient wrong. Yes, the patient may be irrational. Still, you may know less about the patient's situation than the patient. The patient has gone through many unverbalized subtleties that you may never realize. Do not presume that the patient will not understand how you see things or how things should be seen. Do not assume the patient will not understand what you are trying to explain about the illness. Lecturing neither induces nor improves insight. If there is any misunderstanding in the doctor-patient communication, it is the doctor's responsibility to remedy it. You could have done better, not the patient. If you do not understand what the patient is saying, politely ask to be re-explained. Reiterate your understanding in simple terms and confirm with them if you understood it correctly. But, if you do not get adequate clarifications, do not stubbornly persist. Move on with what you have.

#5 Don't Make it Ugly.

Diseases have existed since humankind. But cures and doctors have not. Historically, humans have stayed away from medical doctors. It is only since the establishment of the germ theory of disease that humans have regarded medical doctors as a predominant option for treating physical illnesses. Success in treating acutely catastrophic conditions such as trauma, burns, cardiac arrests, stroke, etc., has reinforced the position of modern medical practice. In chronic disease states, people seek non-medical remedies more readily than medical measures to alleviate their suffering. The reason behind this historical aversion to doctors is the possibility that the doctor could make things worse! Medical treatment may complicate the situation, expedite the inevitable, or both.

This concern is actual and accurate. Yes, we could make things worse. And a single worse development could deter your personal and professional progress more than a hundred good outcomes could. This is an undiscussed open secret – The medical literature discusses 'indications' and 'contraindications'. It does not discuss 'patient selection'. What it means is that – even if a patient meets the indications for treatment, should *you* do it? Can *you* handle it? Can *you* handle it if it does not produce the intended outcome?

There is a tendency to decide to start therapy on a patient when the diagnosis and the benefits of treatment are obvious. There is a tendency to ignore the possibility of complications because they have been taught to you as 'minor' or 'rare'. But can you handle them if they were to happen? Have you discussed with the patient the possibility of such adverse outcomes? If you cannot handle discussing such adverse outcomes with them or think you cannot handle the complications, seek help from a senior colleague before starting treatment. You could refer it to them, follow along with the other doctor and learn, or seek their guidance every step of the way. Regardless, do not be brash and think you will handle it if it happens. You may get away with it for a while, but not always.

#6 Don't Trespass!

Anytime you win a person's confidence, or if they begin to feel comfortable and protected in your presence, there will be a tendency for such a relationship to grow to the next level. If you have been successful this far and have forged a good rapport with the patient, you will begin to face the problem of the doctor-patient relationship moving to a more personal level. The patient may begin to divulge personal, employment-related, financial, or social details to you. They may ask you favors, invite you to their events, or begin to recognize you as an essential person in their life.

Since psychiatric doctor-patient relationships tend to last for years, it may happen insidiously.

You must actively surveil your boundaries and curtail yourself from wandering off the reservation. No matter how trivial it may seem, avoid interaction outside what is strictly needed for clinical purposes.

#7 Don't Sell.

Recently, there has been plentiful published evidence on the outcomes of any disease. You may be sure about the clinical outcome. Still, don't render a prediction of the outcome to the patient. Do not promise a specific outcome; even if your promise or prediction came true, don't say, 'I told you so'. Even if you are right, such communications are counterproductive in the long run. Your job is to be right, not to prove you're right.

Also, by the nature of our line of work, psychiatrists may rise to very influential positions in the patient's life or the community. Regardless, do not use the potential for influence provided by your work to further your agenda of any kind. This includes professional advancement (such as advertising, 'spreading the word', etc.) or non-professional privileges. Any advancement that benefits you is kosher only if it results from your knowledge or expertise – not the result of your clinical work. Again, this is not ethical advice – but a wise strategy to protect your clinical work in the long run.

#8 Be Noble.

All jobs are not professions, and all professions are not the same. Some become considered 'noble' by the values that drive conduct. Traditionally, the practice of medicine is considered one of the four noble professions (with law, clergy, and teaching being the other three). How so? The rationale is that in these professions, the conduct of the professional is not driven by the client's demand but by benevolence to the client.

For example, if the client asks, a painter may paint the wall with an additional coat. A surgeon must not lay in an additional layer of sutures even if the patient asks for it. The surgeon would put in an additional layer of sutures, even if the patient did not ask for it. The doctor cannot order a test because the patient wants it. A manufacturer prioritizes which orders will be fulfilled based on the most significant order or which client is more valuable. A doctor prioritizes based on who is more sick.

A doctor's profession is considered noble because the doctor's conduct is expected to be subject to intrinsic self-restraint to do what would be benevolent even if it is not asked for or demanded and to refrain from what is not benevolent even if explicitly demanded.

Remember that doctors are not noble; the practice of medicine is considered noble, and only if practiced with the objective of benevolence.

Ignoble behavior could ruin a reputation and dissolve a decades-long clientele in minutes. So, tread carefully.

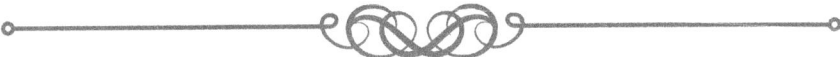

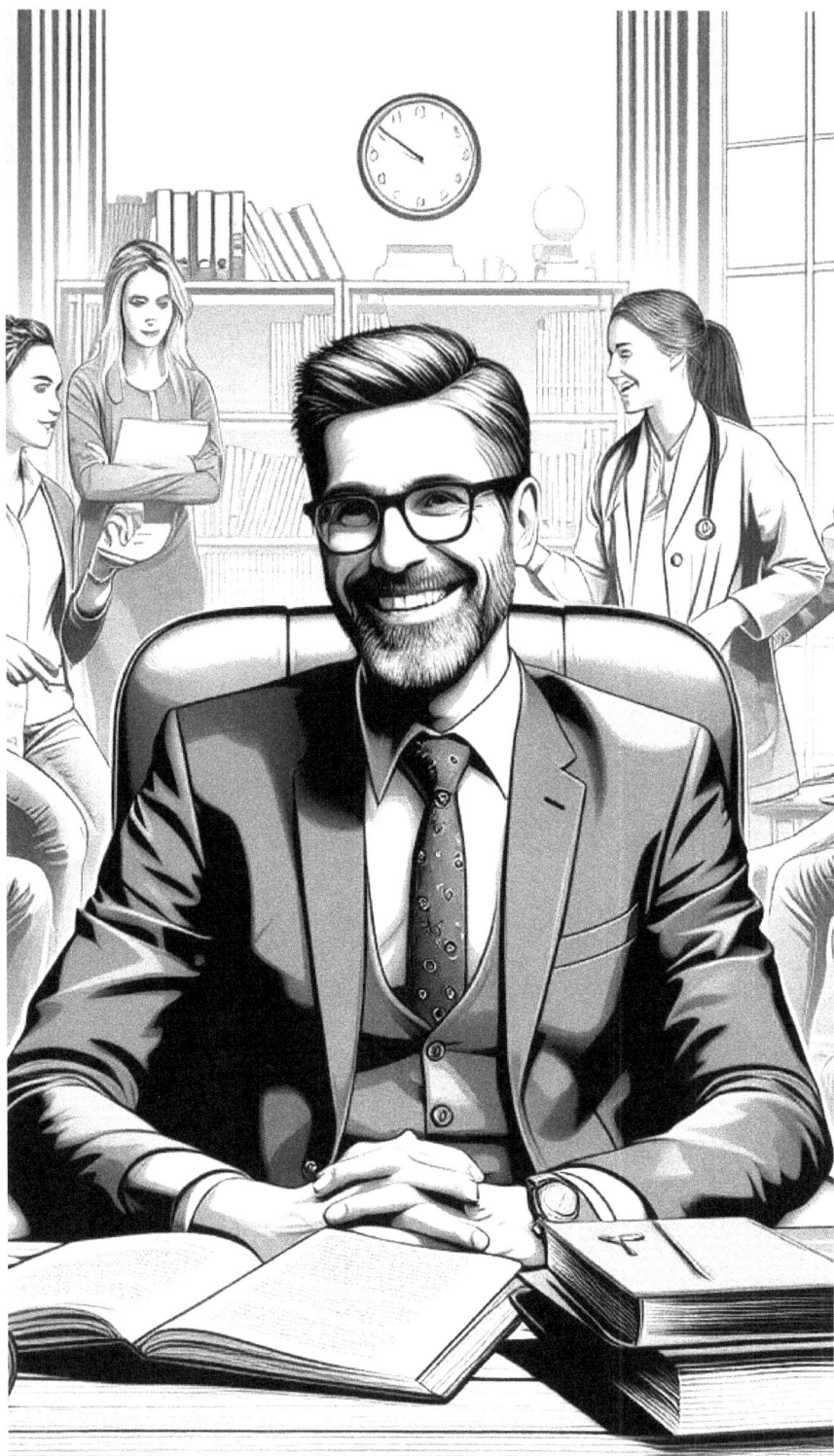

CHAPTER 22

The Joy Of Psychiatry

It is rare to be born human. It is even rarer to spend life unafflicted by disease. Disease is common. Suffering is common. But those who can relieve suffering are rare, very rare.

Among diseases, the worst are those that afflict the mind, and those who can relieve the suffering of these diseases are even rarer. To get to be a psychiatrist is rare for any human. It is a rare gift.

Doctors touch lives like no other. They get exposed to the deepest parts of human life. Psychiatrists get to see the deepest of the trenches. We get trained and licensed to dispense agents that can change how an individual thinks and behaves. It is a rare privilege to be a psychiatrist.

There has never been a better time to be a psychiatrist in human history. And it is only slated to get better. Psychiatry is on its way up. I have been thoroughly fulfilled and personally enriched by being a psychiatrist. I encourage everyone to take a close and serious look at psychiatry before passing it up for another choice of profession.

THE END

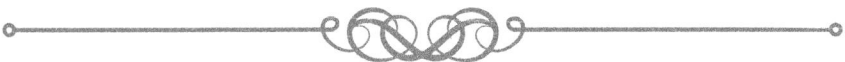

Index

Symbols

5Rs 344

A

Abhorrence 415, 416
Abstraction 148, 149
Academic 116, 289
Acting 369
Adaptability 415
Addiction 315, 318, 321, 323, 335, 357, 358
Addiction triad 321
Affect 105, 135, 185, 198, 203, 228, 264
Aggression 283, 433
Agreeableness 383
Alcohol 109, 248, 266, 296, 335, 336, 339, 340, 342, 410, 412
Alternate seeking 415
Alzheimer 51, 52, 112
Ambivalence 343
Amphetamine 111
Anchorage 416
Anger 433
Angst 202, 204
Anhedonia 197, 201, 202, 203
Antisocial PD 390, 399
Anxiety...
.........xxv, xxviii, 105, 107, 178, 219, 255, 256, 257, 258, 259, 263, 267, 268, 273, 295
Appetite 196, 202
Approach-withdrawal 161
Appropriate affect 186, 212
Approximation 141
Argumentative 449
Aristotle 50, 92
Attention 104, 137, 147, 164
Auditory hallucinations 248
Autism 104
Autoscopic 145
Avoidant PD 397, 400

I

B

Beck Depression 207
Big 9 123
Binge drinking 338, 340
BMI 76, 133
Borderline PD 392, 400
Businessman 224, 225

C

Cannabis 109, 248, 325
Cardinal 202, 399
Catatonia 104
Chief complaint 125
Child abuse 175
Child harm 205
Chronological 172, 332
Circumstantial 139, 399
Clean OCD 282
Clomipramine 296
Cluster A 113, 387, 388
Cluster B 113, 387, 427
Cluster C 113, 388
Cocaine 111, 413
Cognitive .... xxv, xxvii, xxviii, 34, 138, 197, 240, 262, 366, 374
Coherence 139
Command 145
Complex 145, 284, 347
Compliance 416
Comprehensive Textbook of Psychiatry 85
Compulsion 271
Compulsive drinking 338
Concentration 137, 196, 198, 340
Conditioning 28
Conflict 19, 70
Congruence 82
Congruent 82
Conscientiousness 383
Constitutionally cyclical 226, 227
Constitutionally depressive 226
Constitutionally elated 226
Constitutionally irritable 226, 227

Constitutional temperament 225
Constriction 409
Conversion 107, 369, 371, 372
Core 445
Counseling 116, 250, 332
Crash 326
Craving 322, 353, 355
Cultural factors 377
Custody 169

D

Dangerousness 422, 444
De-addiction 328
Delayed PTSD 305
Deliberate self-harm 100, 451
Delusion 141
Delusions of reference 247
Demographic 125
Dependence 325
Dependent PD 396, 400
Depersonalization 106, 146, 277
Depression 34, 185, 188, 191, 192, 196, 205, 207, 208, 211, 296, 326, 413
Derealization 106, 146
Descartes 50, 51, 52, 68, 361
Detoxification 327
Dismissible 82
Dispensable 98
Dissociation 372
Doctor-patient 328
Documentation 250
Doubt OCD 284
Dualism 362
Dystonia 114

E

Echolalia 141
Ego 14, 15, 16, 18, 20, 21, 22, 26
Elated 212, 213
Electroconvulsive therapy 32, 234
Elementary 145
Encapsulated delusion 142
Endogenous ....xxviii, 192, 193

Erik Erikson 88
Erotomanic 142
Etiology 352
Extremeness 385
Extroversion 382

F

Facial expression 262
Factitious 107, 369, 370
Failure 318, 338, 343, 362, 378, 415
Family 114, 129, 130, 175, 223, 264, 280, 309, 352, 452
Family history 130, 223, 264, 280
Fatigue 190, 196, 197
First person hallucination 145
Flight 140, 218
Focus 91, 205, 370, 442
Folie Du Doute 285
Freud   xvi, 5, 6, 10, 11, 12, 13, 14, 15, 18, 23, 24, 25, 26, 27, 28, 29, 63, 86, 153, 289, 295, 301, 361, 374
Freudian 5, 6, 7, 8, 25, 26, 28, 29, 34, 302, 371, 384
Fusion 140

G

Gambling 111, 348
Games 168, 348, 349, 350
Gaming 347, 348, 349, 350, 351, 356, 357, 358
Generalized Anxiety Disorder .... xxv, 105, 256, 268
Geriatric 330, 447, 448
Grandoise 142
Guilt 196, 197, 199, 342
Gustatory 145

H

Hades 49
Hallucination 144
Hamilton 208
Haptic 145
Harmful use 338
History of present illness 127
History of Presenting Problem 170
Histrionic PD 394

Home 128, 228, 344, 378
Homelessness 116
Hopelessness 410, 411
Housewife 224
Hunger 202
Hypervigilance 366
Hypnogogic 145, 181
Hypnopompic 145
Hypochondriasis 373, 374, 376, 378
Hypomania 214

I

Ian Pavlov 27, 28, 29
Iatrogenic 376
Ictal 145
Id 14, 15, 16, 17, 18, 19, 22, 23, 24, 25, 26
Identity 106
Illness 107, 364, 365
Illness behavior 365
Illusion 144
Immediate recall 148
Impulsivity 213, 407, 410
Incongruent 82
Indispensable 98, 99
Indulgent 243, 246
Insight 97, 149, 150, 244, 264, 275, 285
Intellect 58, 80, 82, 104, 112, 146, 448
Intoxication 109, 110, 111, 325, 326
Introversion 382
Irrelevancy 139

J

James Trefil 55, 56
Jealousy 12
Judgment 149
Justice x

K

Knowledge 386

L

Learned helplessness 309
Learning ....iv, 27, 165, 173
Legal history 130, 331
Leo Kanner 153
Lethality 410
Libidinal 10
Libido 10, 201
Living situation 416
Long-term recall 148
Loosening 140

M

Major depressive disorder 292, 390
Malingering 117, 369
Mananalam ..... iii, xiii, xxi, 82, 85, 123, 150, 177, 186, 195, 198, 212, 213, 217, 224,
         239, 246, 266, 267, 271, 272, 287, 289, 290, 295, 299, 300, 321, 323, 330,
         366, 377, 385, 386, 399, 400, 416, 421, 425, 427, 434, 443, 449, 453
Mananalam Clinic Experience .... xxi, 82, 123, 150, 177, 186, 195,
         198, 212, 213, 217, 224, 239, 266, 267, 271, 272, 287, 290, 299, 300, 321,
         323, 330, 366, 377, 399, 400, 416, 421, 427, 434, 443, 449
Manas 41, 43, 57, 58
Mania 214, 215
Martin E. Seligman 88
Maturity 89, 156
Memory 137, 148, 216
Mental health ....xv, 62, 63, 64, 66, 67, 70, 85, 86, 96, 100, 122, 124
Mentally healthy 65
Mentally ill 65, 66, 101, 102
Mentally not healthy 65, 101
Mentally unhealthy 65, 101, 102, 122
Mental retardation 167
Migrainous 145
Mind ....x, 1, 2, 37, 39, 46, 69
Mischievousness 217
Misidentification 143
Model G 93
Mood . 33, 58, 60, 78, 82, 105, 106, 135, 136, 185, 186, 188, 217, 221, 337, 355, 455
Mood contagion 188, 221
Mood imbalance 355

Moral model 317
Moral OCD 282
Muddling 140
Mutism 105

N

Narcissistic PD 400
Nazi 6, 302
Neat OCD 280
Negative symptoms 234
Neurobiology 353
Neurosis 273
Neurotic 192
Neuroticism 383, 384
Nihilistic 143
Nissil's granules 52
Normal 73, 74, 75, 78, 79, 80, 81, 82, 87
Normality 76

O

Objective mood 135, 136
Obsession 271, 292
Olfactory 145
Openness 382, 383
Opioids 325
Oppositional Defiant Disorder 109
Overdose 325, 326
Overinclusive thinking 140

P

Paranoid 113, 390, 399
Paranoid PD 390, 399
Parasuicide 406
Passivity 143, 247
Pathophysiology 277, 308
Pavlov 27, 28, 29, 51
Perception 110, 137, 145, 243
Perceptual disturbances 191
Periodicity 127
Persecutory 143

Perseveration 140

Personality ......xxvii, 67, 104, 109, 113, 132, 375, 376, 381, 384, 385, 386, 387, 388, 398, 402, 437

Personality disorder 402

Pervasiveness 385

Phobia 105, 144, 266, 267, 287

Phobioids 287

Plato 49, 50

Pleasure 12

Polysubstance abuse 325, 326, 413

Positive symptoms 234

Postpartum 193

Posturing 134

Pre-mania 214, 215

Premenstrual 105, 193

Premorbid 132, 241

Preoccupation 240, 351, 354, 374

Primary ....xii, 192

Progenial history 132

Pseudologica fantastica 140

Psychache 408, 409, 411

Psyche 68

Psychopathology 319, 353

Psychosis 231, 232, 233, 234, 239

Psychosomatic 369

Psychotic 104, 192, 193, 219, 287

Q

Quarreling 449

R

Rage 12

Reactive 192, 193, 434

Reactivity 161

Recreational drugs 326

Reference 143

Relapse 332, 355

Resilience 90, 91

Rigidity 385

Ripe OCD 293

Ritual 286

Rosenhan 43, 44, 45, 47, 64, 70, 71, 86

Rumination 107, 204

S

Sadism 113
Salience 354
Schizoid PD 388, 399
Schizophrenia 102, 104, 232, 233, 274, 413
Schizotypal PD 389, 399
Screen time 350, 355
Seasonal 193
Secondary 192
Second person hallucination 145
Seductive 221
Self-mutilation 240, 419
Self-regulation 161
Separation anxiety 260, 282
Sex 9, 116, 201, 279, 438
Short-term recall 148
Shut-down 205
Sibling 114, 166
Somatic 85, 107, 143, 167, 262, 356, 366
Somatoform 361, 366, 369
Speech 218, 389, 395
Spending 223, 224
Step-parent 181
Stigma 86, 122, 124, 233, 329
Stimulants 324
Stoicism 415
Stranger anxiety 163
Subconscious mind 21
Substance-induced 193, 235, 324
Substance use 222, 264, 316, 318, 324
Success 165, 457
Suffering 188, 463
Suicidality 294
Suicide 196, 223, 405, 406, 407, 408, 411, 412, 413, 415, 417, 426, 429, 430
Suicide attempters 417
Superego 14, 15, 18, 19, 22, 23, 25, 26
Symbolic thought 163
Symptomatic alcoholic 338
Systematized delusions 142

T

Tangential 139
Tearful 206
Temperament 133, 160, 194, 226
Therapeutic alliance 414
Third person hallucination 145
Thirukkural 62, 85, 149
Thought...
.................58, 79, 82, 104, 106, 107, 108, 109, 110, 111, 113, 136, 140, 218, 247, 248, 264
Thought block 140, 248
Thought insertion 247
Thought withdrawal 247
Tics 284
Tolerance 324, 325, 351, 354
Toys 168
Trait 381
Trauma 106, 117, 299, 305, 310
Traumatic event 299
Traumatic experience 300
Traumatic trigger 300
Tremor 114

U

Ulan .... xxi, 41, 42, 78, 80, 81, 92, 96, 97, 98, 103, 104, 122,
        124, 128, 132, 134, 135, 136, 137, 138, 139, 140, 141, 144, 146, 148, 150, 187,
        189, 190, 191, 204, 214, 216, 231, 243, 256, 271, 272, 275, 276, 286, 287, 291,
        300, 306, 307, 308, 309, 321, 337, 362, 363, 385, 386, 387, 388, 448, 452
Unipolar 193
Urge 321
Utilitarian 43, 96, 391

V

Violence 115, 433, 434, 435, 437, 438, 439, 440, 443

W

Whip 129
Withdrawal 109, 110, 111, 325, 326, 351

www.ingramcontent.com/pod-product-compliance
Lightning Source LLC
Chambersburg PA
CBHW071314210326
41597CB00015B/1225